HANDBOOK OF PSYCHOLOGY

AND DIABETES

HANDBOOK OF PSYCHOLOGY
AND DIABETES

*A guide to psychological measurement
in diabetes research and practice*

Edited by

Clare Bradley

*Diabetes Research Group, Royal Holloway
University of London, UK*

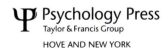

Psychology Press
Taylor & Francis Group

HOVE AND NEW YORK

First published 1994 by Harwood Academic Publishers
Amsteldijk 166, 1st Floor, 1079 LH Amsterdam,
The Netherlands

Reprinted 1996 and 2001

Reprinted 2003 and 2006 by Psychology Press
27 Church Road, Hove, East Sussex BN3 2FA
270 Madison Ave, New York, NY 10016

Psychology Press is an imprint of the Taylor & Francis Group, an informa business

Copyright © 1994 OPA (Overseas Publishers Association) NV. Published by licence
under Psychology Press

Printed and bound in Great Britain by TJI Digital, Padstow, Cornwall

---

Library of Congress Cataloging-in-Publication Data

Handbook of psychology and diabetes : a guide to psychological measurements in
    diabetes research and management / edited by Clare Bradley.
        p. cm.
    Includes index.
    ISBN 3-7186-5562-4 (hc).
    1. Diabetes—Psychological aspects. 2. Psychological tests.
  1.   Bradley Clare, 1952–
    [DNLM: 1. Diabetes Mellitus—psychology—handbooks.
  2.   Psychological Tests—handbooks. 3. Attitude to Health—handbooks. 4. Health
Behavior—handbooks.   WK 39 H2367 1994]
    RC660. H364 1994
    616.4'62'0019—dc20
    DNLM/DLC
    for Library of Congress   94-4391
                                   CIP
    ISBN 13: 978-3-7186-5562-5

To Peggy and John Bradley
who, as parents, teachers, colleagues and friends, have provided
all the inspiration, encouragement and support
that I could wish for.

CONTENTS

LIST OF CONTRIBUTORS

LINDA J. BEENEY, NH and MRC Postgraduate Scholar, Medical Psychology Unit, Department of Medicine, University of Sydney, NSW 2006, Australia

CLARE BRADLEY, PhD, Reader in Health Psychology, Director Diabetes Research Group, Department of Psychology, Royal Holloway, University of London, Egham Hill, Egham, Surrey TW20 0EX, UK

DANIEL J. COX, PhD, Professor/Director, Behavioral Medicine Center, Box 223, University of Virginia Health Sciences Center, Charlottesville, Virginia, VA 22901, USA

DIABETES CONTROL and COMPLICATIONS TRIAL (DCCT) RESEARCH GROUP, USA

STEWART M. DUNN, PhD, Associate Professor, Director Medical Psychology Unit, Departments of Medicine and Psychiatry, Royal Prince Alfred Hospital and Department of Medicine, University of Sydney, NSW 2006, Australia

RUSSELL E. GLASGOW, PhD, Research Scientist, Oregon Research Institute, 1899 Williamette, Eugene, Oregon, OR 97401-7716, USA

LINDA GONDER-FREDERICK, PhD, Research Associate Professor, Department of Behavioral Medicine and Psychiatry, Blue Ridge Hospital, Drawer F, Charlottesville, Virginia, VA 22901, USA

AUDREY IRVINE, PhD, Research Associate Professor, Department of Behavioral Medicine and Psychiatry, Blue Ridge Hospital, Drawer F, Charlottesville, Virginia, VA, 22901, USA

ALAN M. JACOBSON, MD, Associate Professor in Psychiatry, Harvard Medical School, Director Mental Health Unit, Joslin Diabetes Center, One Joslin Place, Boston, Massachusetts, MA 02215, USA

KATHRYN S. LEWIS, PhD, Department of Psychology, University of Sheffield, P.O. Box 603, Western Bank, Sheffield S10 2UR, UK

TINA N. POSNER, PhD, Senior Research Fellow, Centre for Mental Health Nursing Research, School of Nursing, Queensland University of Technology, Kelvin Grove Campus, Locked Bag No 2, Red Hill, Queensland 4059, Australia

CHRISTOPHER M. RYAN, PhD, Associate Professor of Psychiatry, Department of Psychiatry, Western Psychiatric Institute and Clinic, University of Pittsburgh School of Medicine, 3811 O'Hara Street, Pittsburgh, PA 15213, USA

CHRIS TODD, PhD, Department of Community Medicine, Institute of Public Health, University of Cambridge, Forvie Site, Robinson Way, Cambridge CB2 2SR, UK

DEBORAH TOOBERT, PhD, Research Scientist, Oregon Research Institute, 1899 Williamette, Eugene, Oregon, OR 97401-7716, USA

GARRY WELCH, PhD, National Institutes of Health Postdoctoral Fellow, Mental Health Unit, Joslin Diabetes Centre, One Joslin Place, Boston, Massachusetts, MA 02215, USA

PREFACE

This *Handbook* provides access to a wide selection of psychological measures for use in diabetes research and clinical practice. The *Handbook* is designed to help researchers and clinicians a) to select scales suitable for their purposes b) to administer and score the scales and c) to interpret the results appropriately. It brings together information about the reliability, validity, scoring, norms, and use (and abuse) of a series of well-known instruments. Most of the chapters are each dedicated to a specific scale. Scales included provide measures of a wide range of psychological issues concerning diabetes and its management including quality of life, well-being, satisfaction with treatment, fear of hypoglycaemia, knowledge of diabetes, adjustment to diabetes, beliefs about diabetes, perceptions of control over diabetes, barriers to self-care, and assessment of self-care. The development and use of each scale is discussed by the invited contributors who were the originators of the scales they describe.

Most, though not all, of the scales included in the Handbook explicitly focus on diabetes. The scales have all been developed with populations of people with diabetes. However, the scales in the Well-being Questionnaire may be appropriate for use with other chronic illness populations. Other scales, such as the Diabetes Treatment Satisfaction Questionnaire and the Perceived Control of Diabetes Scale, would appear to be readily modifiable for use with other groups. The final chapter of the book considers the advantages and drawbacks of modifying scales and decribes the procedures needed to investigate the psychometric consequences of using modified scales or unmodified instruments with new populations.

Diabetes research has attracted many psychologists who have recognised the need for reliable and valid measures of the psychological phenomena they are researching. Most of these psychologists, myself included, became involved in the design and development of measurement instruments not as an end in itself but in order to facilitate research into some aspect of diabetes and its management. Although the original scale development work is published in journals, subsequent publications reporting on results of using the measures may be scattered through the social science and medical literature and in theses and reports that are not always easy to obtain. Other researchers wishing to use a particular scale are faced with a daunting task of piecing together information from a variety of sources. Often they contact the author of the scale for help. In order to provide essential information and advice for users and potential users of scales developed by my research group it became clear that the *Handbook* was needed.

The scales selected for inclusion in this *Handbook* have initial psychometric development information published in journal papers. The contributors are active in the field of diabetes research and wish to encourage appropriate use of their scales. There are many other scales that would meet these inclusion criteria and reference to many of these may be found in the introductions to specific chapters. There are also more recently designed scales and interview schedules that have yet to be widely used or have little or no published evidence about their psychometric properties. A selection of these more recent measures, particularly those which are designed to fill a need that is not addressed by the scales described in detail in the main text, is documented in the Appendix.

My purpose in editing and contributing to this *Handbook* has been to make readily accessible to fellow researchers comprehensive and up-to-date information on scales and other psychological measures. Potential users of scales can see which measures look appropriate for their purposes and can assess the possibilities of those that look suitable without having to search the wide flung literature or write to each author of the scales for details. The scales are not usually published in their entirety elsewhere. In addition to providing readily available information about their scales, contributors to the book have been asked to search out information about studies where their scales have been used (perhaps by following up requests to use the scales) and to review the findings of these studies so that they can provide further information about the value and limitations of their measures as they become more widely used.

In most cases the authors of the scales continue to develop the instruments as they work with them and they may modify them to improve their reliability or validity. Potential users of the scales are therefore advised to contact the copyright owner, who is usually the senior author of a chapter describing the scales, not only to request a version of the scales that they may take copies from and permission to make a specified number of copies, but also to find out whether the scales or scoring recommendations have been updated since publication of this *Handbook*. The authors of the scales included in this Handbook have given their permission and information freely and generously in the past and would hope to be able to continue to do so in the future. In return, many users of the scales have shared their data or provided feedback on the use of the scales, including much validity information. Such communication and exchange of views and information is vitally important to the continuing process of scale validation and for the development of new ideas and initiatives.

In addition to the chapters concerned with scales developed specifically for use with people with diabetes, a further chapter focuses on the measurement of acute and chronic changes in cognitive function associated with diabetes and the application of measures developed elsewhere in this important and expanding field of research and clinical concern. Other chapters provide guidance on evaluating the design and psychometric development of the measures included, guidance on translating and evaluating translations for use in different languages and cultures and, in the final chapter, the circumstances are described under which scales may require modification and the psychometric consequences of such modifications are considered. A chapter on qualitative methodologies provides an introduction to alternative approaches that may well be more appropriate than scales for certain purposes and equally appropriate for others. Qualitative methodologies have been employed in the early stages of questionnaire design by many designers of scales intended for quantitative research and the advantages and limitations of both methodologies are discussed.

I would like to thank all contributors for their very considerable efforts to meet the many demands made of them including the requirements for producing the 'disc manuscripts'. I thank all those colleagues who read and offered valuable criticism and encouraging comments on manuscripts. Those who have helped in this way include Peggy Bradley, Chris Todd, Elaine Funnell, Mary Alice Flint, Valerie Kent, Anne-Louise Kinmonth, Philip Home, Sarah Hirst, and Cathy Coombs, as well as Nadine Thibult whose essential contributions are acknowledged in two of my chapters. Several members of my Diabetes Research Group have made valuable contributions to the work of editing the *Handbook*. I thank everyone for their help, direct and indirect, with special thanks to Janet Cerely for her secretarial support, Liz Symonds for helping to edit several chapters and appendix entries; Kathryn Lewis and Rosalind Plowright for providing data; Julie Cheesman for her skills and accuracy in editing disc manuscripts on a variety of word processing systems and for her ability to spot ambiguity, contradictions and confusions which has been of great benefit in many of the chapters in this *Handbook*; Rosalind Plowright also provided invaluable help in the last stages of preparing the manuscript and appendix entries for the publishers. Finally, my thanks go to my family, especially my husband, Jonathan Gilbride, for his forbearance and support while I have been writing and editing the *Handbook*.

I have learnt a great deal about scales, diabetes, psychometrics, and the contributors in the process of editing this volume. My own research group has already found the draft manuscript to be a valuable resource that facilitates our research. The availability of the published *Handbook* to other researchers and health professionals will promote more widespread and appropriate use of the scales and this greater use will in turn provide useful information about validity. I see publishing this volume not as a final product but as documentation of a stage reached in a continuing process of developing our understanding and appreciation of people who have diabetes.

Clare Bradley

SECTION 1

AN INTRODUCTION TO
ISSUES AND CHOICES

CHAPTER 1

AN INTRODUCTION TO THE GUIDE TO PSYCHOLOGICAL MEASUREMENT IN DIABETES RESEARCH AND PRACTICE

CLARE BRADLEY

Department of Psychology, Royal Holloway, University of London, Egham, Surrey, TW20 0EX, UK

REASONS FOR DEVELOPING AND USING DIABETES-SPECIFIC MEASURES

Designing and developing a new scale is costly in time and resources and is not a task to be undertaken lightly. There are arguments for using well-known generic measures in order to try and provide comparative data that might be used to make national health policies or local decisions about resource allocation. So why develop a diabetes-specific quality of life measure such as the DQOL described by Alan Jacobson and the DCCT research group in Chapter 5 or the Diabetes Treatment Satisfaction Questionnaire that I have described in Chapter 7? Why have we not used the ubiquitous SF-36 and other generic measures? In answering such questions it is worth considering why we don't expect one set of physiological or biochemical outcome measures to be suitable for all patients regardless of the nature of their problems and treatments. Peak flow measures may be useful in asthma management but they have little or no relevance for diabetes management. Measures of blood glucose control will be of no value in asthma management. Neither measure would be relevant for people with arthritis where measures of mobility would be more useful. Similarly, where psychological processes and outcomes are concerned the same measure will not be equally relevant for patients with different disorders. The experience of pain is a central concern for people with arthritis but is not an issue for most people with insulin dependent diabetes for whom fear of hypoglycaemia may be a dominant concern. Thus when designing measures specifically for people with diabetes we can focus on those issues which are especially important for them and avoid irrelevancies that will cloud the picture. In this way we can produce diabetes-specific measures that have greater sensitivity than generic measures.

When we come to consider the measurement of well-being it might seem that the conditions of depressed mood, anxiety, energy and positive well-being (subscales in the Well-being questionnaire presented in Chapter 6) are of global relevance not just in diabetes but in other conditions and indeed they may well be. However, indicators of depression, anxiety, energy and positive well-being do not remain constant across all conditions. Many of the indicators of depression in the general population that are included in commonly used measures such as the Beck Depression Inventory (Beck *et al.*, 1961) are likely to be confounded with symptoms of hyperglycaemia, hypoglycaemia or chronic complications in people with diabetes. Such symptoms include appetite disturbances, weight loss, tiredness, and loss of libido. With other conditions such as asthma or arthritis other symptoms, such as sleep disturbances, included in the Beck may be directly attributable to the physical disorder and may not be valid indicators of depression. Thus we need to consider not just the relevance of the mood state to be measured but the precise way in which it is being measured. Use of the same instrument with different populations cannot be assumed to be measuring the same psychological phenomenon. Chapter 16 considers appropriate ways of using questionnaires with new populations. Developing apparently generic measures of, for example, depression, with specific populations such as people with diabetes increases the likelihood that the instrument concerned will provide a valid measure of what it is intended to measure (depression) rather than unintentionally providing a proxy measure of metabolic control.

There is increasing recognition of the value of condition-specific measures and a rapidly expanding literature on health-related psychological measures. In 1987 McDowell and Newell wrote a valuable guide to a wide range of generic health status instruments. Other excellent texts followed with more specific purposes in view. Several of these have been specifically concerned with measurement of particular psychological constructs such as quality of life (e.g. Fallowfield, 1990; Spilker, 1990; Bowling, 1991; Walker and Rosser, 1993) or patient satisfaction (Fitzpatrick and Hopkins, 1993). Most of the quality of life texts devote specific chapters to consideration of quality of life measurement in specific diseases and conditions. Other books have been concerned with the measurement of a variety of constructs in a particular health-related setting such as primary care (Wilkin *et al.*, 1992). A recent volume edited by McGee and Bradley (1994) focuses on quality of life in patients with end stage renal disease who depend on high technology medicine for their survival. That edited volume includes a substantial contribution from Welch reviewing the use of generic and disease-specific measurement instruments for use with patients with end stage renal disease. Some of the texts have included example items or sections from the instruments they review (e.g. Wilkin *et al.*, 1992) or, most usefully of all, have reproduced measurement scales in their entirety (e.g. Fallowfield, 1990). In most cases the authors or contributors are users of scales or reviewers of such work rather than the designers and developers of such scales though there are notable exceptions including several of the well-known contributors to Walker and Rosser's (1993) edited collection. The present *Handbook* is concerned with the measurement of a much wider range of psychological phenomena than the forerunners mentioned above. It also differs in having a specific focus on one disorder, diabetes, its management and complications. The contributors to the *Handbook* have been actively involved in diabetes research, designing, developing and/or using scales to measure the psychological issues they have been researching. The *Handbook* provides the means of pulling together the expertise gained during the 1980s and into the 1990s and provides access to the measures developed and associated information on their use.

THE PURPOSE OF THE *HANDBOOK*

Many of the scales relevant to diabetes are presented or referred to in this *Handbook*. Others may be discovered by a careful search of the literature. A new scale should be designed only as a last resort. It is important to make a thorough investigation of existing measures to avoid duplication of work. Measures may already be in use which serve the same purpose as your projected measure. When I started designing new measures in 1982 there was only a handful of psychologists involved in research in diabetes around the world, now there are hundreds of researchers at work and the chances of there already being a suitable measure are much greater. Available measures in your own language may not be quite appropriate for your purposes and may require adapting and thereafter treating as new instruments (see Chapter 16 on adapting scales and procedures and the limits of reliability and validity) but this is preferable to reinventing the wheel.

This *Handbook* is intended to facilitate access not only to the diabetes-specific scales presented here but also to the information concerning the reliability and validity of the scales and evidence for their suitability for different purposes. Chapter 2 by Todd and Bradley provides an introduction to psychometric design and development for those with little or no experience of the processes involved. The intention is to help readers to evaluate the information provided about the scales.

The scales described in detail in the *Handbook* chapters have been shown to satisfy criteria for many of the important aspects of reliability and validity outlined in Chapter 2. However, the process of developing scales is not a finite one. Information on some aspects of predictive validity may take years to collect and its measurement may only prove possible when a suitable study is funded for a different primary purpose and the study can also provide evidence concerning the predictive validity of the questionnaire. The task of design and development of the scales produced by my own research group has not until recently attracted funding in its own right but has been piggy-backed onto other studies evaluating new technologies, education or other management programmes for diabetes care. Scale developers may not have had resources specifically to support the development process and it may therefore not be surprising if information on some aspects of reliability or validity is patchy or non-existent. Sometimes the data are or were available but some potentially informative analyses have yet to be done. It will be interesting to see whether, for example, the Quality of Life scale described in Chapter 5 does factor naturally into the theoretically conceived subscales when the data are explored using factor analysis or whether such empirical testing identifies an alternative structure for the scales. In the meantime, the alpha coefficients of internal consistency for the current subscales provide support for the current scoring recommendations. Where all the scales in this *Handbook* are concerned, however, the development process is a continuing one. Many well-known and highly regarded questionnaires in general use (rather than specifically in diabetes research) cannot claim to have been subjected to most of the tests of reliability and validity addressed in this *Handbook*.

LAYOUT OF CHAPTERS

Contributors of chapters describing specific scales have been asked to follow a standard ordering of contents to help readers to find their way around the book and locate what they are looking for with greater ease. The scales themselves can always be found as the first figure presented in each chapter with additional figures showing any short form which might be available (as with Welch *et al.*s' ATT19 short form of the ATT39 in Chapter 11) or parallel forms (as with the knowledge scales in Beeney *et al.*s' Chapter 9). Two versions of the Health Beliefs and Perceived Control scales are provided in Chapters 12 and 13, one for insulin-treated and one for tablet-treated patients. The scheme outlined in Table 1 shows the ordering of headings that have, where possible, been followed in the chapters describing scales. Chapter 2 by Todd and Bradley provides information on the concepts of reliability and validity listed in Table 1 and associated methods of assessment.

Table 1 Guidelines to content organisation of *Handbook* chapters

INTRODUCTION	Describes the original purpose of the scale and the range of uses to which the scale has been put by users
THE SCALE	
Design	The latest version of the scale(s) is presented in a figure or figures. The design of the scale is described including any theoretical underpin and/or account of clinical observations/interview or other source material which influenced the design of the scales.
Scoring	Details of the scoring procedures recommended.
SCALE DEVELOPMENT	
Subject Sample(s) and Procedures	Details are given of sample selection and sample(s) on which the measure has been developed. Details of administration procedures followed and instructions and information given to patients were also asked for here. Any written instructions given to subjects should be presented along with the scales themselves in the figure(s).
Statistical Methods and Qualitative Judgements	The methods/criteria for determining which items were retained in the measure and which were dropped are outlined and referenced.
Structure of Scale	Evidence for the structure of the scale might include some kind of factor analysis for multidimensional scales.
Reliability	Includes *Internal consistency: Test-retest reliability.*
Validity	Includes *Face and Content validity: Concurrent validity: Construct validity: Predictive validity: Discriminant validity: Convergent validity: Extreme Groups validity.*
SHORT FORMS	Where available these are described and evaluated.
DISCUSSION	Includes consideration of the limitations as well as the advantages of the measure.
SUMMARY	Summarises the purpose of the measure and its scope and recommendations for future use.

In addition to those aspects of reliability and validity listed in Table 1 there are several further criteria which can be useful in choosing between instruments and these include sensitivity to change, discriminatory power, and standardisation and norms.

Sensitivity to Change

If changes across time are a focus of interest of the study then a measure will only be useful if it is sensitive to the kind of changes that are expected to occur. Ceiling and floor effects can be important here. For example, use of a measure of depression in a study evaluating the use of Continuous Subcutaneous Insulin Infusion (CSII) pumps is likely to be too blunt an instrument to be sensitive to change following a period of CSII use. Depression scores will generally be low to begin with so there will be little room for improvement (a floor effect), only room for deterioration. The measure will therefore only serve to check that this specific psychological consequence (increase in depressed mood) will not follow CSII use. No psychological advantages of CSII use will be detectable with this measure. As shown in Chapters 5 and 6, measures of Positive Well-being, Energy and Satisfaction with Treatment proved to be far more sensitive to change than were measures of Depression and Anxiety in studies evaluating CSII pumps.

The chapter by Ryan draws particular attention to those tests of cognitive function that have proved sensitive to changes in diabetes control as well as to those tests that differentiated between extreme groups such as those with complications versus those without.

Discriminatory Power

A measure needs to achieve a good spread of scores. The measure will be useless if every respondent scores the same. There are, however, limits to the spread that will give meaningful results. Generally it has been found that respondents can hold in mind up to nine categories when they are marking or rating a scale. More intelligent subjects are generally able to make use of a greater number of categories than less intelligent subjects. The scales presented in the *Handbook* mostly use five or six-point scales with seven-point scales being the maximum and four-point scales the minimum. Four-point scales when combined to form a scale varying from 0 to 36 as with the Depression, Anxiety and Positive Well-being subscales of the Well-being Questionnaire presented in Chapter 6 provide a much greater spread of scores than would be obtained with the separate items though the skewed distributions of the Depression subscale in particular will limit the discriminatory power.

Standardization and Norms

Norms are sets of scores from clearly defined samples and the procedures for obtaining these scores constitute the test standardization. If norms are available it is possible to interpret the scores of individuals meaningfully. However, norms are only as useful as the appropriateness and size of the sample. If the sample is too small the norms may be misleading. Norms are most valuable in the practical application of tests where a clinician wants to assess individual patients. Where research is concerned, raw test scores are used and norms are not usually needed. The scales included in the *Handbook* have predominantly been developed in a research context and the only norms available are the descriptive statistics for the particular sample populations studied. These can, however provide a useful guide to the kind of results that might be expected. The continuing and more widespread use of the scales in the future will supply normative data of value in clinical applications of the scales.

CHOOSING MEASURES FOR SPECIFIC PURPOSES

Questionnaires can be a valuable and straightforward method of obtaining quantifiable information reliably. Although the design and development of questionnaires requires special skills and experience, they can be administered and scored by individuals who simply have access to the questionnaire and associated scoring instructions and who have no need of special training. This method of measurement is often preferred to more time-consuming interview and observational methods that require specially trained interviewers or observers. However, there is danger that off-the-peg scales are overused and misused in inappropriate circumstances because they are readily available, inexpensive and easy and the user does not stop to ask "Is it appropriate for my purposes?".

A questionnaire designed to measure knowledge of diabetes in adults will not be appropriate for use in a paediatric clinic if it asks about the effects of moderate exercise on blood glucose levels and gives the example of "gardening" as gardening is not a common activity among children. A similar measure designed in America may give the example of "yardwork" which will be incomprehensible to most adults with diabetes in the UK. Even within the same country and within the same age group of patients, clinics differ and individual health care professionals differ in the knowledge that they believe is required and even in the knowledge that they believe is correct. I have yet to hear of a diabetes care team where members have been given one of the several multiple-choice knowledge of diabetes questionnaires available and have agreed among themselves about which answers are correct. The thrashing out of disagreements between team members with a view to reaching a consensus about what patients should be taught and why, is a potentially very valuable use for diabetes knowledge measures and an essential first step in deciding whether a questionnaire is appropriate for use in assessing patients' knowledge in a particular clinic. The DKN scales cannot be expected to detect improvements in knowledge following a diabetes education programme if patients on that programme are taught, for example, that the normal range of blood glucose is 6–10 which is not one of the options offered in the questionnaire.

Even if scales have been developed with the same clinic population you are working with, important changes may have occurred which affect responses to the instrument. Patients' and doctors' and other health professionals' knowledge changes, monitoring and screening procedures change, feedback to patients and education programmes change and any of these may reduce the 'face validity' of a questionnaire (especially one intended to measure knowledge) which previously may have been quite appropriate. Decisions to use questionnaires to measure self-care activities and barriers to self-care will need to be made in the context of information about local recommendations for diabetes care.

Given the variation in practice of diabetes management between clinics in the UK and my observations of even greater variation between UK clinics and those I have visited in the USA, Scandinavia and Europe, I am not surprised at the differences in the patterns of responses found in samples from different countries to the attitude statements included in the ATT39 described by Welch *et al.* in Chapter 11. Such differences, if not attributable to the linguistic translation process, may well reflect real differences in attitudes towards diabetes and its management in different countries which in turn may reflect differences in health professionals' attitudes and behaviour, and health care policies. It is clear that users of the ATT39 cannot rely on previous work to tell them the nature of the responses indicative of good adjustment to diabetes but instead need to explore and give careful thought to the meaning of the data collected in their own clinic. It appears that the short form of the ATT39, the ATT19, which is also described by Welch *et al.* in Chapter 11, provides a selection of attitude statements which constitute a more replicable core of the longer questionnaire. However, while the ATT39 is able to boast more large scale studies than any of the other questionnaires included in this *Handbook*, it continues to raise more questions than it can answer. The ATT39 should be regarded as a stimulus to research and thought about the complexities of attitudes towards diabetes and adjustment to the condition and should not be expected to provide any simple answers.

When there are differences between your own population of patients with diabetes and those involved with developing a questionnaire you are interested in using, you will need to decide whether the differences are likely to be important or not. This is a matter of judgement but it is also empirically testable once you have collected sufficient data using the questionnaire in your clinic. Just looking at a questionnaire that is explicitly designed for insulin users and refers to insulin use will tell you that it cannot be given to tablet and/or diet-treated patients in its present form. However, if the questionnaire looks equally appropriate for patients treated with diet alone but has not previously been used with such patients (e.g. the Well-being Questionnaire described in Chapter 6) your new data may be explored to establish whether the new population of respondents is using the subscales in the same way as the earlier populations studied. Such an exploration might involve factor analysis or simply a correlation matrix looking at the relationships between the items in the questionnaire. Methods of checking the structure, reliability and validity of a questionnaire used in a new context or with a different population are considered in more detail in Chapter 16 which is concerned with adapting scales and the limits of reliability and validity. Some of the key questions to consider when choosing a questionnaire are summarised in Table 2. Pilot work may well be needed before these questions can be answered.

Table 2 Questions to consider when choosing a questionnaire

- Is it appropriate for my population of patients, judging from the appearance of the questions and my experience of the patients?
- Is it appropriate in my particular clinic?
- Is it appropriate given the views/behaviours of my diabetes care team?
- Has it been shown to be reliable with a similar population?
- Is there good reason to think it will be reliable with my population?
- Is it likely to be sensitive to the changes I expect or hope to find?
- How will I handle the data generated? (see final section of Chapter 16).

CONSIDERING ALTERNATIVE METHODS

Scales are only one method of measurement. Other methods may be preferable or may provide a useful addition. For example, if you are looking for a measure of quality of life to include in a study evaluating different treatments for diabetes, you may well expect the particular treatments you are evaluating to affect particular aspects of life. You may want to ask about those aspects in more detail than is allowed for in a standard measure such as the DQOL presented in Chapter 5. You might then, as Alan Jacobson and the DCCT research group suggest in Chapter 5, add on a series of specific questions to suit your needs. These additional items should be analysed and interpreted separately from the original DQOL items.

It may be that you have reason to believe that individual differences in the importance of different domains in a person's life are too great to give equal weight to each domain in the way that the Impact subscale of the DQOL would do. To explore such individual differences may require qualitative methods such as those described by Tina Posner in Chapter 4 or a structured interview technique for quantifying individual differences in quality of life devised by McGee *et al.* (1991) which has recently been adapted and used for the first time in diabetes research (Walker, 1993).

MODIFYING OR TRANSLATING EXISTING SCALES

In cases where an existing scale could be appropriate for use given certain modifications, the reader is referred to Chapter 16. That chapter considers the advantages and disadvantages of adapting scales, the precautions which can sometimes be taken to protect reliability and the checks that are needed to establish the psychometric properties of the adapted measure which, depending on the nature of the adaptations, may well need to be treated as if it were a new instrument.

A translation into a new language can all too easily distort the intended meaning of items in the questionnaire and such a translation should be treated as a new instrument with the reliability and validity to be established. Chapter 3 offers recommendations for linguistic and psychometric procedures to be followed to increase the chances of producing a translation that works as well as the original questionnaire from which it was derived.

CLINICAL APPLICATIONS OF THE MEASURES

There is increasing interest in using many of the measures presented in the *Handbook* for direct clinical applications rather than restricting them to research use. The DKN measures developed by Stewart Dunn's group in Australia and described by Beeney *et al.* in Chapter 9, have been used clinically by diabetes health care professionals in the UK. The Barriers to Diabetes Self-Care instrument developed by Russ Glasgow (Chapter 14) and the Summary of Diabetes Self-Care Activities Questionnaire presented by Deborah Toobert and Russ Glasgow in Chapter 15 are both likely to have direct clinical uses in identifying difficulties or potential problems with diabetes treatment regimens with a view to modifying the regimen to improve self-care.

The Well-being Questionnaire and Diabetes Treatment Satisfaction Questionnaires developed by my own research group are now being widely used for purposes of clinical audit of diabetes care in the UK and around Europe. We cannot, on the basis of the currently available research data, answer all of the new questions which will arise with clinical use of the measures. In particular, clinically oriented research is needed in order to advise on cut-off points for identifying patients with high scores on the Depression and Anxiety subscales who might benefit from intervention. Research is also needed to determine the most appropriate forms of intervention for individual patients.

The Fear of Hypoglycaemia Scale described by Irvine *et al.* in Chapter 8 is likely to become a useful clinical tool. The DCCT Quality of Life scale presented by Alan Jacobson may be regarded by many health professionals as too long for routine clinical use though its use in a research context may well inform clinical decisions. Clinical applications of the scales are to be welcomed wherever they are appropriate and conducted within a context of continuing evaluation that facilitates further development of the measures as needed. Developers of scales welcome feedback from clinicians who have experience of using their scales and, when they have the resources to process extra data sets, may also welcome offers to share data.

RECOGNISING THE LIMITATIONS OF MEASURES

Contributors to the *Handbook* were invited to consider critically the value and limitations of the measure(s) they presented in the various studies/clinical settings/circumstances in which research has been conducted. They were invited to comment on any problems that may have arisen in studies. For example, response rates may be affected by different circumstances, patient acceptability may vary. Where appropriate contributors were asked to recommend certain procedures and warn against others as a result of the lessons learned. Likely errors of interpretation and any pitfalls to be avoided were other possible problems that might usefully be made explicit in a way that is often too risky to attempt in manuscripts submitted to journals where reviewers and editors may be disinclined to publish scale-development papers which acknowledge problems with the measure however specific and remediable those problems may be. It is not easy to be openly critical of a measure you have designed and developed and it is natural to focus on its successes and minimise its shortcomings. However, it is preferable to specify the limitations of a measure and reduce the number of times the measure is inappropriately used by other researchers than to have the measure misused and blamed when it proves unreliable or insensitive to change under such circumstances.

No measure is perfect and diabetes research and clinical practice is likely to be best served by recognising the limitations of the measures used whether they be psychological scales or physical measurements such as the also-far-from-perfect indicators of blood glucose control — fructosamine, glycosylated haemoglobin (GHb) and HbA_1 measures. These measures of blood glucose only provide an average of blood glucose levels over particular time periods and give no indication of variation in blood glucose. The same measure of GHb may be obtained from someone with blood glucose varying only slightly around a mean of 8 mmols/L with no episodes of hypoglycaemia as is obtained from another patient who has experienced repeated episodes of hypoglycaemia with occasional periods of hyperglycaemia. Unfortunately some doctors overlook the limitations of GHb and other such "objective" measures and give them undue emphasis in assessing diabetes control and in evaluating treatments while failing to take appropriate account of the patients' reports of hypoglycaemia.

While personally advocating the value of recognising the limitations as well as the advantages of measurement methods, I also recognise the risk involved when health professionals are inappropriately reluctant to use scales about which the developers are cautious. The countributors to the *Handbook* would like to see greater recognition of the importance of considering psychological processes and outcomes in diabetes care. Just as GHb measures can be of great value in facilitating diabetes management despite their limitations, so too can the psychological scales described in this *Handbook*. Constructive recognition of the limitations of the scales should serve to encourage careful thought in interpretation of results obtained and to encourage further research and development of improved measurement instruments.

COPYRIGHT AND USE OF SCALES

Copyright of the each of the scales included in full in the *Handbook* is owned by one or more of the authors of the chapter describing the particular scale. The publishing agreement does not allow authors of the scales to give permission to potential users to photocopy the scales directly from the *Handbook* itself which is subject to the usual copyright restrictions. When readers identify a scale that they wish to use, they should write to the authors named in the copyright statement on the instrument requesting a copy of the instrument published in this *Handbook* and permission to reproduce it a specified number of times for a purpose which should also be specified. The authors will then be able to inform potential users of any updates to the scales or scoring procedures and alert them to any new developments that may be useful for their purposes.

SUMMARY

This chapter outlines the reasons for developing measures specifically for use in diabetes research and practice rather than using generic measures developed with other populations. The purpose of the *Handbook* is described as one of facilitating access to the scales themselves and to the information needed to encourage appropriate use of the measures. The organisation of material within the chapters is described and Table 1 provides a ready guide to the ordering of material within the *Handbook* chapters. The section on choosing measures for specific purposes provides some examples of inappropriate uses of scales and suggests questions that need to be asked when choosing between scales (see Table 2) or when considering alternatives which may include qualitative methods described in Chapter 4. Readers wishing to translate questionnaires are referred to Chapter 3 while those wishing to adapt questionnaires in other ways are referred to Chapter 16. Clinical applications of measures within a framework of continuing evaluation are considered. Constructive recognition of the limitations of the scales is encouraged with a view to promoting careful data interpretation and recognition of the need for continuing development.

REFERENCES

Beck, A. T., Ward, C. H., Mendelson, M., Mock, J. and Erbaugh, J. (1961) An inventory for measuring depression. *Archives of General Psychiatry,* 4, 561–571

Bowling, A. (1991) *Measuring Health: a Review of Quality of Life Measurement Scales.* Buckingham: Open University Press

Fallowfield, L. (1990) *The Quality of Life: the missing dimension in health care.* London: Souvenir Press

Fitzpatrick, R. and Hopkins, A. (1993) *Measurement of patients' satisfaction with their care.* London: Royal College of Physicians of London

McDowell, I. and Newell, C. (1987) *Measuring Health: A Guide to rating scales and questionnaires.* Oxford: Oxford University Press

McGee, H. M. and Bradley, C. (eds) (1994) *Quality of Life Following Renal Replacement: psychosocial challenges accompanying high technology medicine.* Harwood Academic (in press)

McGee, H. M., O'Boyle, C. A., Hickey, A., O'Malley, K. M. and Joyce, C. R. B. (1991) Assessing the quality of life of the individual: the SEIQoL with a healthy and a gastroenterology unit population. *Psychological Medicine*, **21**, 749–759

McHorney, C. A., Ware, J. E. and Raczek, A. B. (1993) The MOS 36-item Short-Form Health Survey (SF-36): II. Psychometric and clinical tests of validity in measuring physical and mental health constructs. *Medical Care*, **31**, 247–263

Spilker, B. (ed.) (1990) *Quality of Life Assessments in Clinical Trials.* New York: Raven Press

Walker, J. (1993) Assessing quality of life in adolescents with diabetes: a comparison of patients' and nurses' assessments using two different methods of quality of life measurement (the DQOL and the SEIQoL). Unpublished psychology undergraduate project. Royal Holloway, University of London

Walker, S. R. and Rosser, R. M. (eds) (1993) *Quality of Life Assessment: Key Issues in the 1990s.* Lancaster: Kluwer Academic Publishers.

Wilkin, D., Hallam, L. and Doggett, M-A. (1992) *Measures of Need and Outcome for Primary Health Care.* New York: Oxford University Press

CHAPTER 2

EVALUATING THE DESIGN AND DEVELOPMENT OF PSYCHOLOGICAL SCALES

CHRIS TODD and CLARE BRADLEY

Health Services Research Group, Department of Community Medicine, Institute of Public Health, University of Cambridge, Forvie Site, Robinson Way, Cambridge, CB2 2SR, UK.

Department of Psychology, Royal Holloway , University of London, Egham Hill, Egham, Surrey, TW20 0EX, UK.

INTRODUCTION: THE QUANTIFICATION OF THE PSYCHOSOCIAL

Measurement is central to the scientific endeavour. Whilst, perhaps mistakenly, measurement has not routinely been considered problematic in clinical laboratory sciences, the measurement of subjectivity is often viewed in a quite different light. A central theme of the *Handbook of Psychology and Diabetes* is the measurement of subjective responses to diabetes mellitus. The *Handbook* presents a series of measures specifically designed for use with people with diabetes. Most of these measures are of use under specific circumstances, but not necessarily under all. Rather than being aimed solely at psychologists with an interest in psychometrics, it is hoped that this volume will prove a resource for clinicians and researchers from a variety of disciplines with little or no expertise in the use of psychological measures. Such clinicians and researchers who have had no training in psychometrics may find it difficult to assess the quality of the measurement instruments available. The present chapter aims to lay out the ground rules for developing psychological measures and identify criteria which should be met when choosing between tests for use in practice.

As Kline has pointed out: "it remains an unfortunate fact that a huge majority of psychological tests are both invalid and unreliable" (Kline, 1986; p. 207). All too often, it seems that if some lip service is paid to psychometric development an instrument can enter the literature and be taken up by further researchers to answer applied questions. However, uninformed acceptance of instruments can result in spurious answers and wasted effort and resources. Furthermore, it needs to be recognised that there are several different kinds of reliability and many different forms of validity. It is rarely the case that a measure has been shown to be reliable and valid in all respects and the potential user needs sufficient understanding of psychometric concepts to make informed decisions about the likely value of instruments. Whilst this chapter aims to provide an introduction to the psychometric concepts used throughout the book, this chapter will not suffice as a guide to those wishing to develop a test of their own. Any such readers are referred to more detailed and extensive texts such as Kline (1979, 1986), Streiner and Norman (1989) or Rust and Golombok (1989).

Whilst we will be describing the "science" of psychometrics, there is also an "art" (Kline, 1979). The art of test development is to be found in the initial formulation of the items which constitute the instrument and in the judgements made in choosing between them. Psychological tests may be designed to measure all manner of psychological attributes; ranging from those used in "pure" research to those which are more applied in nature; intelligence, ability, personality, attitudes, mood and state, motivation or occupational assessment. Perhaps the best known (most notorious) sorts of test are the so called Projective Tests, such as the Rorschach Test and Thematic Apperception Test. These require that individuals respond to ambiguous images which are designed with a view to revealing their underlying concerns. Such tests require not only design of the stimulus, but also interpretation of the results by the individual tester. It is the need for such interpretation that has brought these instruments into scientific disrepute and these techniques will not be discussed further here.

Most of the measures described in this *Handbook* require that subjects respond to a stimulus, but the scoring system is fixed and based on statistical inference rather than the judgment of the tester. Although non-verbal tests of cognitive function are discussed in one of the chapters (Ryan, Chapter 10), most of the other measures described are questionnaires. In these questionnaires subjects are required to follow explicit instructions and respond to some form of verbal statement. Such statements are descriptions of behaviours, attitudes, feelings and the like. Subjects are asked to indicate the extent to which the description is true of him or her, the extent to which she or he agrees with the statement, etc. Table 1 presents a number of questions and response sets from this *Handbook* which are typical for diabetes and health-related measures.

Such items are not just made up and put into the questionnaire at random. They should have been carefully chosen, worded, pilot tested and selected on the basis of empirical data to contain certain properties such as the ability to discriminate between specific groups. Before going on to describe how such items are generated we should note an important distinguishing characteristic between scales; the level of measurement which they attain and therefore the statistical tests which are appropriate. Measurement theory refers to four levels of measurement and the allowable operations (and thus statistics) to which the numbers may be subjected: nominal, ordinal, interval and ratio scales. Asking questions that result in yes/no answers provides responses that are purely categorical and hence nominal in nature. At the other extreme physicists are often, (but not always) justified in assuming that the numbers they use are isomorphic with the physical properties being measured, and hence use ratio level scales. Medical science ranges between these two extremes and care should always be given to identify the level of measurement attained. An important point for the present purposes is that when a rating is made on a five-point scale the resultant numbers do not necessarily attain the

Table 1 Typical questions and response options from scales presented in this volume

Scale and question	Response					
Diabetes Quality of Life (Ch 5)						
How often are you embarrassed having to deal with your diabetes in public?	Never	very seldom	sometimes	often	all the time	
How often do you feel physically ill?	Never	very seldom	sometimes	often	all the time	

Well Being Questionnaire (Ch 6)

	all the time			not at all	
I enjoy the things I do	3	2	1	0	
I feel dull or sluggish	3	2	1	0	

Diabetes Treatment Satisfaction Questionnaire (Ch 7)

	very convenient						very inconvenient	
How convenient have you found your treatment to be recently?		6	5	4	3	2	1	0

Hypoglycaemia Fear Scale (Ch 8)

	never	rarely	sometimes	often	always
I worry about... Passing out in public	0	1	2	3	4
I worry about... Getting a bad evaluation or being criticized	0	1	2	3	4

Diabetes Knowledge Scale (Ch 9)

The presence of ketones in the urine is	A	A good sign
	B	A bad sign
	C	A usual finding in diabetes
	D	I don't know

Attitudes to Diabetes (Ch 11)

	I disagree completely DC	I disagree D	I don't know ?	I agree A	I agree completely AC
Talking to my doctor about my diabetes usually makes me feel better	DC	D	?	A	AC
I dislike being referred to as "A DIABETIC"	DC	D	?	A	AC

Health Beliefs Scale (Ch 12)

	strongly agree					strongly disagree
It is just not possible to control my diabetes properly and live in a way that is acceptable to me	6	5	4	3	2	1	0
Regular controlled exercise helps in the management of my diabetes	6	5	4	3	2	1	0

Barriers to Adherence Scale (Ch 14)

	very rarely or never	once per month	twice per month	once per week	twice per week	more than weekly	daily
I don't feel well	1	2	3	4	5	6	7
I'll say to myself that it won't matter if I don't follow my diet	1	2	3	4	5	6	7

properties required of an interval scale and may well require non-parametric statistical analysis (Siegel, 1956). These issues are discussed in any standard statistical text (e.g. Howell, 1987; Altman, 1991).

ITEM DESIGN

The Origin of Items

The first thing an instrument designer will have to do is collect a series of individual items from which the instrument is to be constructed. Such items will (classically) consist of individual statements which respondents have to endorse in some way, for example by indicating the extent to which they agree or disagree. Initially the questionnaire designer will want to compile a pool of potential items and this list may be derived from a number of sources.

Clinical experience and observation

Items in a health-related questionnaire are often developed from clinical sources. A diabetes questionnaire, for example, may relate to clinical observations which distinguish between groups. Thus, observations by a clinician that people who have better control of their diabetes appear to lead more ordered and less stressful lives may suggest a number of potential scale items. Some clinical observations turn out to be spurious when subjected to careful investigation but such observations are an important source of the first inklings of an hypothesis or theory to be tested.

Theory

A theoretical position is another important starting point in questionnaire design. The design of Health Belief Scales described by Lewis and Bradley (Chapter 12) was guided by the Health Belief Model. Items were constructed to measure four theoretical components of the model adapted to apply specifically to diabetes management: perceived barriers to treatment, perceived benefits of treatment, perceived vulnerability to the complications of diabetes and perceived severity of those complications. The Perceived Control of Diabetes scales described by Bradley in Chapter 13 provide a second example of a questionnaire where the design was strongly influenced by a particular theoretical position, in this case, attribution theory.

Previous research

In addition to providing the basis for hypotheses, the research literature can also be a great source of potential items. Published scales may include certain themes appropriate to particular needs even though the questionnaire as a whole might be inappropriate. Providing copyright is not infringed, due credit is given to the original authors of the items, and providing the new users do not make unwarranted assumptions that items taken from a longer questionnaire will retain the psychometric properties of that questionnaire, such recycling of items is an acceptable and time saving practice.

Expert opinion

It is quite common for items to be devised by discussion with other experts in the subject area. Such expert opinion may be sought in a number of ways with differing degrees of formality. On occasion one may suspect that the experts were canvassed very informally, often over a beer at a conference perhaps! Sometimes it is clear that a more formal procedure is used, formal interviews may have been conducted with selected experts; expert committees may have been consulted (e.g. Williams *et al.*, 1992) or formal written communication may take place with experts. Questionnaires to measure knowledge of diabetes (see Beeney *et al.*, Chapter 9) are usually constructed on the basis of expert opinion. A formal technique for canvassing expert opinion which has to date not been greatly used in questionnaire development is the **Delphi panel** (Linstone and Turoff, 1977; Reid, 1988). The Delphi technique is named after the Greek oracle and was originally developed to estimate the effects of atomic warfare. The Delphi technique is essentially a survey method whereby individual members of the panel are asked for written information which is then fed back to the panel as a whole for further comment with the intention of reaching a consensus. It is thus especially useful when attempting to design items where there is uncertainty concerning the "correct" answer, for example, diabetes knowledge items. As such it can be conceptualised as a committee meeting by post with the test designer acting as chairperson. An important aspect of Delphi is that the panel is anonymous even to other members, thereby removing those components of a committee meeting which depend heavily on personal interaction (for example the postgraduate student deferring to the professor). A disadvantage of the technique is that the developer (the delphic priestess Pythia) may have unwarranted powers of interpretation of the views of the experts, even if the mechanisms are formalised (Mullen, 1983). The technique deserves greater use in instrument development than it has received to date and the development of electronic mail systems using networks such as JANET, INTERNET and BITNET, greatly enhances the viability of the Delphi technique.

The population of interest

A very important source of items is the population that is to be studied. A valuable strategy is to interview a sample of the population for which the instrument is being developed to identify their concerns. Although this is a classic method of developing questionnaire or survey instruments (Cannell and Kahn, 1968), it is surprisingly infrequently used in instrument development. In addition, samples of the survey population can sometimes be directly asked what items they would include in an instrument such as a questionnaire to identify aspects of the diabetes care service with which patients are less than satisfied. However, if patients only have experience of one kind of treatment they may not be the best judges of, for example, appropriate satisfaction items to differentiate between treatment groups. Nevertheless, they may be able to say what they find unsatisfactory with the clinic. Under all circumstances, individuals from the target population should be used for piloting the instrument at an early stage. The Diabetes Health Profile developed by Keith Meadows and Peter Wise presented in the appendix of this *Handbook* was developed on the basis of in-depth interviews with a series of patients.

In overview it is often preferable to use a number of these approaches when designing and selecting items. In practice these different approaches often interlink. Clinicians' experience feeds into the development process. Theoretical positions are held by researchers, who also keep up to date with the literature. Patients are canvassed for their views. What is most important is that these processes are formally constituted, and that pilot studies are conducted with respondents from the target population. Since there is both an art and a science to psychometrics it is not clear whether the best scales would be produced by a newcomer to the field who carefully reviews the literature, uses Delphi panels and interviews people with diabetes or whether scales produced "on the back of an envelope" by an experienced researcher who has years of overview of the subject would be better. What is clear, however, is that an experienced researcher, with a good feel for the area who conducts interviews with patients, reviews literature, obtains expert opinions formally and bases his or her work on theory is most likely to produce credible instruments.

In first judging the likely value of an instrument for a particular purpose there are a number of questions one can answer just by looking at the items. Some measures may be judged to be entirely inappropriate on the basis of an "eyeball" test. Those measures that seem 'on the face of it' to be satisfactory may then be considered in more detail and the more general validity and reliability data scrutinised. Specific questions asked when eye-balling the measure will depend on the nature of the specific issue being investigated but may include the following:

(a) Are the attributes or behaviours (or whatever) represented those which would be expected from clinical experience and/or the literature?
(b) Is each attitude/behaviour represented by multiple items?
(c) Are items written in a clear and unambiguous style?
(d) Are the response alternatives suitable for each item?
(e) Are response alternatives clear and unambiguous and have terms such as "frequently" been adequately defined?
(f) Do items refer to specific behaviours rather than generalities, (as the latter may be responded to in an ambiguous way?)
(g) Finally (and perhaps most importantly) can items be easily answered?

Often one would also want to ask whether the items are double-barrelled, that is do they ask two or more questions at once? However, there are occasions when such phrases are quite allowable and they have a special meaning (e.g. are you tired and emotional?). Such phrases may prove problematic in translation (see Chapter 3). There are also a number of issues concerning the way in which respondents give socially desirable responses, or respond in ways that are biased by general psychological processes, which may need to be taken into account when "eyeballing" a scale. For example does the item format guard against extreme or middle category responding? Such effects, which are more fully discussed by Streiner and Norman (1989), can be avoided by knowledge of likely biases against which to guard and careful wording of items. For example, putting items into the negative in order to reverse the polarity of the response set is one technique used to overcome response biases such as the tendency to make global judgements (the so called "halo" effect).

When first considering an instrument "off the shelf" for a study three further important issues should be considered: standardisation of scores and the existence of normative data, discriminatory power and sensitivity to change. These are discussed in more detail by Bradley in her introductory chapter to this *Handbook*. Often scoring systems for instruments will be such as to standardise scores so that individual scores are expressed in standard deviation units, which can facilitate interpretation. Existence of normative data is clearly important to permit comparison of one's own samples with population norms. Discriminatory power is important since we often use instruments to discriminate between individuals and spread them out across some continuum. Unless the instrument is able to do this, even if it can dichotomise between cases and non-cases accurately, it may be of little use for our purposes. Finally it is clear that the instrument should be sensitive to changes that occur due to treatment and this can be estimated in a number of ways (Streiner and Norman, 1989; Van Belle *et al.*, 1990; Fitzpatrick *et al.*, 1992).

Item Selection and the Structure of Scales

Kline (1979) referred to the art of test construction as that part concerned with the initial formulation of the items, the instructions to subjects about how to complete the instrument and the response types offered. Once data have been collected on the initial pool of items the science can begin, testing them out, subjecting them to validity and reliability tests and using multivariate analysis (especially factor analysis) techniques to inform the construction of scales. Factor analysis can be used to reduce the number of variables to those few that most clearly define a construct. In essence the technique is based on pair-wise correlations between items. The analysis identifies "*factors*", or patterns in the data where that pattern which accounts for the greatest variation in the data set is labelled factor 1. The pattern accounting for the next greatest variation is factor 2 and so on. Each item has a value or loading on each factor. The higher the loading the more important is the item in defining or characterising that factor. Loading values can range from +1 to -1. A loading close to zero indicates that the item does not load on the factor and is therefore unimportant in defining the factor. A cut off point of 0.4 (disregarding the +/-) is often taken to identify items loading highly enough to be important in characterising the factor. The signs in front of the loadings indicate the direction of relationships between the items in much the same way as the sign in front of a correlation coefficient. Imagine, for example, factor analysis was used to select high-loading items designed to measure anxiety. Items were statements with which respondents indicated extent of agreement/disagreement on a four-point scale. Some items were worded as statements describing feelings of tension and stress while others described feelings of calm and relaxation. We would expect those items describing states of anxiety to have the same sign, (it could be + or - depending on the way the items were scored), while items describing state of calm would have loadings with the opposite sign. The factor analysis of the Well-being Questionnaire presented in Chapter 6 demonstrates the relevance of the signs of the loadings quite clearly.

Some measures include a single question to assess a construct (e.g. the two blood glucose items of the Diabetes Treatment Satisfaction Questionnaire are treated as separate items). More often, however, a number of items are used to tap the same underlying construct, or factor. Once multiple questions are used to assess a factor some questions may be more important than others, and hence require weighting, and some items may tap more than one factor. Once a factor is identified it represents whatever the group of items have in common and it should be named in a way to reflect this commonality. Sometimes there may be a "general factor" as well as "specific factors" apparent in a scale. Whether such factors are clarified can depend on the parameters of the analysis set by the researcher. For example, items in a well-being scale may load highly together on a single factor if a one-factor solution is forced. But if no constraints are made by the researcher on the number of factors sought the items may divide up to load on several different factors representing different aspects of well-being. Streiner and Norman (1989) and Kline (1986) are recommended for further general discussion. Kline (1979) gives an overview of statistical techniques in psychometrics and Lawley and Maxwell (1971) present a more specialised introduction to factor analysis.

READABILITY

When constructing psychological scales it is always important to remember that the people completing the questionnaire may not be as literate as those who wrote it. Unless respondents can comprehend the instructions and understand the questions they are being asked the results will have little validity or reliability. It may be worth recalling that tabloid newspapers such as *The Sun* in the UK, *Die Bildzeitung* in Germany and *National Enquirer* in the USA represent the literacy level of many members of our societies.

There are a number of ways in which readability may be assessed. These can be roughly split up into:

1. Subjective assessments
2. Question and answer techniques
3. Ready reckoners
4. Sentence completion and "cloze" techniques
5. Readability formulae

Each of these approaches have their advantages and disadvantages.

Subjective Assessments

Clearly we all make subjective assessments of the style and content of things we read and when choosing a test this will have some influence on a decision as to whether or not to use this test. Multiple readers could be used to grade text and the extent of agreement of these grades checked to give some idea of their reliability. Such subjective judgements are important because as we shall see, objective readability quotients are based on word and sentence length and word familiarity. Thus they are unable to take into account factors such as sentence structure, or motivational factors such as interest, or aesthetic factors. We would recommend that test developers always allow for subjective judgements to be made by respondents about the meaning of items during the early piloting of their measures. Furthermore, such views should be sought from members of the target population, not just easily accessible samples such as undergraduates and colleagues. We would also recommend potential users of "off the shelf" instruments during pilot work to ask their patients to give their views about an instrument. These views may alert the researcher at an early stage to any problems with the acceptability of a measure to her or his subjects. One questionnaire or even one question that causes offence among a battery of questionnaires could result in refusal to complete the series, to say nothing of the personal and professional ramifications it may have.

Question and Answer Techniques

Here independent readers are required to read the text and answer questions on the text. This is done in much the same way as school comprehension tests and précis exercises. There are a number of problems with such comprehension tests, not least of which is that it is not clear what is being assessed. The readability of the text, the ability of the readers to answer questions, the readability of the questions, and the ability to identify redundant words are all factors that may influence responses.

Ready Reckoner Techniques

A number of such techniques have been developed. In general these require counting up the number of sentences, words, syllables or letters in samples of text and consulting preconstructed tables or graphs to interpret the results (Fry, 1968; Mugford, 1969). Whilst such techniques may have the advantage of simplicity this advantage is at the expense of exactitude which reduces the attractiveness of such ready reckoners. Moreover, the time consuming part of the exercise tends to be counting up the number of words and syllables, not the computation of the readability index using a readability formula. It is thus unfortunate to lose information by using the approximations offered by "ready reckoner" techniques, especially now that computers cut out the more tedious parts of the analysis (see below).

Sentence Completion and "Cloze" Techniques

These techniques require that words are left out of the text and respondents fill in the gaps. Simple sentence completion has been modified to the "cloze" procedure by Taylor (1953). "Cloze" requires removal of, usually, some 20% of the words in a text, either at random or systematically. Readability is assessed by having subjects fill in the gaps and then scores are calculated on the basis of the correct responses. Higher scores reflect simpler, more readable texts. Such techniques appear to be of considerable value (Klare, 1963, 1976). They are particularly useful since they take account of both the nature of the text and reader performance. "Cloze" may also be of use for fairly small samples of text, such as may be found in psychometric tests. To date the "cloze" technique has not been greatly used in the development of psychometric instruments. One reason may be that this approach involves running a study with subjects performing the "cloze" procedure rather than the less time consuming use of formulae. Further "cloze" should be used with readers from the population for which the questionnaire has been developed. This methodology will require some development and evaluation, given the lack of contextual cues that questionnaires provide in comparison to longer narratives.

Readability Formulae

A number of formulae have been proposed over the years to assess readability. The Flesch Reading Ease Formula (Flesch, 1948), the Estimated Reading Grade (Dale and Chall, 1948), the "Fog Index" (Gunning, 1952) and the "SMOG" Grading (McLaughlin, 1969) are the most common. We describe the two most frequently used in health-related research the "Flesch" and "Fog" formulae. It is worth noting that the Microsoft Word (Word for Windows) word processing package applies a number of these readability formulae on text as part of its grammar checking procedure.

Flesch formula

Reading Ease (RE) is calculated by selecting samples of 100 words from the text at random, and by counting up to calculate the average number of syllables per 100 words (WL) and the average number of words per sentence (SL) in the selected samples.

$$RE = 206.835 - 0.846 \, WL - 1.015 \, SL$$

The reading ease of the text can then be assessed by reference to Table 2.

Table 2 Interpretation of Flesch Reading Ease Scores

Reading Ease Score	Verbal description	Typical text	Estimated % who would understand	
			aged 25+	aged 65+
90–100	Very easy	Comics	97	91
80–90	Easy	Pulp fiction	95	88
70–80	Fairly easy	Slick fiction	90	77
60–70	Standard	Digests		
50–60	Fairly hard	Quality	77	50
30–50	Difficult	Academic	31	17
0–30	Very hard	Scientific	7	3

Adapted from Ley (1988)

Flesch (1948) also described a "Human Interest" formula to assess personal and motivational characteristics of the text. This requires counting up the number of personal statements in the text, but this approach is not recommended as it can be misleading with many sorts of text.

The Fog Index

The Fog Index (Gunning, 1952) requires first selecting 100 word sample passages. The average sentence length in words (SL) is calculated and the number of "hard" words (HW) counted up. "Hard" is defined as words of three or more syllables but excluding proper nouns, compound words (e.g. bodyweight), verbs that become polysyllabic when conjugated (e.g. dividing), and words very familiar to the reader such as jargon (e.g. insulin). This reading score (FI) is then calculated using the formula.

$$FI = 0.4 \, (SL + HW)$$

Albert and Chadwick (1992) reported Fog Index scores for various types of writing (Table 3).

In overview there appear to be reasonable correlations between these different formulae and other methods of assessing readability (Klare, 1963, 1974, 1976; Gilliland, 1972; Ley, 1977, 1988). Gilliland (1972) reported that the Fog Test tends to

Table 3 Reading scores of various forms of writing using the "Fog" score

	"Fog" Score
Wordsworth ("Upon Westminster Bridge"; repunctuated)	6
Arthur Hailey (*Strong Medicine*)	7
Sunday People (news story)	10
Kingsley Amis (*The Old Devils*)	11
Medical information leaflets (mean of 79 leaflets)	12
Daily Mail (news story)	12
BMJ article (on audit)	16
Times leader	17
Insurance policy	20

Adapted from Albert and Chadwick (1992)

give slightly higher scores (i.e. indicating that the text is less readable) than the Dale and Chall or the SMOG tests. We would recommend that potential users assess the readability of questionnaires using one of these simple techniques, if the readability is not already reported in the literature. This is especially important if the instrument is to be used with a new population. We have recently submitted the instructions and items of a variety of the measures presented in this *Handbook* to Fog testing. The results are presented in Table 4, suggesting that the majority of the scales do not demand particularly sophisticated reading skills, despite the specialist language often used. For comparison it may interest the reader to know that this chapter is not surprisingly a somewhat harder read, with a "Fog" score of 16.5.

Table 4 "Fog" scores for scales presented in the volume

Scale	*(Chapter)*		*"Fog" Score*
DCCT Quality of Life Scale	(5)		9.8
Diabetes Well-being Scale	(6)		6.9
Diabetes Treatment Satisfaction Questionnaire	(7)		11.6
Hypoglycaemia Fear Scale	(8)		6.7
DKN IDDM Scales	(9)	A	8.9
		B	9.4
		C	11.0
ATT39	(11)		10.1
IDDM Health Beliefs Scale	(12)		10.7
NIDDM Health Beliefs Scale	(12)		10.2
IDDM Perceived Control Scale	(13)		10.8
NIDDM Perceived Control Scale	(13)		11.2
Barriers to Adherence Scale	(14)		9.0
Diabetes Self-Care Activities Questionnaire	(15)		12.0

RELIABILITY

Reliability may be more familiar to medical practitioners and scientists in the guise of repeatability. When referring to the reproducibility of test scores, reliability is as applicable to a thermometer or blood glucose assay as it is to a psychometric scale. This is however only one aspect of reliability as it is understood in psychometrics. The second aspect of reliability of a psychometric instrument refers to its internal consistency. These two forms of reliability are dealt with below in turn.

Reliability as Repeatability

The most widely seen forms of reliability *qua* repeatability are test-retest reliability and intercoder reliability. Parallel forms reliability is a less commonly encountered form of reliability, but one that is offered by the Diabetes Knowledge scales described in Chapter 9.

Test-retest reliability

This assesses the stability of test results over time. The instrument is readministered to the same participants after a specified time period, with the expectation that the two sets of scores will be similar, unless there is some *a priori* reason to believe otherwise. The results of the first testing are then correlated with those of the second and a highly reliable test will result in a correlation coefficient approaching +1. If the two sets of scores correlate poorly this is likely to be interpreted as indicative of poor reliability, but it may also indicate that the phenomenon being measured changes over time. This is a difficult issue and in part has to be evaluated on the basis of knowledge of the qualities being measured.

A couple of important points need to be considered in interpreting test-retest results. The first is the test-retest interval. If the test-retest interval is too short, respondents will recall their previous responses and, wishing to appear consistent, may reproduce their earlier responses. Minimising the test-retest interval reduces the opportunity for the to-be-measured quality (e.g. anxiety or beliefs) to change. But it also increases the probability that replies on the second occasion may reflect memory rather than the stability of the actual attribute. Thus whilst evaluating the test-retest reliability of a new blood-glucose assay may be best done by minimising the inter-test interval so as to be sure that the actual levels have not changed, this is not necessarily the case for psychological measures. A high test-retest reliability score over a short time period for a psychological variable is likely to reflect nothing more than participants recalling how they responded previously. On the other hand lower test-retest reliability over longer periods may (as in the case of a blood glucose assay) reflect changing values of the quality being measured. Furthermore, lower test-retest correlations could be good evidence for the *validity* of a measure. This might be the case for measures of state anxiety which one expects to change over time since the measure must possess sensitivity to change. This is especially the case if there are reasons to expect changes in anxiety, (Spielberger *et al.*, 1970) or for that matter blood-glucose levels, which are not expected to remain static across the day. Thus test-retest reliability assessment needs to reach a compromise between these conflicting forces. Furthermore whether or not such assessment is appropriate and how it is interpreted will depend upon theoretical expectations.

Parallel-forms reliability

Although one does not see parallel-forms reliability in the literature very often, it is worth mentioning because test-retest is not always appropriate and some diabetes-related scales exist in parallel forms. One way of overcoming the effects of memory (or learning) is to develop parallel versions of the test rather than giving exactly the same test on repeated occasions. This is especially important for tests of ability or cognitive function (e.g. measures of knowledge of diabetes (Beeney *et al.*, Chapter 9) or measures of cognitive function (Ryan, Chapter 10)). To set the same school exam each year would clearly be ridiculous even though one tries to test the same things annually. So to overcome the problems in examinations new exams are set, but as long as the curriculum does not change the exams are intended to access the same underlying competence and knowledge. Thus, in one version, addition may be tested by "12+4=?" whilst in the parallel version the question is "11+5=?". The same principle can be applied to psychometric scales. Product moment correlations are calculated then between the two sets of scores for the different versions of the tests to examine their reliability. Some authors consider parallel forms reliability to be the best form of reliability (e.g. Rust and Golombok, 1989), but there are problems with this form of reliability. First, it is not always clear that the alternative versions of the test are really parallel. The items may in fact vary in difficulty. Second, there are major practical difficulties in developing multiple versions of a test. Third, some items might be better than others in terms of various aspects of their validity and reliability. In practice they are often incorporated into a single best version of the test (rather than have two less good versions). The Stanford-Binet IQ test is a well-known example of this phenomenon.

Inter-coder or inter-rater reliability

This form of reliability is of major importance in tests which are not self-completed by the individual, for example the Present State Examination (Wing *et al.*, 1974). In essence this form of reliability is assessing the agreement between independent observers of a phenomenon. In test development it is likely to be used if one is attempting to ensure that the scoring procedures for a test are unambiguous. Alternatively as part of a construct-validation exercise one may wish to associate test scores with observed behaviour. One would need to ensure that the behaviour was itself reliably observed and thus one would use inter-rater reliability techniques to do this. In such cases a measure of agreement such as Cohen's Kappa statistic (Cohen, 1960) is usually appropriate. The Kappa statistic ranges from −1 to +1 and results in excess of +0.60 are usually accepted as indicative of reasonable reliability, although this judgement will need to be made in the light of the number of variables and coders being used. Landis and Koch (1977) proposed benchmark terms for Kappa values, (Table 5). Percentage agreement methods should not normally be accepted as measures of inter-coder reliability as these give an inflated impression of agreement (Fleiss, 1973). However a number of authors have suggested that intraclass correlational techniques may under some circumstances be used in preference to Kappa (Maclure and Willett, 1987; Streiner and Norman, 1989). In addition Bland and Altman (1986) proposed a series of simple-to-use methods for continuous data based on graphical presentation.

Table 5 Kappa value benchmarks (Landis and Koch, 1977)

Kappa value	Description
−1.00 – 0.00	"poor"
0.00 – 0.20	"slight"
0.21 – 0.40	"fair"
0.41 – 0.60	"moderate"
0.61 – 0.80	"substantial"
0.81 – 1.00	"almost perfect"

Reliability as Internal Consistency

Reliability is also used to refer to the internal characteristics of a test, specifically its internal consistency. In this approach the homogeneity of the test is being investigated; that is whether the different items that make up a scale are measuring the same thing. Such reliability is measured by item-total correlation, split-half reliability and internal consistency coefficients such as Cronbach's alpha (Cronbach, 1951) or the Kuder-Richardson formulae the KR-20 or less frequently the KR-21 (Kuder and Richardson, 1937; Gulliksen, 1950).

Item-total correlations

In the item-total correlation technique each item is correlated with the total score of the scale with that item omitted. (Nunnally, 1970, 1978). This process requires a series of correlations between each item and the scale scores with that item omitted. This technique is particularly important when attempting to identify specific items that predict the final score well, when for example attempting to shorten a scale. The item's contribution to the total scale score must be removed from the total score as otherwise it will inflate the correlation since it is being correlated with itself.

Split-half reliability

In the split-half technique the instrument is split in half (usually by selecting items at random) and the results of the two half scales are correlated. It is not hard to see that if the scale has internal consistency these two halves should correlate highly. There are a number of draw-backs with this approach however. Perhaps the most important are that (i) split-half reliability tends to underestimate the total reliability of a scale, (ii) there are many ways to split a test in half and not all splits are equal or under all circumstances appropriate and (iii) a single split-half reliability test does not help to identify which items in the scale are contributing to low reliability.

Cronbach's alpha coefficient and the Kuder-Richardson measures of internal consistency

Conceptually Cronbach's alpha and the KR-20 techniques calculate the average of all possible split-half reliabilities of the scale. The advantage of these techniques is that by repeating the operation leaving out different items they permit identification of those items which contribute to low reliability. The correlation techniques needed for calculation are fairly accessible (e.g. Pearson's product moment correlation) and Cronbach's alpha can be calculated using a number of readily available statistical packages (e.g. SPSS/PC+ (Norusis/SPSS Inc, 1990a)). Cronbach's alpha normally varies from 0 to 1, so that the higher the score the greater the internal consistency indicated. However, negative values of alpha can be obtained when the items are not positively correlated with each other and the reliability model is violated (Norusis/SPSS Inc, 1990b).

Interpretation of alpha depends on the number of items. The greater the number of items the higher the alpha coefficient needed to indicate adequate internal consistency. For a three-item scale an alpha coefficient of 0.5 might be regarded as quite sufficient, but inadequate for a ten item scale where an alpha coefficient closer to 0.7 would be sought. It should be noted that alpha coefficients can be artificially elevated by including reworded versions of the same item in a scale. Thus when interpreting alpha coefficients the nature of the items should also be examined. Very high alpha coefficients of 0.9 or greater may indicate that items are being duplicated (e.g. redundancy) and the scale could be shortened. For these reasons then, we normally aim for internal consistency coefficients (such as Cronbach's alpha) of in the region of 0.7 to 0.8 for a scale of ten items or more. This is of course a judgement. However, alphas of much in excess of 0.8 are usually indicative of redundancy within the scale, whilst alphas less than 0.7 may indicate too diffuse a scale (Kline, 1986). The KR-20 is appropriate when the response set is dichotomous (e.g. yes or no). The formula is similar to that for calculations of alpha and is based on the proportion of positive responses to each question and the total score standard deviation. The KR-21 is easier to calculate than KR-20 since it requires only the number of items, the test mean and variance. Whilst KR-21 does give a lower bound for reliability it makes the further assumption that all items are equally difficult.

Whilst both Cronbach's alpha and the KR-20 are relatively easy to calculate and data for their calculation can be obtained on single administration of the instrument, they are unable to take into account variation over time or between raters and are often considered over-optimistic measures of reliability. Such measures must therefore be interpreted in the context of other information about the instrument.

Sample sizes

A number of authors give rules of thumb for the estimation of sample size requirements for reliability studies. Kline (1986) recommended a minimum of 200 participants, but this overgeneralises the sample requirements which will vary with the nature of the measure, and the study design.

For a 95% confidence interval the sample size of a group is normally taken to be $N=(1.96/CI)^2+1$ where CI is the width of the confidence interval. Gore in her series on assessing clinical trials in the *British Medical Journal* gives clear advice about sample size calculation (Gore, 1981). Armitage and Berry (1987) also give a complete overview. Streiner and Norman (1989) present a graph from which it is possible to read off sample size requirements given the bounds of the acceptable confidence intervals. The above texts outline specific techniques for different designs, most importantly depending on estimates of the size of the effect one is measuring. There is an important point to take into account when estimating sample size for any study which is often overlooked. This is that the sample size relates to the numbers of subjects required for analysis rather than to how many people are asked to take part in the study. Thus one should also estimate the refusal and drop-out rates so as to identify sufficient subjects to give a final sample size of the required magnitude. It is always worth rounding up in this circumstance and not being blinded by the apparent precision of the sample size estimate one calculates.

Questions to ask of reliability testing

In overview when considering reliability one should ask a number of questions. These include:
(a) What was the logic of testing reliability in this way?
(b) Would one expect the attribute to be stable?
(c) Has test-retest reliability been assessed over a reasonable time period?
(d) Has the reliability been tested on a reasonable sample?
(e) Is the population sampled similar to the one of interest?
(f) Is the internal consistency reported reasonable?
(g) Is there excessive redundancy?

VALIDITY

At its simplest the validity of an instrument refers to whether or not it measures the qualities it purports to measure. To the medically trained this may be reminiscent of the *specificity* and *sensitivity* of a diagnostic or screening test. Sensitivity is the proportion of truly diseased individuals in the population who are identified by the test, it is thus a measure of the probability of correct diagnosis of a case (true positive rate). Sensitivity is of course directly related to specificity, which is the proportion of truly non-diseased individuals so identified by a test. Thus specificity is a measure of the probability of correctly identifying a non-diseased person (true negative rate) (Last, 1988).

Whilst with a diagnosis it is taken for granted that there is a true prevalence of the disease which a screening test is attempting to identify, it is perhaps not so straightforward when attempting to measure psychological processes or entities such as "fear of hypoglycaemia" or "well-being". One way of conceptualising validity is to identify what it is we are attempting to do when testing individuals. For example, only the most jaded of teachers or university lecturers see examinations as an end in themselves. Exams are designed to tap students' knowledge of a subject area, their skill in solving problems and the like. These abilities in themselves are seen only as surrogates for identifying which individuals may be permitted to go on to a university education or to practise medicine (or whatever) within the accepted bounds of competence. A test then is designed to permit us to make judgements or inferences about the people who complete it. It is only of use in so far as it is accurate. This is the essence of validity testing. Whilst validity and reliability are distinct concepts they are in fact related. To be valid a test needs also to be reliable. Higher validity is associated with higher reliability (the maximum validity of a test equals the square root of its reliability coefficient) although there is one important exception to this which we will describe later. The reverse is not always the case: higher reliability is not necessarily associated with greater validity. A test may be highly reliable while not measuring accurately what it purports to measure. Thus a scale purporting to measure depressed mood may include items concerned with physical symptoms (such as fatigue and weight loss) that can be indicators of depression in the general population. Even if such a measure proves to be reliable when used with people who have Type 1 diabetes (and it may not), its validity as a measure of depression in this group is in doubt. This is because items which reflect the physical symptoms of depression in the general population may be due to high blood glucose levels in someone with Type 1 diabetes. As with reliability testing it is also necessary to assess whether the sample sizes used in the validation exercises are large enough. Since validity testing is essentially hypothesis testing there are no simple rules of thumb. Each study will have to be considered on the basis of its own merits. The earlier references given on sample size calculation will prove of use here also.

Validity is a heterogeneous concept. For any one instrument, a number of aspects of validity will be relevant, and these can sometimes be mutually exclusive or at least antagonistic. Below, the main sorts of validity are described. However, when assessing validity one must always consider for oneself the logic that underlies the use of the different forms of validity for any instrument. Most important is to ask the question "why did the test constructors test validity in this way?" It is unfortunate that on occasion the designers of the instrument will not have asked themselves this fundamental question before proceeding, but instead may have followed some "cookbook" and ritualistic approach to scale development. A second point should also be borne in mind. Even once you are satisfied that the validity of an instrument has been demonstrated it cannot be assumed that it will generalise to all populations or users. For example the Diabetes Quality of Life instrument described by Jacobson in Chapter 5 of this volume was initially developed for use with young insulin users. For use with older patients with Type 2 diabetes its psychometric properties have needed to be reassessed and were found to be rather less satisfactory.

Face Validity

Face validity refers to how an instrument looks: does the scale appear to measure what it claims to measure? Thus one asks whether "on the face of it" the scale appears to measure the qualities it is intended to measure. Face validity may bear little relation to the other more formal aspects of validity but it is not trivial since it relates to the motivation of participants completing the test. If face validity is low respondents may refuse to do a "stupid test". Alternatively, face validity may be good but not supported by other aspects of validity. Consider, for example, a hypothetical scale that is designed to distinguish between patients who follow their doctor's advice in the treatment of their diabetes and those who do not. Such a scale which consists of items which ask patients whether they always do as their doctor advises, whether they listen to their doctor, etc. may have good face validity. However, it may not actually be measuring this aspect of their behaviour at all, but rather some aspect of their social conformity. The ability of the scale to predict behaviour may be poor even though face validity appears to be good. Face validity is not only of importance to participants completing questionnaires. It is often also an important factor in users' decisions as to whether or not to use an instrument and we referred to this earlier as "eye-balling" an instrument. While it is important to satisfy face validity concerns, choosing an instrument solely on this basis would be rather like buying a motor car on the basis of its colour, rather than its ability to start, fuel consumption and other less immediately obvious attributes. One problem with face validity is that with some tests, the purpose of the test may be hidden from respondents intentionally, perhaps in order to minimise faking. Such an aim will be antagonistic to the aims of face validity and must be carefully considered when choosing a test. An important practical issue here relates to how the scale is administered and how to maximise response rates. It may be possible to sacrifice the advantages of high face validity if there are other ways to ensure good response rates. However, postal surveys are particularly influenced by face validity in the maintenance of response rates, (see Miller (1992) for ways of improving response rates for mail surveys). A slightly different but related point is that when administering instruments one should avoid poor quality photocopies or poorly laid out questionnaires as these will influence the way in which they are filled out, or whether they are filled out at all.

Content Validity

Content validity refers to whether or not all relevant topics are sampled by an instrument. Content validity is most easily exemplified when the subject area is clearly defined. An instrument measuring "diabetes knowledge" which failed to include items about blood glucose levels would have little content validity, even if to the patients completing the test it had high face validity. Content validity then refers to the representativeness of the selection of questions included. As well as ensuring all relevant parts of the construct are represented within the scale, there is a need to ensure that no extraneous questions are asked.

As Streiner and Norman (1989) argued there are also implications for the sorts of inferences one can draw on the basis of the content validity of the instrument. When measuring relatively broad constructs such as satisfaction with the diabetes care service provided, if some aspects of the construct are not covered by the instrument then the inferences we make from the scores on the scales may on occasion be wrong. Thus a satisfaction scale that focused on doctors' communication skills would not be sufficient to permit accurate inferences about other aspects of patient satisfaction (length of wait, privacy, competence of doctor, acceptability of regimen). On the other hand an over-inclusive satisfaction scale that included items about job satisfaction or family relationships may be just as misleading, but in a different way.

Content validity is the one area of validity testing where there can be conflict between the aims of obtaining high reliability, in the form of internal consistency, and validity. The reason for this is easy to see when one considers that internal consistency is also related to redundancy. A scale which had perfect internal consistency would suffer from redundancy. In this case every item would be measuring exactly the same thing and therefore all but one of the items are redundant. This may also imply that the overall scale is highly specific and hence does not address all aspects of a construct and therefore has low content validity. High internal consistency therefore has its own disadvantages and should be treated as subsidiary to the goals of content validity and reducing redundancy. It is for these reasons as we argued earlier that one should usually aim for alpha coefficients of approximately 0.7 – 0.8 for ten or more item scales.

Criterion-Related Validity

This is the classic concept of validity. To validate the instrument it is compared to some other criterion, some "gold standard". One problem worth thinking about when looking at a new instrument is that if there is a "gold-standard" why is it necessary to develop another test. One answer is that the "gold standard" may be too long for everyday purposes, but there are a number of other reasons one might develop a new test, not all of which relate to the science (e.g. owning the copyright and being able to use the test freely). Criterion-related validity(also called external validity) is often thought of as being of two varieties; concurrent and predictive validity (see below).

When developing a practical scale of diabetes-related beliefs or knowledge, the test developer is probably not centrally concerned with individuals' scores in terms of his or her knowledge, but with the influence the knowledge or beliefs have on behaviour and the clinical outcomes associated with this behaviour. For example, for it to be of any practical use, a measure of foot-care procedures in diabetes should be predictive of future complications of the feet and amputation. Whilst it makes certain assumptions about the causal relationship between foot-care knowledge and amputation it would be reasonable to predict that patients who score poorly on a "foot-care scale" would be more likely in future to require amputation. This is, in theory, a simple enough hypothesis to test. But in practice it is more problematic for two reasons. First, there is a time delay inherent in this approach since amputation would be a long-term outcome of poor foot care. Second, there is the ethical consideration of what one does when an individual is identified as being at high risk of some adverse outcome. Whilst such considerations may not be of paramount importance in, for example, prediction of consumer behaviour for purchasing one soap powder as opposed to another, the prediction of health outcomes - or expectation that there will be a poor outcome - will be used to make intervention decisions. Thus in our "foot-care scale" example a poor score would perhaps result in the patient receiving some remedial foot-care education. This is in essence a violation of the "blindness" of the study and such contamination will result in a poor study at least in scientific terms. Such **criterion contamination** is probably most common in clinical practice because of the need to intervene and classic examples are to be found in the suicide prediction literature (Todd, 1992). If, for example, when developing a new instrument to measure "self-care behaviour" the results from the administration of the instrument are used in the clinical or diagnostic process the criterion group will be contaminated. Similar problems regularly occur in our education systems, but a slightly different problem can also be clarified by considering education. If students' entry to university, is made on the basis of an exam result and then these exam results are used to predict how well they will fare with their degree, often we will be disappointed with the low correlations between the two sets of scores. In part this is because we have used the original exam data to permit our students to enter university thus truncating the distribution of scores on the first exam. This has the consequence of reducing the correlation of the first exam with the second. The first exam was designed to be discriminating across a broader distribution than just those who actually entered for the second exam who will have all scored in the top range of the marks awarded.

Construct Validity

Psychometricians often talk of measuring a "construct" and we have already used the term on a number of occasions in this chapter. The concept of "construct validity" was introduced into the literature nearly forty years ago (Cronbach and Meehl, 1955). A construct is a hypothetical entity which underlies the responses obtained. It is something which itself is not observable directly. This may seem a strange notion to people educated in medicine, used to measuring physiological processes such as blood pressure and heart rate. It is however a fundamental problem for psychology where the very objects of interest have no physical existence. Where are intelligence, depression, anxiety, or extroversion? In this sense intelligence is a hypothetical construct which is powerful enough to explain a number of more directly observable behaviours. The problem is also to be found in the physical sciences. In quantum mechanics, force-carrying particles are in this sense constructs, they cannot be directly detected by a particle detector but they are known to exist because of their measurable effects.

As Streiner and Norman (1989) pointed out, in clinical medicine the syndrome is a very similar entity to the construct. A cluster of signs and symptoms may come to be recognised as a typical clinical manifestation for which there is no clear causal pathogen or mechanism. It is impossible to prove that an individual has the syndrome by a test, but other diagnoses can be excluded. The syndrome is used to explain the observed symptoms, and tying "them together conceptually by postulating an underlying disorder which cannot be measured directly." (Streiner and Norman, 1989, p.114). As such, a syndrome may be a "disease-in-waiting", although it may be something quite different. A construct then can be thought of as a theory (one that we may even take for granted as we do "intelligence") which explains the data (or experience). In attempting to measure construct validity one should be able to identify a number of variables and hypothesise relationships between them.

Construct validity testing is perhaps best explained by example. To validate a measure of "fear of hypoglycaemia" one might generate a number of hypotheses and experiments to test these. If an individual has low fear of hypoglycaemia then we would expect them to score low on a more general fear scale, be less anxious and thus score low on a trait anxiety measure or have higher scores on a self-confidence measure than a person with high fear of hypoglycaemia. We might hypothesise only moderate correlations as the other measures are either not very good ones or they measure a more general notion of affect than our specific measure. It would not be hard to think up a number of testable hypothetical relationships between fear of hypoglycaemia and other psychological attributes or behaviours, such as frequency of blood glucose monitoring. Perhaps, also one could think up a number of situations by which to test the hypothetical construct. People with high fear of hypoglycaemia may be hypothesised to be more likely to carry glucose tablets than people who had low hypoglycaemia fear. They may be hypothesised to behave differently if told to prepare for a long wait in an isolated location. Experiments can be designed to test these hypothesis. Such an experiment, or series of experiments, would go some way towards validating the construct. However a Popperian would argue that one cannot prove the hypothesis to be correct. Popper (1959, 1963) argued that we learn more to advance science by the falsification of hypotheses than we do by their confirmation. According to this view in order to learn anything we need to falsify the hypothesis, which is at odds with the inductive logic of this form of test validation. If the expected relationships do not appear it may be because an hypothesis or prediction is erroneous or the measure inadequate, or the theory (the construct) on which our testing is based is incorrect. However it is generally accepted that construct validity is a powerful approach to validity demonstration, whereby rather than considering a single result we simultaneously take into account a set of results. Given that in practice the results are seldom clear cut, when reviewing instruments validated in this way, one must carefully consider the logic of the tests and be willing to be critical of their interpretation.

Concurrent Validity

Concurrent validity, which is an aspect of criterion-related validity, involves administrating the measure under development at the same time as a "gold standard" or criterion measure of the same attribute. The choice of criterion measure may be problematic, but one should aim to identify a well validated and accepted measure of the attribute. This concurrent administration of measures permits comparison and correlations to be calculated. For example, if one was developing a short measure of global neuropsychological function for routine clinical use with diabetic patients, one may administer this short measure alongside the "gold standard" Halstead-Reitan Neuropsychological Battery (HRNB) (described by Ryan in Chapter 10) to a series of subjects. One would then correlate the results from the new test and its subscales with those from the HRNB and its subscales to assess concurrent validity.

Predictive Validity

Predictive validity, another aspect of criterion-related validity, assesses whether the scale permits prediction of some future event. For example, is IQ at eleven years of age a good predictor of university achievement? Do health beliefs and perceptions of control over diabetes predict blood glucose control twelve months later? Do they predict ketoacidosis? Do they predict the development of the long term complications of diabetes? Clearly numerous hypotheses could be generated about such constructs and then tested.

Discriminant Validity

When demonstrating construct validity one should attempt to demonstrate what a test does not measure as well as what it does. This is an important notion and is known as discriminant validity. The scale measuring the construct should not correlate with scales measuring dissimilar constructs. In the case of the measure of "fear of hypoglycaemia" we would not expect any relationship with intelligence. Thus if during the validation studies we demonstrated little or no correlation between intelligence and "fear of hypoglycaemia" this would be evidence of discriminant validity. However, there can sometimes be confounding relationships between constructs and one must formulate hypotheses with considerable care. Readers should also be aware that there is some confusion in the literature since some authors use the term "discriminant validity" to refer to what is here called "extreme groups validity".

Convergent Validity

Convergent validity is, as it were, the concurrent validity of construct validation. An attempt is made to demonstrate how well the new scale relates (converges) with other measures of either the same construct, or other related constructs. Whilst in practice the procedures for assessing concurrent and convergent validity are very similar, the distinction is conceptually and theoretically important. Concurrent validation assesses how the new instrument measures up against a "gold standard". Convergent validation assesses whether the measure taps an underlying construct successfully by comparing it to another (presumably imperfect but accepted) assessment of the construct.

Extreme groups validity

This approach (sometimes called criterion groups validity) is perhaps one of the most obvious ways to test the validity of an instrument. Some authors refer to it as "discriminant validity". Extreme groups validation consists of administering the instrument to different groups whom one hypothesises will have different total scores or patterns of scores on the instrument. Thus, for example, a "fear of hypoglycaemia" scale should elicit different responses from a group of insulin users leaving a casualty department following a "hypo" than from a similar group of people who have not experienced a "hypo".

Overview

In overview, validity testing requires an hypothesis testing approach, for which there is no single cookbook recipe. In many ways, validity testing tests the ingenuity of the test developer to set up hypotheses and test them in novel ways. To some degree validity testing does consist of "pulling oneself up by one's bootstraps" and can be in danger of tautological argument. As such, there are risks that confounding variables have not been adequately teased out or taken into account. As a reader and potential user.it is up to you to question the logic of the designers and not just take at face value a plethora of numbers and claims that a measure is valid.

While it is essential that new scales be developed psychometrically, no single scale can be expected to demonstrate all aspects of reliability and validity. Scales that have been in widespread use for decades may be expected to have evidence for most kinds of reliability and validity. Newly developed scales cannot be expected to have evidence for more than a limited range of acceptable properties which might include (where appropriate) internal consistency, face, content and construct validity and factor analytic evidence for any hypothesised subscales. Forms of reliability and validity testing that require the passage of time, such as test-retest reliability and predictive validity might be tested at a later date. Opportunities for testing extreme groups validity and sensitivity to change may arise in other researchers' studies and gradually a fuller range of psychometric properties are established and can be pieced together. At the beginning of this chapter we quoted from Kline (1986) to the effect that psychometric scales are not always as well validated as one may hope. It is hoped that the present chapter has given some insight into the processes of instrument development so that in future there will be less chance of unreliable scales entering the literature and being blindly accepted by readers. This is a particular problem in health research because there is currently such demand for psychosocial scales to measure outcomes of care and so few reviewers of specialist medical journals with the knowledge and expertise to sort the wheat from the chaff; itself a good psychometric project.

SUMMARY

In this chapter we have given an introduction to the art and science of test development, concentrating on the principles of designing "paper and pencil" self-report instruments of the kind described in this *Handbook*. We have described the origin of items that go to make up such measures and have stressed that test designers not only need insight into the issues but that clinical experience, observation, theory, previous research, expert opinion (by formal methods such as the Delphi technique) and the views of people with diabetes (the population of interest) should all be considered in building up a pool of items for any new measure. Such items are then tested with groups of subjects in order to identify underlying factors and to ascertain the other formal psychometric properties of the new instrument. We emphasise the importance of readability and reviewed readability assessment methods. "Fog" testing is suggested as a straightforward and accessible method of identifying the readability of a text. The measures presented in this *Handbook* have been "Fog" tested and found to be for the most part on a level with the euphemistic "easy read".

The range of formal psychometric properties which a measure should possess include aspects of reliability and validity. Reliability refers not only to the property of the measure to give the same or similar results on repeated administrations, but also to internal characteristics of the measure (internal consistency). When deciding to adopt a test from the literature, evaluating a journal paper or a chapter in this *Handbook* readers are advised to consider carefully the logic of the reliability testing presented, the nature of the statistics presented and the size and composition of the samples upon which the studies are based. Internal consistency testing is one of those cases where a larger value does not necessarily mean better, since it may just indicate redundancy in items. Validity refers to whether or not a measure actually measures the qualities it purports to measure. Face validity refers to how an instrument appears, content validity to how representative the questions are, criterion validity to its relationship to some "gold standard". Since there is seldom a "gold standard" we argue that the most important initial approach is to assess the construct validity along with face and content validity and the internal consistency reliability of the instrument.

REFERENCES

Albert, T. and Chadwick, S. (1992) How readable are practice leaflets? *British Medical Journal*, **305**, 1266–1268

Altman, D. G. (1991) *Practical statistics for medical research*. London: Chapman and Hall

Armitage, P. and Berry, G. (1987) *Statistical methods in medical research*. Oxford: Blackwell Scientific

Bland, J. M. and Altman, D. G. (1986) Statistical methods for assessing agreement between two methods of clinical measurement *The Lancet*, **1**, (Feb 8th), 307-310

Cannell, C. F. and Kahn, R. L. (1968) Interviewing. In G. Lindzey and E. Aronson (eds) *The handbook of social psychology*. Reading, Mass: Addison Wesley

Cohen, J. (1960) A coefficient of agreement for nominal scales, *Educational and Psychological Measurement*, **20**, 37–46

Cronbach, L. J. (1951) Coefficient alpha and the internal structure of tests, *Psychometrika*, **16**, 297–334

Cronbach, L. J. and Meehl, P. E. (1955) Construct validity in psychological tests, *Psychological Bulletin*, **52**, 281–302

Dale, E. and Chall, J. S. (1948) A formula for predicting readability *Educational Research Bulletin*, 27 Jan, 11-20 and Feb, 37–54

Fitzpatrick, R., Fletcher, A., Gore, S., Jones, D., Spiegelhalter, D. and Cox, D. (1992) Quality of life measures in health care. I: Applications and issues in assessment *British Medical Journal*, **305**, 1074–7

Fleiss, J. L. (1971) Measuring nominal scale agreement among many raters *Psychological Bulletin*, **76**, 378–382

Fleiss, J. L. (1973) *Statistical methods for rates and proportions*. London: Wiley

Flesch, R. F. (1948) A new readability yardstick *Journal of Applied Psychology*, **32**, 221–233

Fry, E. A. (1968) A readability formula that saves time, *Journal of Reading*, **11**, 513–516

Gilliland, J. (1972) *Readability*. London: University of London and UK Reading Association

Gore, S. M. (1981) Trial size *British Medical Journal*, **282**, 1687-1689. Reprinted in S.M. Gore and

D.G. Altman (1982) *Statistics in practice.* London: British Medical Association

Gulliksen, H. (1950) *Theory of mental tests.* New York: Wiley

Gunning, R. (1952) *The technique of clear writing.* New York: McGraw Hill

Howell, D. C. (1987) *Statistical methods for psychology.* (2nd Edition). Boston: Duxbury

Klare, G. R. (1963) *The measurement of readability.* Iowa: Iowa State University Press

Klare, G. R. (1974) Assessing readability *Reading Research Quarterly,* 1, 62–102

Klare, G. R. (1976) A second look at the validity of readability formulae *Journal of Reading Behaviour,* 8, 129–152

Kline, P. (1979) *Psychometrics and psychology.* London: Academic Press

Kline, P. (1986) *A handbook of test construction.* London: Methuen

Kuder, G. F. and Richardson, M.W. (1937) The theory of estimation of test reliability *Psychometrika,* 2, 151–160

Landis, J. R. and Koch, G. G. (1977) The measurement of observer agreement for categorical data, *Biometrics,* 33, 159–174

Last, J. M. (1988) *A dictionary of epidemiology.* (2nd Edition). Oxford: Oxford University Press

Lawley, D. N. and Maxwell, A. E. (1971) *Factor analysis as a statistical method.* London: Butterworth

Ley, P. (1977) Psychological studies of doctor-patient communication. In S. Rachman (ed.) *Contributions to medical psychology. Vol 1.* Oxford: Pergamon

Ley, P. (1988) *Communicating with patients: Improving communication, satisfaction and compliance.* London: Croom Helm

Linstone, H. A. and Turoff, M. (eds) (1977) *The Delphi method: techniques and applications.* Reading, Mass: Addison Wesley

Maclure, M. and Willett, W. C. (1987) Misinterpretation and misuse of the Kappa statistic *American Journal of Epidemiology,* 126, 161–169

McLaughlin, G. H. (1969) The SMOG grading: A new readability formula *Journal of Reading,* 12, 639–646

Miller, D. C. (1992) *Handbook of research design and social measurement.* (5th Edition). London: Sage

Mugford, L. (1969) A new way of predicting readability *Reading,* 4, 31–35

Mullen, P. M. (1983) *Delphi-type studies in the health services: The impact of the scoring system.* University of Birmingham: Health Services Management Centre

Norusis, M. J./SPSS Inc (1990a) *SPSS/PC+4.0 Base Manual.* Chicago: SPSS Inc.

Norusis, M. J./SPSS Inc (1990b) *SPSS Base System User's Guide.* Chicago: SPSS Inc.

Nunnally, J. C. (1970) *Introduction to psychological measurement.* New York: McGraw Hill

Nunnally, J. C. (1978) *Psychometric theory.* New York: McGraw Hill

Popper, K. (1959) *The logic of scientific discovery.* London: Hutchinson

Popper, K. (1963) *Conjectures and refutations.* London: Routledge and Kegan Paul.

Reid, N. (1988) The Delphi technique: Its contribution to the evaluation of professional practice. In R. Ellis (ed.) *Professional competence and quality assurance in the caring professions.* London: Croom Helm

Rust, J. and Golombok, S. (1989) *Modern psychometrics: The science of psychological assessment.* London: Routledge

Siegel, S. (1956) *Non parametric statistics for the behavioural sciences.* New York: McGraw Hill

Spielberger, D. Gorsuch, R.L. and Lushene, R. (1970) *Manual of the State-Trait Anxiety Inventory.* Palo Alto, California: Consulting Psychologists Press

Streiner, D. L. and Norman, G.R. (1989) *Health measurement scales: A practical guide to their development and use.* Oxford: Oxford University Press

Taylor, W. L. (1953) Cloze procedure: A new tool for measuring readability *Journalism Quarterly,* 30, 415–433

Todd, C. J. (1992) Reduction in the incidence of suicide: A health gain objective for the NHS *Psychopharmacology,* 6, 318–324 van Belle G., Uhlmann, R.F., Hughes, J.P. and Larson, E.B. (1990) Reliability of estimates of change in mental status test performance in senile dementia of the Alzheimer type *Journal of Clinical Epidemiology*, **43**,589–595

Williams, D. R. R., Home, P.D. and Members of a Working Group of the Research Unit of the Royal College of Physicians and British Diabetic Association. (1992) A proposal for continuing audit of diabetes services *Diabetic Medicine*, **9**, 759–764

Wing, J. K., Cooper, J. E. and Satorius, N. (1974) *The measurement and classification of psychiatric symptoms: An instruction manual for the Present State Examination and CATEGO programme.* Cambridge: Cambridge University Press

ACKNOWLEDGEMENTS

The authors would like to thank Deborah Morgan, Siobhan Carew and Jennifer Stevens at the Institute of Public Health, University of Cambridge for secretarial assistance in preparation of this chapter.

CHAPTER 3

TRANSLATION OF QUESTIONNAIRES FOR USE IN DIFFERENT LANGUAGES AND CULTURES

CLARE BRADLEY

Department of Psychology, Royal Holloway, University of London, Egham Hill, Egham, Surrey, TW20 0EX, UK

The complexity of the process of translating questionnaires and the skills needed to tackle the task are commonly underestimated. Medical researchers in non-English speaking countries often speak very good English themselves and mistakenly assume that they can rely on their own translation of an English questionnaire into their native language. They often fail to see the need for appropriate checks on their translation and may not appreciate that literal translation cannot ensure equivalence of meaning. Data collection may be proceeded with using an inadequate translation. Translation problems may later come to light if responses to the translation are checked against those associated with the original and found to differ markedly. However, widespread ignorance of the need for such checking is perhaps more likely to lead to the results being accepted as valid and reliable when they are not. At best then, a poorly translated questionnaire will simply be a waste of time as responses are found to be uninterpretable or unreliable. At worst, a poorly translated questionnaire will produce data which are misleading, may undermine patients' confidence, and may be destructive in various other ways if inappropriate management decisions are based upon the results of a faulty translation.

Inadequate translations of questionnaires abound and detecting poor translations is not always a straightforward matter. The unwary user of an existing translation may discover only after collecting all their data and conducting the data analysis that the questionnaire is not working as expected. Before attributing the problem to the questionnaire design, the user should investigate the translation. Better still the procedures used in producing a translation should be determined before using any translation. Although a good translation is only the first step in the successful transfer of a scale from one culture to another it is a vitally important first step and the one on which many translations fall down.

INITIAL LINGUISTIC PROCEDURES

The Individual Translator

It is essential that translators of questionnaires should be fluent in the languages concerned but fluency alone is not a sufficient qualification for the task. The translator needs to understand the purpose of the questionnaire and the intention underlying the design of each item. There are usually many options to choose from when deciding upon the wording of an item being translated. A word-for-word translation, which results in precisely the same meaning as the original, is rarely possible. The translator is often required to construct a new version of the item and hence needs an appreciation of the requirements and pitfalls of item construction and questionnaire design. It is rare to find all these skills in the same person and a compromise usually has to be reached with a linguist working in collaboration with the person who designed and developed the original questionnaire or with someone else experienced in scale development and item construction who is familiar with the details of the design and development of the particular instrument to be translated.

The Committee Approach

One approach to translation of scales is the committee approach described by Simonsen and Mortensen (1990). With this approach, several translations are produced independently by different translators who then meet to discuss discrepancies between their various translations with a view to reaching agreement on the most appropriate translation of each item. Such an approach is likely to identify at an early stage idiosyncratic interpretations of the meaning of items as well as minor inaccuracies. The committee might include the person who constructed the original scale among its members or a selection of individuals who together bring the information, skills and experience needed to tackle the task. The financial resources available would need to be substantial for such a strategy and the logistics of bringing together the necessary committee members would be problematic with a limited budget and several translations to be organised. It is more realistic where only one translation is required, and the linguistic and psychometric expertise is readily available and budgeted for. This committee approach would also be likely to identify and deal with many of the problems of translation that otherwise take much longer to sort out using a series of individual translators and the process of back-translation described below.

Back-translation and Retranslation

Back-translation is a very important second step in the translation process which other writers (e.g. Streiner and Norman, 1989) have noted is frequently omitted. Whether the initial translation is produced by a single translator or by a committee, back-translation is needed to identify any discrepancies between the meaning of the translation and that of the original questionnaire. Back-translation is conducted by one or more translators who have not seen the questionnaire in its original language form and who translate the new translation back into the language of the original. The back-translations are then compared with the original to identify any linguistic inaccuracies. Any poorly translated items identified are then retranslated and subsequently back-translated by a different back-translator. This cycle is repeated until the back-translation is sufficiently similar in meaning to the original instrument.

Combining Methods

Inaccuracies in translation are likely to be less common where a committee approach has been used. Where the translation was created by an individual translator, the process of back-translation and retranslation may have to be repeated more often before satisfactory equivalence is obtained between the back-translation and the original questionnaire. A more economical and realistic alternative to the committee approach might be the Delphi panel approach (Linstone and Turoff, 1977), described by Todd and Bradley elsewhere in this volume. If the Delphi panel technique was applied to the translation process the panel might be equivalent to the committee described above but instead of meeting together they would correspond with the chairperson organising the translation. It is likely that the Delphi panel approach would be most practical and effective if use was also made of back-translations and retranslations which were commented on by panel members.

Choice of Translators, Back-translators and Retranslators

Ideally the back-translators employed should be native speakers of the language in which the original questionnaire was designed and fluent in the language of the translation while the initial translators and retranslators should be native speakers of the language of the new translation and fluent in the language of the original questionnaire.

It is particularly important that the initial translation and any retranslations are conducted by native speakers of the language of the translation in order to increase the likelihood of a translation that reads well and uses colloquialisms where appropriate in addition to having equivalence of meaning. It is not always possible to find back-translators who fit the above criteria. In my own research group's efforts to improve translations of the Well-being scales and the forerunner of the Diabetes Treatment Satisfaction Questionnaire (described in later chapters) it was not possible to find native English speakers who were fluent in some of the languages of translations we were working with such as Albanian. In these cases we employed Albanian translators with fluent English for back-translation.

When questionnaires about diabetes and its management are being translated, terms such as "hypo" referring to hypoglycaemia or "high sugar coma" referring to hyperglycaemic coma may be used. Choice of the appropriate terminology to be used in the translation should be guided by knowledge of the terminology used by the people with diabetes who use the language of the translation. Doctors and nurses involved with diabetes management may be a good source of information about terminology that patients use, another source of information is magazines written for people with diabetes in the language of the translation. In the UK the magazine *Balance* is produced by the British Diabetic Association, in the USA the American Diabetes Association produces *Diabetes Forecast* and there are many European magazines being produced. It is well worth conducting pilot studies of new translations that involve technical terms to reduce the risk of discovering too late in the day that not all patients understood the terminology. A pilot study to check the choice of terminology is appropriate may only require a sample as small as five or six patients if some of the patients are selected from among those most likely to experience comprehension problems. If these patients can define the meaning of the terminology accurately enough and confirm that these are the terms they would use then the translation is likely to be appropriate. If the terminology chosen is inappropriate it will be apparent in discussions with the patients who can then be asked to suggest more appropriate terms.

Review by Potential Users

Once the translators have produced a translation which back-translates well, I recommend that the new translation be sent for review by the potential users of the questionnaire. By users, I am referring here not to the patients who might complete the questionnaires but to the diabetologists, diabetes specialist nurses or psychologists working in diabetes clinics in the country where the language of the translation is spoken. These are the people who will decide whether or not to use the questionnaire. If the questionnaire does not suit their needs and preferences it is unlikely to be used and the translation effort will be wasted. The responses of such users who have been asked to review translations of my research group's Well-being Questionnaire and Diabetes Treatment Satisfaction Questionnaire have varied widely from apparently minor superficial changes, through suggestions for a single but important change to one item to, in an extreme case, the production of three new retranslations within the same language. Even when potential users are informed of the purpose of the questionnaire and any subscales it may have, there is a risk that they will misunderstand the purpose of an item and modifications may distort the meaning away from the original in a manner which is unhelpful. Any changes suggested by users need to be back-translated to ensure that meaning is not changed inappropriately. Where back-translation indicates a problem with the suggested change, the reviewer's reasons for requesting a change need to be explored with a view to reaching a compromise that meets the reviewer's needs while retaining the intended meaning of the item.

The linguistic processes of translating, back-translating, retranslating and reviewing are summarised in a flow diagram in Figure 1.

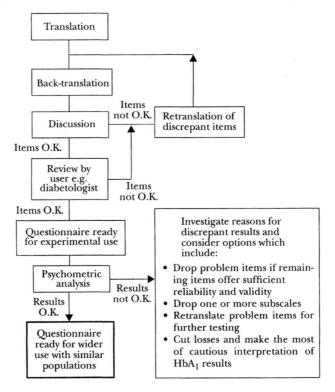

Figure 1: A recommended process for translation of questionnaires

Problems Identifiable by Back-translation and Review

Gross errors of meaning introduced by the translation will mostly be readily visible when comparing the back-translation with the original questionnaire. What are less easily identified are more subtle changes in strength or breadth of meaning which may have a profound effect on respondents' ratings. Some examples are provided below from work by Meadows and Bradley (1991) translating into French and German the Well-being Questionnaire described in a later chapter and the Satisfaction with Treatment scale which was the forerunner of, and closely similar to, the Diabetes Treatment Satisfaction Questionnaire (DTSQ) which I describe elsewhere in this book. The examples give the original English, the back-translation from French or German and a description of our interpretation of the problem.

Examples of mistranslated items identified in the French and German Well-being Questionnaires and DTSQs

1. Original English item   "I feel afraid for no reason at all"
   Back-translated from French as   "I feel uneasy for no reason"

The problem: Feeling "uneasy" for no reason is less strong than the original feeling "afraid". The French are therefore likely to score higher on this item than the English and the difference may be mistakenly interpreted to mean that French respondents are more anxious than English respondents.

2. Original English item   "How satisfied would you be to continue with your present form of treatment?"

   Back-translated from French as   "How satisfied would you be to follow your present form of treatment permanently?"

The problem: The French respondents were being asked to consider a much stronger commitment. Thus they will be likely to have lower scores on this item than the English respondents and the difference may be mistakenly interpreted to mean that the French respondents were less satisfied with their treatment than were the English.

3. Original English item   "I feel that I am useful and needed"
   Back-translated from German as   "I feel that I am useless and am being used"

The problem: The back-translator misread the German. Discussion with other German linguists suggested that the original German was not at fault.

4. Original English item   "My life is pretty full"
   Back-translated from German as   "My life is quite fulfilled"

The problem: The original English item was concerned with keeping occupied or busy. The translated version addresses feelings of achievement and satisfaction with life.

5. Original English item   "How well controlled do you feel your diabetes has been recently?"

   Back-translated from German as   "How do you estimate your metabolic control recently?"

The problem: The translated version gives the impression that patients are being asked for a factual account of blood glucose data rather than perceived feelings of diabetes control. Patients are likely to respond on the basis of their last few blood glucose estimations instead of taking a broader view informed by subjective impression, feedback from doctors and nurses, HbA_1 levels or other measures of diabetes control.

6. Original English item   "I get upset easily or feel panicky"
   Back-translated from German as   "I am easily excited or get panicky"
   Back-translated from French as   "I am easily moved to tears or feelings of panic"

The problem: In the German back-translation, "easily excited" is concerned more with arousal than anxiety and is not suitable for inclusion in measuring an anxiety construct. In the French back-translation, "upset" was back-translated as "moved to tears" which is one specific manifestation of "upset". Use of this more specific wording is likely to introduce sex differences in responses with women scoring higher than men on this item which may give a misleading impression that women are more anxious than men. Other translators have translated the English term upset in terms of other specific manifestations of upset, anger or annoyance, which are more likely to elicit higher scores from men and may give a misleading impression than men are more anxious than women. It seems that few languages have a word that encompasses the breadth of meaning of the English word "upset" which may need to be translated with a series of words meaning "I am easily moved to tears or anger...."

Had the above problems not been identified and dealt with it is not hard to see that the meaning of the construct to be measured would have changed. Most of the subtle changes maintained the face validity of the construct being measured but would be likely to affect the magnitude of the responses elicited. This would have led to differences in the responses of patients in different countries that are attributable to the translation but may be misinterpreted as indications of real differences between the patient groups. The examples given above are examples of questionnaire items where discrepancies occurred. It is important to note that it is equally important to ensure good translation of response options. In the DTSQ discrepancies arose in several translations of the descriptors which anchored the scales such that the term "very undemanding" was mistranslated as "no demands" in one of the translations. It is unlikely that any treatment for insulin dependent diabetes would be viewed by any patient as making no demands though some might see it as very undemanding. Even more crucially, any instructions or preamble at the top of questionnaires must be translated and checked through the same back-translation and retranslation procedures used for the items. Poorly translated instructions may invalidate all the items that follow them, however well translated the individual items may be.

Although many unwanted discrepancies between translations and original questionnaire can be identified by back-translation and review by potential users there are many problems with translations that are less readily detected.

Problems that May Remain Following the Back-translation-retranslation Cycle

Even when back-translation suggests that a translation is equivalent to the original, serious problems may remain. Simonsen and Mortensen (1990) pointed out that apparent equivalence may be created by factors that are unrelated to the quality of the translation: translators may share a set of rules for translating words or phrases that have no direct equivalents and back-translators may be able to make sense out of a poor quality translation.

Streiner and Norman (1989) pointed out that literal translation of phrases may convey very different meanings in the languages of translation and original questionnaires. They gave the example of the colours blue and black being associated respectively with feelings of sadness and depression in their own culture (Canada) while in China, the colour of mourning is white, a shade used to denote purity in some other cultures. Hence a technically accurate translation of "I feel blue" or "The future looks black to me" may nevertheless lead to very different patterns of responding in two different cultures if the same colours carry different meanings. The wider literature on cross-cultural differences in understandings of health and illness, health expectations, labelling of and expectations for symptoms, can help us to see the many ways in which linguistically well-translated items may nevertheless convey substantially different meanings in different cultures (e.g. Zola, 1973; Stainton Rogers, 1991). Furthermore, different subgroups of a population apparently speaking the same language may attach different meanings to an item (see example 6 above).

Well-designed items should be constructed as simply as possible with words in common use by the population for which the questionnaire is intended. It may be that words that are simple and common in one language are only translatable using more complex words in another language. Words that are familiar to a linguist that do not appear to be problematic in the back-translation may nevertheless be unsuitable for use with some respondents who have fewer years of education.

Well-designed items should also be constructed so that they cannot be easily misread. Example 3 given above describes the misreading by the back-translator of the item "I feel that I am useful and needed". Consultation with other linguists suggested that, in this case, the translated item was not particularly easy to misread — no more so than the original English word 'useful' would be misread as 'useless' with the word 'needed' there too, to protect further against misreading. However, when psychometric analyses were conducted on the German translation of the six-item Depression subscale of which "I feel that I am useful and needed" and "My life is pretty full" (example 4 above) were two items, the internal consistency of the German six-item subscale (alpha = 0.58) was found to be substantially lower than the alpha coefficient (alpha = 0.73) for four items, when the two depression subscale items about which there had been questions concerning the translation were excluded from the analysis. This illustration provides one example of the many reasons for conducting psychometric analyses on data obtained from newly translated scales.

Identification of Translation Problems with Psychometric Analyses

The inadequacy of the above linguistic procedures for ensuring appropriate translation of questionnaires has been recognised by cross-cultural psychologists who, in wishing to compare psychological phenomena across cultures, have had to grapple with the methodological problems involved (e.g. Berry, 1969). Cross-cultural psychologists have explored a range of methods such as multidimensional scaling for establishing and improving equivalence of construct measurement, and item response theory for the test and improvement of item and scale equivalence (Hui and Triandis, 1985). The problem faced by cross-cultural psychologists, whose main purpose in translating questionnaires is to make cross-cultural comparisons, requires far greater precision in ensuring construct equivalence than is necessary for the purposes of most psychologists and diabetes health professionals who simply wish to have a translation for use in their own country rather than to make cross-cultural comparisons. Having said this, even a translation that is not intended for cross-cultural comparisons needs to be a reliable and valid measure of the construct it is intended to measure and the linguistic procedures alone cannot ensure this is the case.

A new translation needs to be subjected to the same psychometric procedures that should have been conducted on the original questionnaire in order to check that it is working as originally intended. Similarly, the use of a questionnaire with a sample population that differs in potentially important ways from the population with whom the questionnaire was developed should be investigated psychometrically in much the same way as if it was a newly designed instrument. Thus although the Well-being Questionnaire had been developed and shown to be reliable with tablet-treated patients in Sheffield the psychometric properties could not be assumed when the responses of insulin users were investigated in another study. Psychometric analyses were repeated with the insulin users and data from French and German centres were analysed as well as the data from the English centre (see the chapter on the Well-being Questionnaire). In this case the questionnaires proved to work equally well in insulin users as in tablet-treated patients but evidence that some of the translated items reduced the reliability of certain scales led to some items being dropped from specific translations in order to improve reliability. The Satisfaction with Treatment Questionnaire had to be constructed using some items that differed for insulin users from those that had worked well with tablet-treated patients. The latest version of the DTSQ has modified and selected items to produce a single questionnaire that is equally appropriate for people with all kinds of diabetes (see chapter on DTSQ). The psychometric procedures needed to check the suitability of a new translation or new use of an existing questionnaire are described by Todd and Bradley in Chapter 2 and include factor analysis, reliability analyses and construct validation procedures.

Factor analysis

Factor analysis is a useful way of exploring the structure of a questionnaire that has subscales, provided that the sample size is sufficient for the number of items in the questionnaire (four times the number of subjects as there are items in the questionnaire is the minimum sample size recommended and a larger sample is desirable). If scales such as those in the Well-being Questionnaire, which includes several subscales, have been well translated and the items hold the same meaning for respondents in the translation as they did in the original language, then we would expect the items within a subscale to tend to load highly together on the same factor separately from the items intended for other subscales. If an item does not load highly with other items on the subscale for which it was intended then this could be because translation has distorted the meaning of the item so that it is measuring a rather different construct from that being measured by the other items on its intended subscale. (The reader is referred to the chapter by Todd and Bradley for a more detailed information about factor analysis).

Reliability analyses

Reliability analyses also require a substantial sample size and may be beyond the scope of most researchers (see chapter by Todd and Bradley for further information). However, where it is reasonable to measure Cronbach's alpha coefficient of internal consistency (reliability) this can provide a useful indicator of the extent to which reliability has been preserved following translation and/or use with a new population. If Cronbach's alpha is as high for the translation as it was for the original scale development work in the original language, and if each of the items in the scale contribute positively to maintaining that level of alpha in the original language and in the translation, then this provides good evidence for the reliability of the translation.

Inter-item correlations

Where the sample size is insufficient for factor analysis or reliability analyses it may nevertheless be sufficient to compute a correlation matrix where responses to each item are correlated with responses to all the other items. Items intended for the same subscale would be expected to correlate with each other more strongly than with items intended for different subscales and should correlate in the expected direction. If the developers of the original questionnaire have published an inter-item correlation matrix then a direct comparison can be made and any discrepancies can be considered.

Means, standard deviations and other statistics

The distribution of responses to each item and/or each subscale may have been described by the authors of the original scale development work and presented as means and standard deviations or as medians and ranges and these may be compared with the same statistics calculated for the responses to the translation. Any marked difference should be considered although it does not necessarily indicate that there is a translation problem. Higher Anxiety scores from French respondents than from English may indicate that the French sample were really more anxious. However, other explanations are possible. It may be an indication of a translation discrepancy such as that shown in example 1 above where an item was translated to describe a more mild indicator of anxiety with which respondents

were more inclined to agree. Alternatively it may be that there is a cultural difference, with the French having a greater willingness to express anxiety than the
British. Thus, examination of descriptive statistics of responses to a new translation and comparison with available statistics associated with the original questionnaire may provide reassuring evidence of similarities or may point to differences
that require further investigation and explanation.

Choice of the psychometric analyses that can usefully be conducted on data
from new translations depends in part on the sample size and in part on the nature
of the data and statistics reported on the original questionnaire and available for
comparison. It is most useful to conduct analyses for which there are comparison
results available. Researchers may wish to conduct specific analyses to check certain items that were found to be difficult to translate to determine whether small
changes introduced at translation have influenced the results in any way. Evidence
that the items load as expected in a factor analysis or correlate as expected with
appropriate items in a correlation matrix will be reassuring evidence and provide
a necessary though not sufficient condition for ensuring the reliability and validity
of translations or new uses of existing questionnaires.

TOWARDS IMPROVING THE VALIDITY AND RELIABILITY OF
TRANSLATED SCALES

A summary of procedures that I now aim to adopt whenever supervising the
translation of a questionnaire is provided below. Greater emphasis is here given
to the linguistic procedures and checks than to the psychometric analyses which
are described in the previous chapter by Todd and Bradley.

Guidelines Recommended for Translation of Questionnaires

1. The translation should be done by a native speaker of the language to which
   the translation is being made. This person should be experienced in questionnaire design and development (or closely supervised by someone who is) and
   informed about the structure and purpose of the particular questionnaire to
   be translated (translator A).
2. Back-translation should then be done by translator B who is a native speaker of
   the language used in the original scale and *who has not seen any other versions of
   the questionnaire (including the original)*. Ideally two back-translations should be
   done at this stage by two different back-translators.
3. The back-translation(s) should be sent to the designer of the questionnaire for
   checking or to translator A's supervisor who has experience of questionnaire
   design and development.
4. Any discrepancies should be discussed with the original translator (A) and
   · retranslated as necessary.
5. Any retranslated passages should be sent to a third translator (C) (*who has not*

seen other versions of the questionnaire) for back-translation and so on until there are no discrepancies using a different back-translator on each occasion.

6. The translation should be carefully scrutinised by the native speaker with experience of questionnaire design and psychometric development (translator A or A's supervisor) to ensure that the items remain unambiguous etc.

7. The translated instrument should be treated as a new instrument and subjected to the same psychometric procedures that we would expect of any new instrument or an old one being used with a new population. Thus, when data are first obtained from use of the new translation of the questionnaires the psychometric properties should be checked to ensure that internal consistency and construct validity remain satisfactory, i.e. Cronbach's alpha coefficient of reliability (if the sample size is sufficient) or intercorrelations of items within each subscale should be appropriate (see chapter by Todd and Bradley). Factor analyses should confirm the nature of any expected sub-scales with the required items loading highly on their corresponding subscales. Further analyses of construct validity and other forms of validity and reliability are also desirable.

SUMMARY

The problems of translating questionnaires are outlined and illustrated with examples of errors introduced with translation. Guidelines are offered to encourage appropriate linguistic procedures for translation of psychometric scales. Psychometric analyses are then needed. Although careful attention to the linguistic procedures and checks recommended will increase the likelihood of producing a translation that works as well as the original, it is no guarantee that serious problems have been avoided. The psychometric properties of the new translation cannot be assumed from data on the original questionnaire but need to be established on data obtained using the new translation.

ACKNOWLEDGEMENTS

The author wishes to thank Mr Keith Meadows and Dr Amanda Sowden who were in turn employed as researchers on the project investigating the translations and organising the retranslation of the Well-being and Treatment Satisfaction questionnaries. The author also wishes to thank Nadine Thibult, statistician at the Institut National de la Santé et de la Recherche Médicale (INSERM) who conducted the psychometric analyses of the original translations of the Well-being and Satisfaction questionnaires. The multi-centre European study, of which this work was a part, was organised by Dr Kirsten Staehr Johansen and her colleagues at the WHO, Copenhagen. Keith Meadows and Amanda Sowden were funded by grants to the author from the Diabetes Education Study Group, the World Health Organisation and the British Diabetic Association.

REFERENCES

Berry, J. W. (1969) On Cross-Cultural Comparability. *International Journal of Psychology*, **4**(2), 119–128

Hui, C. H. and Triandis, H. C. (1985) Quantitative methods in cross-cultural research: multidimensional scaling and item response theory. In R. D. Guerrero, *Cross-cultural and National Studies in Social Psychology*. North-Holland: Elsevier Science Publishers BV

Linstone, H.A. and Turoff, M. (eds) (1977) *The Delphi method: techniques and applications*. Reading, Mass: Addison Wesley

Meadows, K. A. and Bradley, C. (1991) The problem of translating questionnaires for use in European studies of diabetes: Towards a set of guidelines. Poster presented at the Diabetes Education Study Group conference, Cambridge, UK

Simonsen, E. and Mortensen, E. L. (1990) Difficulties in translation of personality scales. *Journal of Personality Disorders*, **4**(3), 290–296

Stainton Rogers, W. (1991) *Explaining health and illness: an exploration of diversity*. Hemel Hempstead: Harvester Wheatsheaf

Streiner, D. L. and Norman, G. R. (1989) *Health Measurement Scales: a practical guide to their development and use*. New York: Oxford University Press

Zola, I. (1973) Pathways to the doctor — from person to patient. *Social Science and Medicine*, **7**, 677–689

## CHAPTER 4

QUALITATIVE METHODS IN PSYCHOSOCIAL RESEARCH

TINA POSNER

Centre for Mental Health Nursing Research, Queensland University of Technology, Kelvin Grove Campus, Locked Bag No.2, Red Hill, Queensland 4059, Australia

A researcher is both an active participant in the research process, and, along with the research, part of the social world being studied. While this is generally recognised in relation to qualitative methods of social investigation, this is less often the case in respect of quantitative methods. Acknowledgement of the reflexive nature of all social research carries with it the implication that qualitative and quantitative approaches are not on different sides of an epistemological chasm, as is sometimes suggested, but complementary methods. Quantitative and qualitative approaches were often used side by side by early sociologists and social psychologists, until the ascendancy of logical positivism appeared to give greater status to data derived from experimental and survey research. However, it is recognisably the case that,"While some methods are more structured and selective than others, all research, however exploratory, involves selection and interpretation" (Hammersley and Atkinson, 1983; p. 12). A recent editorial in the *Lancet* (Anon, 1991) discussed the role of subjectivity in data analysis, pointing to the different interpretations of the data collected during the Hispanic Health and Nutrition Examination Survey, the Framingham study and the University Group Diabetes Program. The editorial concluded that "subjectivity in analysis and interpretation is not limited to observational research" and that one can never be sure which analyst holds "the truth".

The focus of qualitative and quantitative research methods tends to differ considerably, with the qualitative approach being applied to social types and forms, and interrelationships between individuals or groups. In typical mode, qualitative research describes the characteristics of social phenomena in terms of acts, activities, meanings, participation, relationships and settings (Lofland, 1971). An attempt to capture the nature of social phenomena may involve a study at one point in time or an investigation of a process extending over time. It may document acts in the actors' own terms and/or the observer's, patterns of activity and participation, relationships, roles, hierarchies, alliances, and systematic interrelationships between actors, as well as whole social settings. These data can result in typologies, models and conceptualisations of stages — observer-constructed patterns which can be checked against participants' accounts to provide further data. The approach attempts to elucidate manifest or latent meanings attributed or attributable to social forms. Such cultural or symbolic analysis takes account of social values, stereotypes, beliefs, attitudes, perspectives and definitions. In short, it seeks to understand people's behaviour in context.

Much qualitative research is based on fieldwork in which the researcher views the phenomena or subjects under study from within the context. A key strength of this sort of research (often termed 'ethnographic' research) is its value in the development of theory, according to Hammersley and Atkinson (1983). A theory, they suggest, "must contain reference to mechanisms or processes by which the relationship among the variables identified is generated" (p. 20). Ethnographic research is a valuable means of describing and elucidating the existence of such intervening variables. Simply to establish a relationship among variables is not enough to constitute a theory, though it may provide a basis for prediction. Hammersley and Atkinson (1983) argued that a weakness of positivism is its reliance on the hypothetico-deductive method in which there is a concentration on testing the 'truth' or 'falsity' of a particular theory in the most rigorous manner possible with little regard to the origins or development of the theory.

In addition, ethnographic research is flexible in its approach so that a research strategy can be adapted according to a changed assessment of what is required to construct a theory. Furthermore, the approach does not depend on a single data source, reducing the risk of results which are peculiar to the method. The use of multiple data sources allows 'triangulation' so that accumulated data can be compared, and result in reinforcement or contradiction. "What is lost in terms of control of variables may be compensated by reduced risk of ecological invalidity" (Hammersley and Atkinson, 1983; p. 24). This reduces the danger of the findings applying only to the research, rather than the everyday situation. Ethnographic research can sometimes be used to test a theory through the use of crucial cases. Thus, qualitative, ethnographic investigation can generate hypotheses about situational, as opposed to dispositional variables, and produce accounts of causes and consequences (intended and unintended). Systematic quantitative comparison is necessary, however, to test such accounts in terms of covariations. The use of some standard tools of qualitative research are described below in order to demonstrate their potential in research on life with diabetes.

OBSERVATION

Observation of subjects in the situation under investigation provides data which can be essential for the formulation of pertinent questions and for understanding the relevant factors at work. It allows information to be gathered which might not be elicited simply by questioning participants. The investigator's questions might otherwise be based on certain assumptions which did not hold, or which failed to cover some pertinent aspects of the situation. The participants' answers might fail to mention such aspects because they had taken them for granted or found them unremarkable. Observation can be a comparatively unselective data-gathering activity which begins the process of developing an analytical scheme for organising relevant material.

Observation in outpatient diabetes clinics in two different hospitals produced evidence of situational variables which would have affected the responses of patients to the interactions. It is unlikely that questions directed to patients or doctors (without prior observation) would have elicited the same amount of useful comparative data. It was observed that the role ascribed to the random blood sugar test as a criterion of control in the two clinics was rather different; one clinic provided a greater degree of privacy for doctor-patient consultations; there were considerable differences between doctors in their interactional styles, for instance in regard to the extent of blame or threat to patients in relation to poor control; and there were differences between doctors in their medical management strategies, for instance, one put more emphasis on diet as an aspect of diabetes control than the others (Posner, 1983, 1988, 1988a). The comparative material gathered by observation in these two clinics could have been used to develop a schema for more systematic investigation of many clinics.

OPEN-ENDED QUESTIONS

Open-ended questions in unstructured or semi-structured interviews allow the authentic expression of subjects' views in their own terms, given that the question is worded appropriately and understood as meant. (In an interview situation, communications can, of course, be checked). Analysis of the answers will give an indication of the range and relative frequencies of different points of view, and is also likely to provide a frequently recurring form of words which can be used to construct a question for use in a less interactive situation such as a self-completion questionnaire.

In a study of self-help activity (Posner, 1988) an interview question asked British Diabetic Association (BDA) branch and group members "What is the best thing about the meetings as far as you are concerned?" The range of answers and forms of expression elicited were analysed for their basic categories and the most frequent form of words used to express each category. One type of answer was related to acquiring information about the medical management of diabetes and was mentioned by people concerned to keep up with the latest developments or in the initial stages of learning to live with diabetes. Many people thought that the fellowship of "people in the same boat" was the best thing about meetings. There were different but interrelated aspects of this fellowship. One was the possibility of sharing experiences and discussing concerns with people who understood; another related to identification with others whether or not there was any exchange; a third was learning that other people with similar problems had coped and how they had done so. A small group of people cited helping other people with diabetes as the best thing about meetings, and this was a separate category of answer from those which focused on the benefit for their own coping with diabetes. Neither the word 'fellowship' nor the word 'identification' was used by interviewees.

Six typical expressions of the benefits spoken about by interviewees were chosen and presented as answers when the question was subsequently used on a postal questionnaire sent to a sample of BDA members. The categories could be used with confidence that most people's answers would fall within one or other of them and that the words used would be relevant. In the analysis, the answers were grouped into three basic types relating to acquiring information, helping others and benefits resulting from fellowship with others 'in the same boat'. Some people gave more than one answer and this was allowed for in the coding since the interest was in making an assessment of the dimensions of the different perceived benefits. The quantitative analysis showed that acquiring information and the fellowship at meetings were frequently perceived benefits (64% and 59% respectively); helping others was less frequently cited as a benefit (18%) (Posner, 1991).

CASE STUDIES

The term 'case study' can be used to refer simply to "the basic descriptive material an observer has assembled by whatever means available about some particular phenomenon or set of events" (Mitchell, 1983, pp. 190–191). The focus of the study may be a single individual, as in the life-history approach, or it may be a set of actors engaged in a sequence of activities over a period of time, a social situation at one point of time, or an event. A distinctive feature of a case study is that it views "a social unit as a whole" (Goode and Hatt, 1952, p. 231), that is, it is an holistic approach. The detailed examination involved in the presentation of a case study can be used to exhibit the operation of some general theoretical principle identified by the analyst. In suggesting that one illuminating case can "make theoretical connections apparent which were formerly obscure", Mitchell (1983, p. 200) argued that this use of case material is dependent on "the validity of the analysis rather than the representativeness of the events" – the inferences are logical rather than statistical.

Looking at how a small group of people with diabetes varied in their orientation to control of the condition produced case studies of different orientations and a suggested typology of variations based on the interview evidence. Mrs P felt that she, in alliance with her doctor, was maintaining control of her diabetic condition when following the medical rules resulted in stability; to Mr Q, the condition seemed out of control, but he could take comfort in his religious beliefs which allowed him to feel prepared for whatever might happen; for Mr R and Mr T, control was in the hands of the eminent hospital doctor and medical science; for Mr S however, having the ability to adapt his treatment to his way of life was crucial to his feeling of being in control of his condition. Mr S was an example of someone who had a strong need for self-reliance, whose confidence depended on acquiring knowledge and skills to allow him to look after his condition with little recourse to medical help and to prevent it from interfering very much in his life. This approach enabled him to feel a sense that he was in control of his diabetes not the other way around, and that life could go on as normal (Posner, 1983, 1988a).

CONTENT ANALYSIS

The content of text of various types can be submitted to systematic analysis. A recent example of such content analysis was a study of letters written to the BDA on the subject of unwanted effects related to the change-over to human insulin. The aim of the investigation was systematically to catalogue the effects - the symptoms and related consequences being reported, and thus to describe the extent and nature of the problem for this group of people living with diabetes. Four main categories of effects were identified from this correspondence: problems with hypoglycaemia, deterioration in diabetic control, in general health and in quality of life. Within each of these dimensions, subcategories were defined. Within the 'problems with hypoglycaemia' category, these subcategories related to the specific aspects of the problem with hypos such as violence, increased frequency, or lack of warnings. In the case of the category mapping deterioration in general health, the subcategories related to the symptoms causing the deterioration. The quality of life dimension of the problem was subcategorized in terms of the problems which pointed to the deterioration in quality of life, for instance, loss of employment or increased dependency because of hypos without warning. Instances of these general and specific effects reported in the correspondence were enumerated, thus allowing a description of the shape of the problem in terms of overall dimensions and proportions within dimensions.

The nature of the data source in the study described above, unsolicited first hand accounts from people living with the problem and motivated enough to write, provided value and relevance at the same time as limitations. Clearly the sample was a self-selected one and not representative of the general diabetic population. Though the data provided material from which to analyse the nature of the problem, where it exists, it did not allow an estimate of the extent of the problem which would require a quantitatively based method. There are clearly similarities between this sort of textual analysis and the process of coding and subsequent listing of frequencies of answers on surveys. In the above case, however, the categories were not presented to the sample but by the sample, the articulation of the problem being entirely in the correspondents' own terms. The researcher's role was to analyse, describe and summmarise – that is to organise and re-present the content of the texts. This method of qualitative analysis has recently become more quantitative in its potential through the use of computer programmes for text searching and categorizing. These programmes have allowed researchers to build complex index structures based on coding categories and to explore concepts and the relationships between them. As Richards and Richards (1991) pointed out, "collections of codes are not theories (but) the act of collecting them may stimulate theory...". In the computer-assisted development of a taxonomy of concepts, qualitative and quantitative methods are jointly aiding the researcher in the generation and construction of theory.

SUMMARY

As a research activity, qualitative methods are complementary to quantitative investigation which they may precede, accompany or follow. Prior qualitative investigation may result in theoretical propositions which subsequently need to be tested quantitatively. A qualitative study accompanying a quantitative investigation may be needed to answer certain sorts of questions and will provide different kinds of data. Alternatively, qualitative investigation may follow quantitative research which has demonstrated an unexplained connection in order to provide further insight into the meaning of the connection. The descriptive and analytical methods of qualitative research are essential both to an understanding of the nature of social phenomena, social types, structures and interrelationships, and to the process of generating theory.

REFERENCES

Anon, (editorial) (1991) Subjectivity in data analysis *The Lancet*, **337**(i), 401–402

Hammersley, M. and Atkinson, P. (1983) *Ethnography: principles in practice* London: Tavistock

Goode, W. and Hatt, P. (1952) *Methods in social research*, New York: McGraw-Hill

Lofland, J. (1971) *Analyzing social settings*, Belmont, California: Wadsworth

Mitchell, J. (1983) Case and situation analysis *The Sociological Review*, **31**(2), 187–211

Posner, T. (1983) The sweet things in life: aspects of the management of diabetic diet. In A. Murcott (ed.) *The Sociology of Food and Eating* Aldershot: Gower

Posner, T. (1988) Sailing single-handed: autonomy in the control of diabetes, *International Disability Studies*, **10**(3), 123–128

Posner, T. (1988a) *A system of medical control: the case of diabetes* London University PhD thesis

Posner, T. (1991) Who are we? *Balance* (Newsletter of the British Diabetic Association), Oct/Nov

Richards, L. and Richards, T. (1991) 'Hard' results from 'soft' data? Computing and qualitative analysis. Paper presented at British Sociological Association Conference: Health and Society, Manchester. See also Richards, L. and Richards, T., Computing in qualitative method: a healthy development? *Qualitative Health Research*, 1, 234–262

SECTION 2

QUALITY OF LIFE, WELL-BEING
AND SATISFACTION MEASURES

CHAPTER 5

THE DIABETES QUALITY OF LIFE MEASURE

ALAN M. JACOBSON and THE DIABETES CONTROL AND
COMPLICATIONS TRIAL RESEARCH GROUP

Chief, Mental Health Unit, Joslin Diabetes Center, Boston, Massachusetts, USA

*The Diabetes Control and Complications Trial Research Group is a collaborative group
of investigators representing 29 clinical centres in the United States and Canada as well
as central laboratories and a statistical centre in collaboration with the
National Institutes of Health.*

The Diabetes Quality of Life Measure (DQOL) was developed in the early 1980s
for use in the Diabetes Control and Complications Trial (DCCT), a controlled,
randomized, clinical trial comparing the efficacy of two alternative treatment regimens on the appearance and development of chronic complications of insulin-
dependent diabetes mellitus (IDDM) (DCCT, 1986, 1987, 1988). Specifically, the
DQOL was designed to evaluate the relative burden of an intensive diabetes treatment regimen, with the goal of maintaining blood glucose levels as close as possible to those of people without diabetes, in comparison to standard diabetes
therapy. Because intensive treatment would carry additional demands such as
extensive reeducation, multiple daily injections of insulin or use of the insulin
pump, frequent blood glucose monitoring, and greater need for cautious adjustment of food, exercise, and insulin doses, it was anticipated that this might affect
the quality of life of patients, and in turn, decrease the willingness of patients and
health care providers to use intensive treatment. Thus, understanding the effects
of the DCCT treatment regimens on quality of life would be potentially useful for
clinical application of the trial's findings.

Prior to the development of the DQOL, there were no available diabetes-specific
or diabetes-oriented quality of life measures. Therefore, the DQOL had to be constructed for use within the trial. However, its structure purposely allowed for a
broader application to other patients with IDDM and even non-insulin-diabetes
mellitus (NIDDM). Thus, the scale items cover a range of issues directly relevant
to diabetes and its treatment (DCCT, 1988).

Approaches to quality of life measurement have been subject to considerable
debate in the literature. Generic measures such as the Sickness Impact Profile
(Bergner *et al.*, 1981), the Medical Outcome Survey (Ware & Sherbourne, 1992),
or the Quality of Well-Being Scale (Bush & Kaplan, 1982) offer ready comparison
across studies and disease groups. Because they must address a wide range of issues, these instruments may not be sensitive to the effects of particular treatments,

especially when the therapeutic effects result in differences in lifestyle rather than functional health status. Alternatively, illness-specific or treatment-specific measures are more likely to be sensitive to the goals of a particular clinical trial (Jacobson et al., 1994). However, they do not allow comparisons between different diseases or facilitate economic comparisons. In general, there is convergence of investigator opinion suggesting that quality of life assessment in clinical trials and clinical treatment should incorporate both generic and treatment- and/or illness-specific measures.

The DQOL has been employed in a variety of recent studies of IDDM and NID-DM (Jacobson et al., 1994; Selam et al., 1992; Nathan et al., 1991; Lloyd et al., 1992). These studies include comparisons of different treatments (Selam et al., 1992; Nathan et al., 1991), the effects of complications of diabetes (Jacobson et al., 1994; Lloyd et al., 1992) and characterization of quality of life in samples of IDDM and NIDDM patients (Jacobson et al., 1994).

THE SCALE

Design

Figure 1 presents the items of the DQOL. It is conceptualized as measuring the patient's personal experience of diabetes care and treatment. Four separate areas are addressed by the measure: satisfaction with treatment, impact of treatment, worry about the future effects of diabetes, and worry about social/vocational issues (DCCT, 1988). There is also a single overall well-being scale that is derived from national surveys of quality of well-being and can, therefore, be used to compare subjects to a wide variety of patients (Howie & Drury, 1978). In addition to these forty-six core items and the well-being scale, the DQOL includes thirteen items to assess adolescent populations who are in school and/or living at home with parents.

The DQOL was initially developed by a working group of the DCCT. This group provided expertise in quality of life scale development, behavioural medicine, psychiatry, diabetology, and nursing. Scale items were derived from patient and clinician input and literature on psychosocial aspects of diabetes. The initial set of items was reviewed by clinicians and selected patients with IDDM for content and relevance. As the instrument was developed, it was repeatedly reviewed by diabetologists, nurses working with diabetic patients, diabetes educators, and mental health professionals familiar with diabetes. After initial professional and patient input, the measure was pre-tested in selected patients with diabetes for ease of use, readability, and self-administration. This process led to substantive changes in the measure. For example, the worry scales were not initially incorporated in the measure. Review by clinicians who treat children suggested that worry about the future was an important element of the life experience of adolescents with diabetes and should be included in the measurement of their quality of life (DCCT, 1988). After final formulation of the DQOL instrument, it was tested for validity and reliability.

SCORING

Responses to questions are made with a five-point Likert scale. Satisfaction is rated from 1 (very satisfied) to 5 (very dissatisfied). Impact and worry scales are rated from 1 (no impact or never worried) to 5 (always affected or always worried). A single item assessing general quality of life was taken from large scale systematic surveys, and therefore, can be used to compare quality of life of patients assessed with the DQOL to patients who have been evaluated in large scale national surveys (Howie & Drury, 1978). It is rated on a four-point scale to maintain continuity with past use. Thirteen additional items that assess schooling, experience, and family relationships for patients living with their parents can be used to provide specific information about the life experiences of adolescent patients.

As initially reported, the method of scoring involved summing the responses to all core items and then dividing by the number of core items in the subscale (DCCT, 1988). Impact items 8 and 16 are reverse scored using this method. All other items would be summed without reverse scoring. The mean scores for each subscale using this method would then be interpreted against a five-point scale where 1 is equivalent to highest quality of life and 5 is considered poorest quality of life. In addition to the scale scores, a total core scale score is derived by summing the responses to all forty-six core items and dividing by the number of core items.

A new method of scoring the forty-six core items that comprise the DQOL has recently been proposed by Jacobson *et al.* (1994). Using this new method, patient responses are reverse scored, with the exception of Impact items 8 and 16, so that positive quality of life is equivalent to a higher score. The core items are then summed into a raw score for each scale. The raw scale score is then translated into a 100 point scale where 0 represents the lowest possible quality of life, and 100 represents the highest possible quality of life. A formula derived from the scoring techniques advocated for the Medical Outcome Survey (SF36) is used to convert raw scores to the 100 point scale (IRC, 1991). In this instance, the patient raw score minus the lowest possible score on each scale is divided by the possible score range and multiplied by 100. It is then rounded off to the nearest whole number. The formula (IRC, 1991) can be written as follows:

$$\text{Transformed scale} = \left[\frac{(\text{Raw score-lowest possible score})}{\text{Raw score range}} \right] *100$$

For example, a patient completing the Satisfaction section has a pre-transformed raw score of 29. After reverse scoring, the transformed raw score is 61. The lowest possible score for the Satisfaction scale, 15, is subtracted from the transformed raw score and the difference, 46, is divided by the subscale raw score range of 60 (highest possible score, 75, minus the lowest possible score, 15). This quotient, .766, is then multiplied by 100 to yield a transformed Satisfaction score of 77. Note, in the original method of scoring, this patient would receive a mean Satisfaction score of 1.93 (29 divided by 15 items), a score indicating high levels of satisfaction. The transformed score of 77 intuitively indicates a high satisfaction score on a 100 point scale. If subjects skip items or mark them as not applicable, the raw score range and the lowest possible score are calculated based on the actual number of core items rated on the 1 to 5 scale. Furthermore, Jacobson *et al.* (1994) have recommended that the entire Diabetes and Social Worry subscales be deleted if two or more of the core items are missing values. For the Satisfaction subscale, up to three of the fifteen core items may be missing while Impact subscale may have up to four of the twenty core items missing. Transforming the scale of the DQOL has the advantage of providing an easy to comprehend scale similar to one of the most widely-used quality of life measures, the Medical Outcome Survey (Ware & Sherbourne, 1992).

SCALE DEVELOPMENT

Subject Sample One

Initially, the reliability and validity of the DQOL was assessed in a study of patients with IDDM who were conventionally treated (DCCT, 1988). For this study, each of the twenty-one participating centres submitted a list of forty non-DCCT patients selected to have similar characteristics to the DCCT research patients in terms of age, duration of diabetes, and level of early vascular complications. The entry criteria for the DCCT and the DQOL study population were:

1) age greater than or equal to 13 and less than 40;
2) pubertal development at or beyond Tanner Stage 2;
3) duration of diabetes greater than or equal to 1 and less than 15 years;
4) treatment with one or two injections of insulin per day;
5) patient was at less than 130% of ideal body weight;
6) for adolescent subjects ages 13 to 17, no history of failure to maintain norma-growth and development during the previous two years;
7) generally good health without advanced complications of diabetes.

Ten subjects were randomly selected from each of the lists and 192 of those 210 subjects consented to participate in the study. Patients from all the twenty-one centres participated.

The sample consisted of 192 patients of whom 136 were adults, ages 18 to 41, and 56 were adolescents, ages 13 to 17.9 years. Demographic information was not obtained from two adults due to clerical error. Of the 190 subjects with complete data, 114 were male and 76 were female. The mean duration of diabetes was eight years. The sample consisted primarily of white subjects from Hollingshead Social Classes one through four. Forty percent of the adult patients were married. None of the adolescents were married. Sixty percent of the adults and 59% of the adolescents were male. The mean age of the adults was twenty eight; the mean age of the adolescents was sixteen.

Subject Sample Two

A second more recent study was undertaken to assess the psychometric properties of the DQOL in a more heterogeneous group of diabetic outpatients followed at a large multi-specialty centre for the treatment of diabetes (Jacobson *et al.*, 1994). In this study, 240 patients were assessed, of whom 111 had IDDM and 129 had NIDDM. Patients could be 18 to 80 years of age and were not excluded if they had diabetic complications. The mean age of the IDDM subjects was 44 and the mean age of the NIDDM subjects was 60. Forty-seven percent of the IDDM and 51% of the NIDDM patients were male. Sixty-three percent and 69% of the IDDM and NIDDM patients, respectively, were married. The mean duration of diabetes was 19 years for IDDM patients and 12 years for the NIDDM patients. All IDDM patients and 53% of the NIDDM patients were treated with insulin. Thirty-eight percent of the NIDDM patients were on an oral-hypoglycaemic agent; nine percent were treated by diet alone. Patients were recruited from consecutive appointments to an outpatient internal medicine clinic over the course of one year.

In both studies the Diabetes Quality of Life Measure was self-administered with a Research Assistant present. The instructions for both studies are presented in Figure 1.

Figure 1   The DQOL and its instructions (The DCCT Research Group, 1987)

Diabetes Quality of Life Measure

Please read each statement carefully. Please indicate how satisfied or dissatisfied you currently are with the aspect of your life described in the statement. Circle the number that best describes how you feel. There are no right or wrong answers to these questions. We are interested in your opinion.

	Very satisfied	Moderately satisfied	Neither	Moderately dissatisfied	Very dissatisfied
Satisfaction - core items:					
1. How satisfied are you with the amount of time it takes to manage your diabetes?	1	2	3	4	5
2. How satisfied are you with the amount of time you spend getting checkups?	1	2	3	4	5
3. How satisfied are you with the time it takes to determine your sugar level?	1	2	3	4	5
4. How satisfied are you with your current treatment?	1	2	3	4	5
5. How satisfied are you with the flexibility you have in your diet?	1	2	3	4	5
6. How satisfied are you with the burden your diabetes is placing on your family?	1	2	3	4	5
7. How satisfied are you with your knowledge about your diabetes?	1	2	3	4	5
8. How satisfied are you with your sleep?	1	2	3	4	5
9. How satisfied are you with your social relationships and friendships?	1	2	3	4	5
10. How satisfied are you with your sex life?	1	2	3	4	5
11. How satisfied are you with your work, school, and household activities?	1	2	3	4	5
12. How satisfied are you with the appearance of your body?	1	2	3	4	5
13. How satisfied are you with the time you spend exercising?	1	2	3	4	5
14. How satisfied are you with your leisure time?	1	2	3	4	5
15. How satisfied are you with with life in general?	1	2	3	4	5

Satisfaction - **adolescent-oriented optional items:**
Answer the next questions if you attend school:

	Very satisfied	Moderately satisfied	Neither	Moderately dissatisfied	Very dissatisfied
16. How satisfied are you with your performance in school?	1	2	3	4	5
17. How satisfied are you with how your classmates treat you?	1	2	3	4	5
18. How satisfied are you with your attendance in school?	1	2	3	4	5

Please indicate how often the following events happen to you. Circle the appropriate number.

	Never	Very seldom	Sometimes	Often	All the time
Impact - core items:					
1. How often do you feel pain associated with the treatment for your diabetes?	1	2	3	4	5
2. How often are you embarrassed by having to deal with your diabetes in public?	1	2	3	4	5
3. How often do you have low blood sugar?	1	2	3	4	5
4. How often do you feel physically ill?	1	2	3	4	5
5. How often does your diabetes interfere with your family life?	1	2	3	4	5
6. How often do you have a bad night's sleep?	1	2	3	4	5
7. How often do you find your diabetes limiting your social relationships and friendships?	1	2	3	4	5
8. How often do you feel good about yourself?	1	2	3	4	5
9. How often do you feel restricted by your diet?	1	2	3	4	5

	Never	Very seldom	Sometimes	Often	All the time
10. How often does your diabetes interfere with your sex life?	1	2	3	4	5
11. How often does your diabetes keep you from driving a car or using a machine (e.g. a typewriter)?	1	2	3	4	5
12. How often does your diabetes interfere with your exercising?	1	2	3	4	5
13. How often do you miss work, school, or household duties because of your diabetes?	1	2	3	4	5
14. How often do you find yourself explaining what it means to have diabetes?	1	2	3	4	5
15. How often do you find that your diabetes interrupts your leisure-time activities?	1	2	3	4	5
16. How often do you tell others about your diabetes?	1	2	3	4	5
17. How often are you teased because you have diabetes?	1	2	3	4	5
18. How often do you feel that because of your diabetes you go to the bathroom more than others?	1	2	3	4	5
19. How often do you find that you eat something you shouldn't rather than tell someone that you have diabetes?	1	2	3	4	5
20. How often do you hide from others the fact that you are having an insulin reaction?	1	2	3	4	5

Answer the next questions if you attend school:

	Never	Very seldom	Sometimes	Often	All the time
Impact - adolescent-oriented optional items:					
21. How often do you find that your diabetes prevents you from participating in school activities (for example, being active in a school play, being on a sports team, being in a school band, etc.)?	1	2	3	4	5
22. How often do you find that your diabetes prevents you from going out to eat with your school friends?	1	2	3	4	5
23. How often do you feel that your diabetes is limiting your career or what you will be able to do in the future?	1	2	3	4	5

Answer the next questions if you are living with your parents:

	Never	Very seldom	Sometimes	Often	All the time
24. How often do you find that your parents are too protective of you?	1	2	3	4	5
25. How often do you feel that your parents worry too much about your diabetes?	1	2	3	4	5
26. How often do you find that close family members (for example brothers, sisters, cousins) tease you about your diabetes?	1	2	3	4	5
27. How often do you find that your parents act like diabetes is their disease, not yours?	1	2	3	4	5

Please indicate how often the following events happen to you. Please circle the number that best describes your feelings. If the question is not relevant to you, circle non-applicable.

	Never	Very seldom	Sometimes	Often	All the time	Does not apply
Social Worry & Diabetes Worry core items:						
1. How often do you worry about whether you will get married?	1	2	3	4	5	0
2. How often do you worry about whether you will have children?	1	2	3	4	5	0
3. How often do you worry about whether you will not get a job you want?	1	2	3	4	5	0
4. How often do you worry about whether you will be denied insurance?	1	2	3	4	5	0
5. How often do you worry about whether you will be able to complete your education?	1	2	3	4	5	0
6. How often do you worry about whether you will miss work?	1	2	3	4	5	0
7. How often do you worry about whether you will be able to take a vacation or a trip?	1	2	3	4	5	0
8. How often do you worry about whether you will pass out?	1	2	3	4	5	0
9. How often do you worry that your body looks differently because you have diabetes?	1	2	3	4	5	0
10. How often do you worry that you will get complications from your diabetes?	1	2	3	4	5	0
11. How often do you worry about whether someone will not go out with you because you have diabetes?	1	2	3	4	5	0

Answer the next questions if you attend school:

	Never	Very seldom	Sometimes	Often	All the time	Does not apply
Social Worry — adolescent-oriented optional items:						
12. How often do you worry that your teachers treat you differently because of your diabetes?	1	2	3	4	5	0
13. How often do you worry that your diabetes will disrupt something you are currently doing in school (for example, act in a play, continue on a sports team, be in the school band, etc.)?	1	2	3	4	5	0
14. How often do you worry that because of your diabetes you are behind in terms of dating, going to parties, and keeping up with your friends?	1	2	3	4	5	0

Individual general item:

Compared to other people your age, would you say your health is: (circle one)

1. Excellent
2. Good
3. Fair
4. Poor

© DCCT Research Group, c/o Dr. A. M. Jacobson, Joslin Diabetes Center, One Joslin Place, Boston, MA 02215, USA.

Reliability

Table 1 presents the intercorrelations of subscales and Cronbach alpha coefficients derived from the initial study by the DCCT research group (DCCT, 1988) and similar data from Jacobson *et al.* (1994) for adults with IDDM and NIDDM. As can be seen, the level of the internal consistency of the scales and of the total score were similar in both IDDM populations and NIDDM populations studied by the DCCT (1988) and Jacobson *et al.* (1994). The subscale correlations were found to be similar in both studies.

The test-retest reliability was evaluated by the DCCT research group (1988). As shown in Table 2, both adults and adolescents with IDDM had high test-retest correlations in the .78 to .92 range (DCCT, 1988). This was based on retest results approximately one week after the original test. The one week interval was selected with the expectation that quality of life would be unlikely to change in that period, but that any shorter time period would elicit responses that were recalled from prior testing. The actual mean time interval between the two measurements was nine days with a median of seven days. Eighty percent of the sample took the second DQOL within six to fourteen days of the first DQOL test.

Validity

Validation of any measure is an iterative process that involves systematically planned assessments of scales as well as the use of data gathered for other purposes to lend support to the validity of a measure. Two studies were specifically designed to validate the DQOL measure (DCCT, 1988; Jacobson *et al.*, 1994). In addition, other studies using the DQOL provide information about aspects of the measure's validity (Selam *et al.*, 1992; Nathan *et al.*, 1991; Lloyd *et al.*, 1992).

Face validity

Face validity was addressed in the initial development of the measure. The DQOL was developed, as noted above, by reviewing the relevant psychosocial literature in diabetes, utilizing the expertise of diabetes nurses, physicians and behavioural scientists, and by review and pretesting of patients with IDDM. These groups addressed issues as to the relevance of the content to quality of life issues in diabetes. Indeed the process led to an expansion of the measure from its original intent to include an area not usually incorporated in quality of life assessment, that is, worries about the future (DCCT, 1988).

Table 1 Internal consistency (Cronbach alpha) and intercorrelations of the DQOL and its core subscales for adults and adolescents from the DCCT Research Group (1987) and among adult patients with IDDM and NIDDM from Jacobson, *et al.* (1994)

	CRONBACH ALPHA		INTERCORRELATIONS							
			Total Score[a]		Satisfaction		Impact		Worry D - R.	
	Study 1	Study 2	Study1	Study 2	Study 1	Study 2	Study 1	Study 2	Study 1	Study 2
IDDM:										
Adult:										
DQOL Total	.92	.83								
Satisfaction	.88	.87	.	.89**						
Impact	.77	.81	.	.89**	.60**	.62**				
Worry:										
Diabetes-related	.67	.77	.	.66**	.26	.44**	.58**	.62**		
Worry:										
Social/Vocational	.83	.47	.	.75**	.37	.57**	.52**	.42*	.68**	.57*
IDDM:										
Adolescents:										
DQOL Total	.92	.	.	.						
Satisfaction	.86	.	.	.						
Impact	.85	.	.	.	.64**	.				
Worry:										
Diabetes-related	.66	.	.	.	.27	.	.54**	.		
Worry:										
Social/Vocational	.87	.	.	.	.34	.	.41	.	.54**	.
NIDDM:										
Adult:										
DQOL Total	.	.70								
Satisfaction	.	.87	.	.93**						
Impact	.	.78	.	.88**	.	.66**				
Worry:										
Diabetes-related	.	.70	.	.61**	.	.49**	.	.46**		
Worry:										
Social/Vocational	.	.49	.	.52*	.	.49*	.	.17	.	.17

[a]Total DQOL to subscale correlations are not available from published data presented by the DCCT Research Group (1987).
*p ≤ .01 ** p ≤ .0001

Table 2 Test-retest correlations of the DQOL Total Score and the subscales from the DCCT
Research Group (1987)

	Adults	Adolescents
DQOL TOTAL	.92*	.92*
Satisfaction	.89*	.86*
Impact	.89*	.89*
Worry: Diabetes-related	.80*	.88*
Worry: Social/Vocational	.78*	.88*

* p ≤ .0001

Construct validity

The first formal assessments of the validity of the DQOL by the DCCT Research
Group (DCCT, 1988) addressed the construct validity of the DQOL. The DCCT
Research Group identified a subset of measures that addressed issues relevant to
quality of life in patients with diabetes. Specifically, the study examined the relationship of the DQOL to three measures. These were the Symptom Checklist 90-
R (Derogatis *et al.*, 1983), the Bradburn Affect Balance Scale (Bradburn, 1969),
and the Psychosocial Adjustment to Illness Scale (Derogatis, 1983). The SCL-90
and the Affect Balance Scale together with the psychological distress subscale of
the PAIS addressed issues that were especially relevant to a patient's satisfaction
with diabetes as well as worries about diabetes-related and social-vocational
related issues. Subscales of the PAIS also addressed a range of possible impacts of
illness on patients. These included: health-care relationships, domestic relationships, sexual experience, and social environment.

   Table 3 presents the results of these comparisons for the adults and adolescents
separately. As can be seen, there were moderately strong, consistent correlations
of the total DQOL score with the SCL-90, Affect Balance Scale, and the PAIS subscales. The strongest correlations were found with the Psychological Distress Subscale of the PAIS, the Global Severity Index of the SCL-90, the Affect Balance
Scale, the Health Care Orientation Scale, and the Domestic Environment Scale of
the PAIS. Similar patterns of correlation were found for each of the DQOL subscales, with the Satisfaction Scale and Impact Scale showing the most consistent
correlations with the validating measures. The pattern of correlations suggested
that the Worry scales indexed issues primarily related to psychological distress and
symptomatology. This differentiation of the Worry scales was anticipated by the hypotheses of the initial investigators. The authors concluded that the Satisfaction
and Impact scales serve as broad gauges of diabetes-related quality of life, while
the Worry scales address concerns more specific to patient perceptions of their diabetes-related psychological distress (DCCT, 1988). The level of the correlations
found from this study is consistent with the assumption of the investigators that
they would generally fall in the range of .3 to .7 indicating that diabetes quality of

Table 3 Correlations of DQOL scores of adults and adolescents with scores of other scales: from the DCCT Research Group (1987)

	DQOL Total		Satisfaction		Impact		Worry: Diabetes–related		Worry: Social/Vocational	
	Adults	Adol.	Adults	Adol.	Adults	Adol.	Adults	Adol.	Adults	Adol.
SCL										
Global Severity Index	.60*	.77*	.49*	.59*	.50*	.66*	.40*	.49*	.50*	.66*
ABSa	-.57*	-.67*	-.55*	-.60*	-.47*	-.54*	-.27	-.25	-.28	-.55*
PAIS										
Health-care orient.	.53*	.74*	.57*	.80*	.40*	.65*	.25	.24	.25	.26
Vocational environ.	.53*	.44	.47*	.30	.51*	.34	.25	.39	.28	.26
Domestic environ.	.58*	.72*	.51*	.62*	.58*	.68*	.23	.29	.28	.44
Sexualb relat.	.35*	.36	.33	.23	.40*	.25	.08	.35	.06	.53
Extended family relat.	.34*	.38	.28	.30	.35*	.34	.06	.08	.21	.38
Social environ.	.46*	.59*	.42*	.52*	.44*	.54*	.12	.35	.29	.29
Psychol. distress	.63*	.81*	.51*	.61*	.55*	.71*	.46*	.59*	.46*	.67*

DQOL, Diabetes Quality of Life measure; SCL, Symptom Checklist; ABS, Affect Balance Scale; PAIS, Psychosocial Adjustment to Illness Scale

*p<.0001

aBecause of direction of scoring, the negative correlations signify positive relationships between the ABS and DQOL

bA small sample (N=20) of adolescents responded to the PAIS Sexual relationship questions. It was not applicable to all other adolescents. Therefore, conclusions drawn from the correlations with the PAIS and other scales must take into consideration this small subsample

life is related, but not identical, to psychological well-being, affective balance, and adjustment to illness.

The study by Jacobson *et al.* (1994) presented further information about construct validity of the DQOL by examining its relationship to a generic quality of life measure, the Medical Outcome Survey and extended prior observations to adults with NIDDM. The correlations between the Medical Outcome Survey (SF36) and the DQOL were examined separately for adults with IDDM and NIDDM (see Table 4). Overall, the patterns of correlation were similar to those found in the DCCT study (DCCT, 1988) with the Satisfaction and Impact scales having the strongest relationships overall with the functional health status scales of the Medical Outcome Survey (Jacobson *et al.*, 1994).

External validity

The study by Jacobson, *et al.* (1994), also provided information about external validity with the DQOL. In this study, patients with varying severity and numbers of complications were compared in terms of their diabetes quality of life. As shown in

Table 4 Pearson correlations of Diabetes Quality of Life (DQOL) and the Medical Outcome Survey (SF36) scales for patients with IDDM and NIDDM: from Jacobson et al. (1994)

IDDM

SF36

		Physical functioning	Social functioning	Role functioning	Pain score	General health score
D	Total	.38**	.56**	.51**	-33*	.60**
Q	Impact	.37**	.59**	.49**	.30*	.58**
O	Satisfaction	.30*	.43**	.44**	.28*	.50**
O	Diab. Worry	.12	.34*	.26*	.16	.44**
L	Social Worry	.21	.46*	.31	.13	.31

NIDDM

SF36

		Physical functioning	Social functioning	Role functioning	Pain score	General health score
D	Total	.35**	.34**	.40**	.38**	.43**
Q	Impact	.35**	.32*	.34**	.39**	.41**
O	Satisfaction	.33*	.37**	.42**	.36**	.42**
O	Diab. Worry	.08	.19	.26*	.19	.23
L	Social Worry	.001	.05	.17	-.003	.17

*p<.01   **p<.0001

Table 5, increasing severity and number of complications were associated with lower levels of satisfaction and greater impact of diabetes, even after taking into account other relevant demographic data (age and marital status and treatment type for NIDDM patients). The Worry scales were less sensitive to complications. The effect of number of complications was more pronounced among patients with IDDM. This may reflect the small number of NIDDM patients with three complications.

Figure 2 shows the effect of number of complications on quality of life for the patients with IDDM. This graph provides an indication of the relative impact of having up to three of the classic microvascular complications (symptomatic neuropathy, proliferative retinopathy, nephropathy requiring treatment). The effects of complications are cumulative so that having all three leads to a twenty five point drop in overall DQOL score.

Finally, external validity was examined by comparing patients with NIDDM using three different treatment regimens: insulin, oral agents, and diet alone (Jacobson et al., 1994). Patients who used insulin reported less satisfaction (F=3.96, p<.05) and greater impact (F=14.84, p≤ .0001) of diabetes than patients taking an oral agent or on diet management alone. Strikingly, a different pattern was found regarding patient worries: patients taking oral agents appeared to have more worries about their diabetes than patients who were taking insulin or were on diet alone (F=5.55,

Table 5 Hierarchical regression analyses examining the effect of number or severity of complications on quality of life for patients with IDDM and NIDDM: from Jacobson et al. (1994)

Number of complications

DQOL	Model 1 R^{2a}	Change in R^{2b}	$Fobs^c$	$Significance^c$
IDDM				
Total	.01	.16	10.2	.005
Impact	.02	.09	5.86	.05
Satisfaction	.04	.24	18.06	.005
Diabetes Worry	.002	.002	.09	NS
Social Worry	.06	.11	1.81	NS
NIDDM				
Total	.32	.06	2.73	NS
Impact	.29	.04	2.09	NS
Satisfaction	.17	.09	4.42	.05
Diabetes Worry	.08	.04	1.32	NS
Social Worry	.14	.37	3.08	NS

Severity of complications

DQOL	Model 1 R^{2a}	Change in R^{2b}	$Fobs^c$	$Significance^c$
IDDM				
Total	.03	.17	21.6	.005
Impact	.005	.16	19.74	.005
Satisfaction	.09	.14	18.17	.005
Diabetes Worry	.003	.05	5.54	.05
Social Worry	.17	.03	1.28	NS
NIDDM				
Total	.13	.05	7.19	.01
Impact	.08	.09	12.21	.005
Satisfaction	.14	.05	6.55	.05
Diabetes Worry	.04	.009	1.05	NS
Social Worry	.26	.002	.05	NS

[a]Model 1 includes age and marital status for patients with IDDM and age, marital status, and treatment type for patients with NIDDM
[b]Change in R^2 when the number or severity of complications score is added to Model 1
[c]F test and significance level is indicated for change in variance when the complications variable is added to the model

p<.05). This may reflect the anticipatory concerns of a patient knowing that their diabetes has demanded more intensive treatment than diet and that they are on the road to insulin treatment, something that patients connect with having a more serious illness. This would be expected to lead to further worries. Together with the findings about the effect of complications on worry, these results seem to suggest that worries about diabetes detect a different aspect of patient views of diabe-

Figure 2 The effect of microvascular complications (neuropathy, nephropathy, retinopathy) on DQOL scores among patients with IDDM (Jacobson *et al.*, 1994)

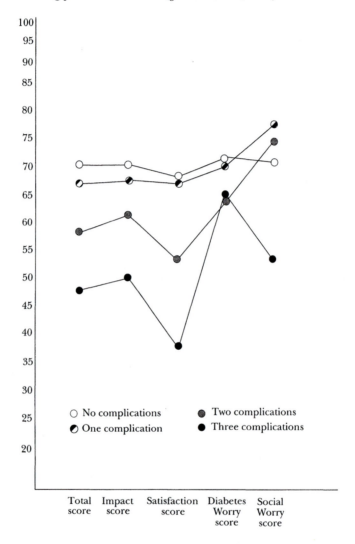

tes. As such, further information is needed to characterise the Worry scales. These data suggest that the Worry scales may be useful in understanding the effects of changes in regimen early in the course of illness. For example they may be useful in studying the effects of initial treatment of NIDDM. The Worry scales may also be useful in examining the impact of early treatments of IDDM such as those used to decrease the auto-immune destruction of the pancreatic Beta cell. Treatment failure, followed by transfer to insulin treatment might lead to increased worries without necessarily being reflected by other aspects of quality of life. It should be noted that the Social and Diabetes Worry scales, because they are designed for use with adolescents, are less relevant for adults who are settled in their lives.

A study by Lloyd and colleagues provides additional evidence for external validity using the DQOL (Lloyd *et al.*, 1992). In this study, patients with differing numbers of complications were compared in terms of quality of life, depressive symptoms, and Type A behaviour. The study population consisted of participants in the Epidemiology of Diabetes Complications Study. All patients (N=175) had IDDM for at least twenty-five years at the time of examination. They were carefully assessed as to presence of: proliferative retinopathy, overt nephropathy, symptomatic neuropathy, and clinically evident macrovascular complications. The results were similar to those reported by Jacobson *et al.* (1994). Those patients having more complications had worse quality of life. This was particularly evident in patients with three or more complications. While this study was not designed specifically to assess the validity of the measure it lends support for the ability of the DQOL to differentiate between patients at different levels of health status. It also underlines the resilience of adults with IDDM in that patients with fewer than three complications showed minimal change in their quality of life.

Sensitivity to Change

All quality of life measures must eventually be evaluated in terms of their ability to capture important clinical changes in patient functioning. However, this is typically the last property of a quality of life scale to be evaluated because it necessarily involves longitudinal follow-up. There are two studies that provide information relevant to this question. Nathan *et al.* (1991) evaluated patients who had long-term diabetes with severe nephropathic complications such that they all required treatment for end-stage renal disease. Patients were given either a kidney transplant or a combined pancreas/kidney transplant and followed over a one year period. The investigators found that there was a distinct improvement in the quality of life as measured by the DQOL total score and all subscales among patients who had received the combined kidney/pancreas transplant, while there was no improvement in quality of life for those patients who received the kidney transplant alone. The only clinical differences in the two groups were in terms of improved glycaemic control in the patients receiving the pancreas transplant and the lifestyle change reflecting the freedom from daily self-care of diabetes. Thus, the change in quality of life reflected the freedom from diabetes self-care activities rather than differences in morbidity.

In a second study, the quality of life of patients who received an implantable pump was compared to usual insulin treatment (Selam *et al.*, 1992). This pump required periodic attention and did not relieve the patient from the need for regular daily glucose monitoring. Furthermore, patients had to continue to programme the pump to give themselves insulin. Finally, the pump reservoir had to be filled with insulin on a monthly basis. The pump was associated with a decrease in the frequency of hypoglycaemia and a slight improvement in overall metabolic control. Evaluations of the patients with the DQOL showed an improvement in the Satisfaction subscale of the DQOL but no other changes (Selam *et al.*, 1992).

These two studies provide an indication of the sensitivity of the DQOL to change. In the first instance, the treatment led to a substantial alteration in the patient's lifestyle as it related to diabetes. In essence, for a time, these patients were relieved from the metabolic disequilibrium of diabetes and its treatment demands. This was reflected in a large change in DQOL ratings even though the patients still had substantial complications of long-term diabetes. In the second study, the method of treatment led to a very modest change in lifestyle plus reduction in hypoglycaemic frequency. This was reflected in a smaller improvement in quality of life detected only in the satisfaction scale. Therefore, these two studies provide an indication of the DQOL's sensitivity to meaningful changes in the burden of care posed by diabetes.

Alternative Form

Ingersoll and Marrero (1991) have developed a modification of the DQOL measure especially designed for use in adolescent and child populations. This modified measure dropped items of limited value for children and adolescents (for example, the question on worry about denial of health insurance was dropped). Furthermore, items relating to school life and peers were added. The items were field tested among a small group of children aged between eleven and eighteen. Based on this pilot work, the wording of questions was simplified and readability was improved. The revised instrument is composed of a seventeen-item diabetes Life Satisfaction scale, a twenty-three-item Disease Impact scale, and an eleven-item Diabetes-related Worry scale. The general rating of overall health was altered from a four- to five-point Likert index. The Cronbach alpha for the scales ranges from .82 to .85. The investigators found that the three scales were moderately related to the individual self-rated overall health in the .42 to .45 range. No data are available on the test-retest reliability or on the validity of the modified youth scale (Ingersoll & Marrero, 1991).

DISCUSSION

To date, studies of the DQOL provide considerable support for its reliability, validity, and sensitivity to clinical change. It is especially useful for IDDM patients, although the Impact and Satisfaction scales as currently constructed can also be used with NIDDM patients. The Worry scales are most relevant to younger populations, so are best used in studies of patients with IDDM. It would be quite useful to develop specific scales that are more directly relevant to the concerns of elderly adults. Clearly, further work is needed on developing an understanding of what clinical conditions and treatment regimens are most important determinants of change on the DQOL, so that we can better understand its sensitivity to change in clinical trials. Anecdotal observations from the DCCT and from Jacobson *et al.*, (1994) suggest that it is an acceptable and easy-to-use measure that patients have little difficulty understanding.

While the DQOL is a potentially valuable diabetes-specific measure to augment the wide variety of generic quality of life measures that are available, it is important to realise that in any single clinical trial, the assessment of quality of life is best thought of as a three part procedure. 1) In each instance, a broad-range, generic measure of quality of life will be useful in characterising the patient population and will facilitate comparison with other studies across illness groups. These measures also provide a useful gauge of functional health status. 2) An illness-oriented or treatment-specific measure such as the DQOL may provide a more sensitive indicator of change and will address issues that are especially relevant to the illness or treatment under study. 3) It is unlikely that an already-developed illness-specific measure will capture all relevant elements of change anticipated by a clinical study. Therefore, additional questions or questionnaires should be considered in the design of any given study. These may include already available measures of special relevance or specific items designed to capture the special elements of a trial. For example, if it is anticipated that the treatment would have particular impact on the sexual functioning of an individual, neither the DQOL nor any broad gauged, generic quality of life measure would provide specific coverage of this issue. Therefore, it would be helpful to utilise a measure specifically addressing the quality of sexual life. Alternatively, if it is anticipated that a particular treatment might be associated with side effects or lifestyle benefits, not sufficiently covered by the DQOL or other measures available, it is important to develop new questions to augment the quality of life assessment. The DQOL should be considered as part of a package of measures that are carefully selected to capture the range of possible impacts of the treatment or intervention under study.

The new method for scoring the DQOL developed by Jacobson *et al.* (1994) and described in the present chapter, should be considered as an alternative to the original scoring protocol developed by the DCCT. This new scoring strategy provides a more readily interpretable range of scores and should be less confusing for readers.

SUMMARY

The DQOL is intended to evaluate the satisfaction, impact, and worries associated with the treatment of diabetes mellitus. It is most suitable for use in diabetic populations taking insulin though it may be applied to patients with NIDDM who are on diet and oral agent treatment. The Satisfaction and Impact scales can be used with patients age thirteen and older. It is important to note that since the Worry subscale items (e.g. Social and Diabetes Worry) were designed with a young population in mind, they are likely to be less relevant for patients with

Type 2 diabetes. It would be useful to develop a set of scales relevant to the social and diabetes-related worries of adults and especially elderly or retired individuals. No diabetes quality of life scales have been developed with a specific interest in such groups. The DQOL can be used with patients experiencing a wide range of complications. A single general well-being item is also incorporated for comparison with other health-care surveys. Finally, supplemental items that address questions of relevance to adolescents in school and/or living with their families enrich the information gathered from the DQOL. It is readable by patients with a minimum of an eighth grade education (i.e. approximately age thirteen). The DQOL is self-administered with written instructions that should require little additional explanation. The measure provides scores on the Satisfaction, Impact, Diabetes-related Worry, and Social/Vocational Worry subscales as well as a total Quality of Life score that ranges from zero representing worst possible quality of life to 100 representing best possible quality of life on each scale and on the total score.

ACKNOWLEDGMENT

This work is supported by a donation from Herbert G. Graetz and NIH Grants AM27845 and RO1 DK42315. The DCCT is supported by the Division of Diabetes, Endocrinology, and Metabolic Diseases of the National Institute of Diabetes, Digestive and Kidney Disease, NIH, through cooperative agreements and a research contract. Dr. David M. Nathan is the Chairman of the DCCT Editorial Board.

REFERENCES

Bergner, M., Bobbitt, R. A., Carter, W. B. and Gibson, B. S. (1981) The Sickness Impact Profile: Development and final revision of a health status measure. *Medical Care* **19**; 787–805

Bradburn, N. M. (1969) The Structure of Psychological Well-Being. Chicago, IL: Aldine

Bush, J. M. and Kaplan, R.M. (1982) Health-related quality of life measurement *Health Psychol.* **1**; 61–80.

DCCT Research Group (1986) Diabetes Control and Complications Trial (DCCT): Design and methodological considerations for the feasibility phase. *Diabetes* **35**; 530–545

The DCCT Research Group (1987) Diabetes Control and Complications Trial (DCCT): Results of a feasibility study. *Diabetes Care* **10**; 1–19

The DCCT Research Group (1988) Reliability and Validity of a Diabetes Quality of Life Measure for the Diabetes Control and Complication Trial (DCCT) *Diabetes Care* **11**; 725–732

Derogatis, L. R. (1983) The Psychological Adjustment of Illness Scale (PAIS). *J. Psychosom. Res.* **30**; 77–91

Derogatis, L. R., Rickels, K. and Rock, A. (1983) The SCL-90-R. Administration, Scoring, and Procedures Manual II. Baltimore, MD: Clinical Psychometric Research

Howie, L. J. and Drury, T. F. (1978) Current Estimate from the Health Interview Survey: United States –1977. *Vital Health Statistics* **10**; 1–98

Ingersoll, G. M. and Marrero, D.G. (1991) A modified quality of life measure for youths: Psychometric properties. *Diabetes Educator* **17 (2)**; 114–118

International Resource Center (IRC) for Health Care Assessment (1991) How to Score the MOS 36-Item Short-Form Health Survey (SF36). Boston, MA: New England Medical Center Hospitals, Inc

Jacobson, A. M., de Groot, M. and Samson, J. A. (1994) The Evaluation of Two Measures of Quality of Life in Patients with Type I and Type II Diabetes Mellitus. *Diabetes Care* **17** (4) in press

Lloyd, C. E., Matthews, K. A., Wing, R. R. and Orchard, T. J. (1992) Psychosocial factors and complications of IDDM. *Diabetes Care* **15 (2)**; 166–172

Nathan, D. M., Fogel, H., Norman, D., Russell, P. S., Tolkoff-Rubin, N., Delmonico, F. L., Auchinloss, H., Camuso, J. and Cosimi, A. B. (1991) Long-term metabolic and quality of life results with pancreatic/renal transplantation in insulin-dependent diabetes mellitus. *Transplantation* **52** (1); 85–91

Selam, J. L., Micossi, P., Dunn, F. L. and Nathan, D. M. (1992) Clinical trial of programmeable implantable insulin pump for Type I diabetes. *Diabetes Care* **15 (7)**; 877–884

Ware, J. H. and Sherbourne, C. D. (1992) The MOS 36-Item Short Form Health Survey (SF36). I. Conceptual framework and core item selection. *Medical Care* **30**; 473–483

CHAPTER 6

THE WELL-BEING QUESTIONNAIRE

CLARE BRADLEY

Department of Psychology, Royal Holloway, University of London, Egham Hill, Egham, Surrey, TW20 0EX, UK

INTRODUCTION

The Well-being Questionnaire was originally designed in 1982 to provide a measure of depressed mood, anxiety, and various aspects of positive well-being for use in a World Health Organisation study evaluating new treatments for the management of diabetes. Scales were needed which would be sensitive to any increases in anxiety or depression that might be associated with intensified treatment regimens but which would also be sensitive to positive changes in well-being.

During the time these scales have been developed investigators evaluating psychological well-being of people with diabetes and, indeed, other populations with general medical disorders, have used assessment instruments developed for use with psychiatric or with general populations (Friis and Nanjundappa, 1986; Wilkinson *et al.*, 1988; Derogatis, 1986). The problem with using such instruments is that somatic symptoms of depression and anxiety are usually included in the scales and are often similar to the somatic symptoms of illnesses such as diabetes and cancer (Plumb and Holland, 1977). The Beck Depression Inventory (Beck *et al.*, 1961) is one instrument that is often used, inappropriately, with people who have diabetes. Beck's measure includes items concerning tiredness, loss of appetite, loss of libido, and weight loss, which may be symptoms indicative of depressed mood in the general population but in diabetes are more likely to be associated with hyperglycaemia, hypoglycaemia or chronic complications of diabetes. When measures like the Beck are used with people with diabetes, results may suggest the need for referral to clinical psychology or psychiatry services when it may be more appropriate to direct attention to helping them to improve their diabetes control. Although we should also be aware of the risk that physiological signs of a depressive syndrome might be attributed to a patient's diabetes or to unwanted effects of medication, diabetes health care professionals appear to be just as susceptible as everyone else to the form of bias that Ross (1977) termed the "fundamental attribution error". The fundamental attribution error is a common form of bias whereby problems are more likely to be attributed to personal characteristics such as personality and mood factors than to situational characteristics such as the professional advice given and the treatment regimen followed (Gamsu and Bradley, 1987; Gillespie and Bradley, 1988). Another common attribution bias, the so-called "actor-observer bias" (Jones and Nisbett, 1971) leads health professionals (the observers) to be more at risk than patients of overpsychologising in attributing patients' symptoms to dispositional factors in the patient, while the patients (the actors) are more likely to give due weight to situational factors. Thus the risk of health professionals overpsychologising is probably greater than the risk of their overlooking psychological explanations for somatic symptoms.

The present well-being scales were designed to be particularly sensitive to the more cognitive symptoms and to minimize as far as possible the inclusion of somatic symptoms such as weight loss which may be common in poorly controlled insulin-dependent diabetes. Although several items were included to address feelings of tiredness/energy these were not intended for inclusion in the depression subscale.

Since the present well-being scales were first designed, the Hospital Anxiety and Depression (HAD) scale has been developed which is also designed to focus on cognitive symptomatology and avoid somatic symptoms that may confound mood states with physical symptoms in hospital patients with general medical disorders (Zigmond and Snaith, 1983). The HAD scale has been developed with a view to its being used widely with patients from a range of medical specialties but includes only two subscales measuring depression and anxiety and provides no measure of positive mood states. The Well-being scales are designed not only to measure negative mood states and detect changes in such states but also offer the advantage over the HAD scale in that they measure positive effects of treatment changes, or other interventions intended to be improvements in diabetes management.

The Well-being scales were developed from a questionnaire originally designed for use with adults with insulin-treated diabetes but have also been developed with a population of people with tablet-treated diabetes and are probably equally suitable for people with diabetes treated with diet alone. They have been used primarily in studies evaluating the effects of new treatments such as continuous subcutaneous insulin infusion (CSII) pumps compared with conventional injections (Bradley et al., 1992), insulin therapy in patients previously treated with tablets (Bradley and Lewis, 1990; Jennings et al., 1991), and the effects of educational interventions in patients with tablet-treated Type 2 diabetes (Lewis 1994). Increasingly the scales are being used for the purpose of auditing psychological outcomes in diabetes care. One of the subscales is being used in a Royal College of Physicians/British Diabetic Association UK multicentre study of audit of diabetes care (Williams et al., 1992; Bishop et al., 1993). Translations of the scales are available in French and German (Bradley et al., 1992) and untested draft translations in Albanian, Finnish, Hungarian, Serbo-Croat and Spanish (Bradley et al., 1992a). Following a meeting organised by the World Health Organisation and the International Diabetes Federation in Oslo, June 1992, it was decided that scores from the scales are to be included in the basic information sheet designed for the multicentre European Diabcare project which aims to promote continuous quality improvement with a view to meeting and extending the targets of the St Vincent Declaration (Krans et al., 1992). A WHO Regional Office for Europe Consensus Meeting on Quality Assurance Indicators in Mental Health Care endorsed the

Well-being Questionnaire and recommended that it be used more widely (Stockholm, August 1993). Use of the questionnaire not only in diabetes research but also in research into other chronic illnesses was recommended within the context of a programme of continuing development of the measure in its original English and in the translations. It was proposed that the questionnaire be referred to as the WHO (Bradley) Well-being Questionnaire.

THE SCALES

Design

The initial questionnaire consisted of twenty eight items including six depression items, six anxiety items and sixteen potential positive well-being items. The depression and anxiety subscales were taken from a measure already developed on a different population (Warr *et al.*, 1985) while the positive well-being items were put together by the present author following discussions with diabetologists and psychologists at a meeting, organised by the WHO Regional Office for Europe, to plan a multicentre European study evaluating the use of CSII pumps. Thus the scales were intended to be sensitive to any increase in anxiety or depression that might be associated with this more visible and more intensive form of insulin therapy that was intended to improve blood glucose control and hence might increase the risk of hypoglycaemic episodes. The scales were also intended to be sensitive to any positive psychological benefits of CSII therapy and included items concerned with energy levels, personal relationships, sexual relationships, coping, adjustment, happiness and enthusiasm for life. Following psychometric development of the scales in two studies, four subscales were identified and labelled Depression (six items), Anxiety (six items), Positive Well-being (six items) and Energy (four items). The measurement of these four subscales involves twenty two items in total and these are included in the version of the scale shown in Figure 1.

FIGURE 1 WELL-BEING QUESTIONNAIRE

Please circle a number on each of the following scales to indicate how often you feel each phrase has applied to you in the past few weeks:

	all the time			not at all
1. I feel that I am useful and needed	3	2	1	0
2. I have crying spells or feel like it	3	2	1	0
3. I find I can think quite clearly	3	2	1	0
4. My life is pretty full	3	2	1	0
5. I feel downhearted and blue	3	2	1	0
6. I enjoy the things I do	3	2	1	0
7. I feel nervous and anxious	3	2	1	0
8. I feel afraid for no reason at all	3	2	1	0
9. I get upset easily or feel panicky	3	2	1	0
10. I feel like I'm falling apart and going to pieces	3	2	1	0
11. I feel calm and can sit still easily	3	2	1	0
12. I fall asleep easily and get a good night's rest	3	2	1	0
13. I feel energetic, active or vigorous	3	2	1	0
14. I feel dull or sluggish	3	2	1	0
15. I feel tired, worn out, used up, or exhausted	3	2	1	0
16. I have been waking up feeling fresh and rested	3	2	1	0
17. I have been happy, satisfied, or pleased with my personal life	3	2	1	0
18. I have felt well adjusted to my life situation	3	2	1	0
19. I have lived the kind of life I wanted to	3	2	1	0
20. I have felt eager to tackle my daily tasks or make new decisions	3	2	1	0
21. I have felt I could easily handle or cope with any serious problem or major change in my life	3	2	1	0
22. My daily life has been full of things that were interesting to me	3	2	1	0

Please make sure that you have considered each of the 22 statements and have circled a number on each of the 22 scales.

© September 1993; Dr. Clare Bradley, Diabetes Research Group, Royal Holloway, University of London, Egham, Surrey, TW20 0EX.

Scoring

Each item is scored on a 0 to 3 Likert scale where 0 indicates that the respondent felt that the item had applied to them "not at all" over the past few weeks while 3 indicates that it applied "all the time". Scores of 1 and 2 indicate points between the two extremes. Ratings for items on each subscale should be summed after reversing scores where necessary (Depression items 1, 3, 4 and 6: Anxiety items 11 and 12: Energy items 14 and 15). Subscales are scored so that a higher score on each subscale indicates more of the mood described by the subscale label, i.e. Depression, Anxiety, Energy and Positive Well-being. A General Well-being total score can be obtained by summing the subscale scores after reversing the scores on the Depression and Anxiety subscales. Scoring procedures can be summarised as shown in Table 1, which provides formulae which automatically reverse the scores as needed.

Table 1 Formulae for scoring the Well-being scales

Subscale	Items	Scoring procedure
Depression	1 to 6	12 − item 1 + item 2 − item 3− item 4 + item 5 −item 6
Anxiety	7 to 12	6 + item 7 + item 8 + item 9 + item 10 − item 11 − item 12
Energy	13 to 16	6 + item 13 − item 14 − item 15 + item 16
Positive Well-being	17 to 22	Item 17 + item 18 + item 19 + item 20 + item 21 + item 22
Total General Well-being	1 to 22	36 − Depression − Anxiety + Positive Well-being + Energy

SCALE DEVELOPMENT

Subject Samples and Procedures

Study 1: Initial Sheffield scale development study: tablet-treated patients

Respondents were from an initial pool of 239 patients (141 men and 98 women) treated with oral hypoglycaemic agents who had been invited to take part in a study evaluating the management of Type 2 diabetes (Bradley and Lewis, 1990; Jennings *et al.*, 1991). These patients attended one of two outpatient clinics at the Royal Hallamshire Hospital, Sheffield. Ages ranged from forty to sixty five years. Those who were blind or partially sighted were not included. Two hundred and nineteen (92%) patients (132 men and 89 women) agreed to take part and were screened to establish their health status. Participants did not differ from those declining to participate on any of the available measures including sex, age, duration of diabetes or haemoglobin A_1 (HbA$_1$) levels.

At the screening appointment, a booklet of questionnaires, including the undeveloped twenty eight-item Well-being Questionnaire, was given to each participant for completion at home. Each patient was asked to return the booklet, in confidence, direct to the university psychology department within the next two days. Non-responders received a reminder one month following their screening appointment. One hundred and eighty-seven (85%) patients (110 men, 77 women) returned completed questionnaires including 184 completed Well-being Questionnaires. This sample of 184 provided data for the psychometric analyses reported in Bradley and Lewis (1990) and summarised here. There were no significant differences between responders and non-responders to the questionnaires in terms of sex, age, duration of diabetes, HbA_1 or percent ideal body weight.

Study 2: WHO Multicentre European Study of CSII Pump Treatment vs Intensified Injection Therapy

This multicentre European study was organised by the World Health Organisation in 1982 with a view to evaluating the use of continuous subcutaneous insulin infusion (CSII) pumps in comparison with conventional injection therapy (CIT) in the management of Type 1, insulin-dependent diabetes (Staehr Johansen, 1989). A crossover design was used where patients acted as their own controls and the order of the two treatments (CSII and ICT) was allocated at random. Patients used the first treatment allocated to them for six months before crossing over to the second treatment. A run-in period of at least two months preceded the treatment phases. During run-in, injection therapy was optimized and self monitoring of blood glucose levels was introduced. In one of the centres, Hotel Dieu in Paris, patients were introduced to CSII pumps during the run-in period. Previous experience at Hotel Dieu suggested that there would be a high drop-out rate among patients using CSII for the first time. In order to avoid high drop-out rates in the crossover phases of the study, experience of the CSII pump was provided during run-in in the Hotel Dieu centre. Eleven centres in nine countries participated in the study ; Tirana in Albania, Karlsburg in Germany, Helsinki in Finland, Montpellier and Toulouse, as well as Paris in France, Budapest in Hungary, Oslo in Norway, Barcelona in Spain, Sheffield in the United Kingdom and Zagreb in what was then Yugoslavia. The psychometric properties of the Well-being Questionnaire were explored in three of the centres involved in the study, Paris, France; Karlsburg, Germany; Sheffield, UK. Psychometric analysis focused on these three centres because the numbers of patients participating in these centres were greater and/or translation problems with the questionnaires were absent or less apparent than was the case for other centres. Translation problems were first identified during preliminary analysis of the Finnish data (Bradley 1987), were found subsequently to be widespread, and are discussed in Chapter 3 of this volume. Back translation of the French and German translations of the Well-being scales revealed fewer and less substantial translation discrepancies than were apparent in other centres.

Psychometric analyses were conducted on the responses of $N \leq 41$ English, $N \leq 69$ French (Paris only) and $N \leq 40$ German patients who completed the questionnaire at the end of the run-in period, prior to randomisation. The effects of treatment on Well-being subscale scores are reported for N=37 English, N=47 French and N=39 German patients. The ratio of women/men who completed the run-in was 17/24 in the English sample, 34/35 in the French and 10/30 in the German. Mean ages (and standard deviations) were: English 35 years (s.d.10.0); French 37 (10.0); German 30 (9.0). Mean duration of diabetes and standard deviations were: English 12 years (8.0); French 12 (8.0); German 11.5 (7.0) (Thibult, 1990, Table 8a).

The make of pump used varied from centre to centre. All patients in the German centre used the Microjet Bolus 2 while 17% of Hotel Dieu patients used this pump, 47% used a Nordisk pump, 32% used AS8MP, 4% used another make of pump (unspecified) (Thibult, 1990, Table 16). All patients in the UK centre used a Nordisk pump. It should be noted that pen-injector devices (Novopen) became available in the Sheffield, UK, centre during the course of the study and six patients used pen injectors rather than conventional injections in the second treatment phase of the study following a first phase on pump treatment and three patients used a pen-injector instead of a pump during the second phase following a first phase on conventional injections. Furthermore, five patients who used conventional injections during phase 1 continued with these injections instead of crossing over to pump treatment for phase 2. Thus interpretation of treatment effects in the English centre is especially problematic though the pre-randomisation responses to the Well-being Questionnaire used in psychometric analyses were unaffected by these problems.

Interpretation of pre-randomisation data for psychometric development purposes was generally less influenced by protocol differences between centres and deviations within centres than the analysis of treatment effects. However, the experience of pumps obtained in the French sample may well have influenced the data and the kind of patients willing to be recruited into the study may have varied from centre to centre as a result of the different protocols described to them when the study was proposed. Thus the samples needed to be analysed and interpreted separately though similar psychometric characteristics in data from different samples provided strong evidence for characteristics that were robust.

Statistical Methods and Qualitative Judgements

Principal-components factor analysis with varimax rotation (Harman, 1967) was used to confirm the structure of the Depression and Anxiety subscales and explore the stucture of responses to the Positive Well-being items for each of the populations in studies 1 and 2. Selection of the items for the Positive Well-being subscale in study 1 was guided by the factor analysis of the sixteen positive well-being items alone followed by further analyses including the twelve anxiety and depression items. A forced three factor solution was sought to examine the relationship between the anxiety, depression and newly-selected positive well-being items. Reliability was assessed using Cronbach's alpha coefficient of internal consistency (Cronbach, 1951). The distributions of scores on some of the Well-being

scales were skewed, indicating the need for transformation or non-parametric statistical tests in subsequent analyses of these measures. The Sheffield data from
study 1 were analysed using non-parametric tests on SPSSX while the WHO data
from study 2 used non-parametric correlation methods but for the purposes of
analysis of variance, transformed the data so that distributions were statistically
normalised using an SAS procedure. Analysis of the WHO study data was conducted by Nadine Thibult at the Institut National de la Santé et de la Recherche
Médicale (INSERM) near Paris. As the sample size from the Sheffield study was
much greater than that available from any one of the WHO study centres, analyses conducted on the WHO study data were seeking to confirm that the scales
were equally appropriate for insulin users as they had been for patients with tab-
let- treated diabetes. Though an Energy subscale was developed for the first time
using data from the WHO centres, the cluster of items making up the Energy subscale had been noted to load together in factor analyses conducted on the Sheffield data but had not been explored further at that time.

For the purpose of analysing the results of the WHO study, inaccurately translated items which adversely affected the reliability of the German translation were excluded for scoring purposes. These items have since been retranslated but the
results described in this chapter refer to a four-item Depression subscale for the
German translation instead of the full six-item subscale in English and French versions.

Structure of the Scales

Sheffield sample with tablet-treated diabetes

Principal components analysis of the sixteen positive well-being items alone followed by further analyses including the twelve anxiety and depression items,
guided selection of six positive well-being items for use in the final scale. A
forced, three-factor solution, presented in Table 2, showed all six Positive Well-
being items to load on Factor 1 accounting for 40% of the variance. The Anxiety
items loaded primarily on Factor 2 (accounting for 11% of the variance) with
some overlap for the two positively-worded items onto Factor 1. Factor 3 was characterised by the depression items (6% of the variance) though the two negatively-
worded items loaded more highly with the negatively-worded anxiety items on
Factor 2. The overlap between the Anxiety and Depression subscales is not surprising in the context of earlier research suggesting that anxiety and depression
are not entirely separate states but involve a complex interplay of symptoms
(Bramley *et al.*, 1988).

WHO study sample with Type 1 diabetes

Forced and unforced factor analyses were carried out on the positive well-being
items first to confirm the existence of the six-item Positive Well-being scale identi-

Table 2 Forced three-factor solution on data from the Sheffield tablet-treated sample from Bradley and Lewis (1990)

	FACTOR LOADINGS		
	Factor 1	*Factor 2ˑ*	*Factor 3*
Depression			
I feel that I am useful and needed	0.32	0.19	**0.64**
I have crying spells or feel like it	0.10	**0.70**	0.11
I find I can think quite clearly	0.13	0.03	**0.65**
My life is pretty full	0.22	0.12	**0.76**
I feel downhearted and blue	0.23	**0.57**	0.24
I enjoy the things I do	0.35	0.28	**0.50**
Anxiety			
I feel nervous and anxious	0.32	**0.80**	0.02
I feel afraid for no reason at all	-0.04	**0.83**	0.21
I get upset easily or feel panicky	0.25	**0.72**	0.12
I feel like I'm falling apart and going to pieces	0.31	**0.66**	0.04
I feel calm and can sit still easily	**0.44**	0.34	0.20
I fall asleep easily and get a good night's rest	**0.52**	0.26	0.00
Positive Well-being			
I have been happy, satisfied or pleased with my personal life	**0.62**	0.27	0.45
I have felt well adjusted to my life situation	**0.72**	0.18	0.27
I have lived the kind of life I wanted to	**0.74**	0.07	0.25
I have felt eager to tackle my daily tasks or make new decisions	**0.75**	0.18	0.35
I have felt I could easily handle or cope with any serious problem or major change in my life	**0.72**	0.13	0.16
My daily life has been full of things that were interesting to me	**0.63**	0.26	0.41

The magnitude of factor loading indicates degree of relationship to each factor.

fied by Bradley and Lewis (1990) and secondly to explore the possibility of constructing an additional scale. The six positive well-being items loaded on Factor 1 in all three centres with loadings ≥ 0.60 in the English centre, ≥ 0.57 in the French centre and ≥ 0.32 in the German centre. Thus the structure of this subscale was confirmed in the three samples of patients with Type 1 diabetes despite some minor translation discrepancies (Bradley *et al.*, 1992). A second factor emerged with four items loading highly in each of the three centres (loadings were ≥ 0.60 English; ≥ 0.67 French; 0.73 German). The consistency of the factor across centres, together with recognition that this pattern had been apparent though not followed up in the earlier analyses of the Sheffield sample, led to exploration of the psychometric properties of this subscale which was labelled "Energy".

Table 3 Cronbach's alpha coefficients for the original scales with the two study samples of English patients and for the French and German translations used in the WHO study

Subscale	Number of items retained	Type 2 sample English	Type 1 sample (WHO)		
			English	French	German
Depression	6 (or 4*)	0.70	0.67	0.46	0.73*
Anxiety	6	0.80	0.74	0.72	0.65
Energy	4	—.—	0.64	0.78	0.75
Positive Well-being	6	0.88	0.80	0.89	0.66

Factor analyses of the six anxiety items led to single factor solutions for the English (loadings ≥ ± 0.32) and French (loadings ≥ ± 0.40) data though two factors emerged in the German data with three items loading on each factor ≥ ± .68 and ≥ ± .43. Items with the poorest factor loadings identified in the English version were the two positively-worded items "I feel calm and can sit still easily" and "I fall asleep easily and get a good night's rest" with loadings of 0.32 and 0.38 respectively. Interestingly these same two items had the lowest loadings on Factor 2 in the Sheffield study (see Table 2) and the structure of the scale would be more homogenous if it were limited to the four negatively-worded items. Future work might examine the reliablity and validity of such a four-item scale with a view to dropping the two items with lower loadings. It should be noted, however, that all six items of the French version of the scale had very satisfactory factor loadings. In the German version of the subscale, the two items which had low loadings in the English samples emerged on Factor 2 along with "I get upset easily or feel panicky". The translation into German had altered the original English meaning of the three Factor 2 items slightly, but exclusion of all three items would have led to a substantial lowering of the alpha coefficient from 0.65 for the six-item subscale to 0.53 for the three items. Correlation analysis and the satisfactory alpha coefficient indicated that all six items were measuring a variant of an anxiety construct and were therefore retained in a single six-item subscale.

Factor analysis of the six depression items resulted in the emergence of a single factor for each of the English (loadings ± 0.25 to 0.83), French (loadings ± 0.12 to 0.91) and German (loadings ± 0.03 to 0.93) versions. The item with the poorest factor loading was "I feel that I am useful and needed" which had the lowest factor loading for all three versions. The item "I feel downhearted and blue" had a fairly low factor loading of 0.32 on the English version. The item "My life is pretty full" had a very low factor loading of 0.19 on the German version. Due to translation problems with the two items "I feel that I am useful and needed" and "My life is pretty full" and their very low factor loadings (0.03 and 0.19 respectively), these two items were excluded from scoring the German version of the scale for the purposes of the WHO study. The absolute factor loadings for the remaining four items ranged from 0.39 to 0.93, which was considered satisfactory. It is hoped that the problems with the translations will have been solved with the retranslations of the discrepant items in the German version and with the improvements that have also been made to the French translation (Bradley *et al.*, 1992). Only one of the two low loading items for the English version in the WHO sample corresponded with the results of the factor analysis of the Sheffield study of patients with tablet-treated diabetes. The lowest loading item in the WHO data was the positively-worded "I feel that I am useful and needed" item that loaded highly with other positively-worded items in the data from tablet-treated patients. Thus the structure of the Depression subscale is less coherent than that of the other three subscales. To improve coherence of the Depression subscale, additional items are currrently being investigated as potentially better substitutes than those in current use.

Reliability

Internal consistency

Cronbach's alpha coefficients for each of the six-item subscales indicated satisfactory internal consistency as shown in Table 3. The alphas are highly satisfactory for four- or six-item scales.

Validity

Face and content validity

The Depression and Anxiety subscales appear to be much less likely to confound these psychological states with symptoms of poorly-controlled diabetes than is the case with many standard measures that include somatic symptoms as well as cognitive symptoms of depressed and anxious mood. The Positive Well-being and Energy subscales extend the breadth of the well-being domain measured and produce a measure that is designed to be sensitive to positive psychological benefits of treatment programmes as well as to psychological costs such as increased anxiety or depression.

Concurrent validity

No concurrent validity information is presently available though studies are planned. The most appropriate measure for comparison would be the HAD scale (Zigmond and Snaith, 1983) which would allow comparison across the Depression and Anxiety subscales.

Construct validity

Construct validity was assessed by correlating the scales with other variables collected at the time of the studies. Predicted sex differences in Depression and Anxiety were also investigated. Support for scale validity was provided if associations were consistent, predicted and/or intuitively sensible.

Sex differences in Well-being: Bradley and Lewis (1990) reported that as is usually found in the general population, women had significantly higher Depression (p<0.02) and Anxiety (p<0.001) scores than men and lower General Well-being scores (p<0.01) although there were no significant sex differences in the Positive Well-being scores. Means, standard deviations and minimum and maximum scores obtained for each of the subscales are presented in Table 4. Significant differences were also found between men and women in other variables: women had significantly higher HbA_1 levels (p<0.001), were significantly more overweight (p<0.001) and rated their recent diabetes control to be worse than did men (p<0.01). Sex differences were not explored in the WHO data but means for all patients are presented in Table 4.

Table 4 Scale means (s.d.), minimum and maximum scores for total samples and for each sex in the tablet treated sample 1 and for all the insulin dependent patients in Sample 2

	Sample 1: Type 2			Sample 2: Type 1		
	Mean (s.d.)	Min-imum found	Max-imum found	Mean (s.d.) (at baseline)	Range	
Depression						
Men	2.8 (2.8)	0	12			
Women	3.8 (3.0)	0	13			
All patients	3.2 (2.9)	0	13	3.7 (2.1)	0 - 18	
Anxiety						
Men	3.7 (3.5)	0	15			
Women	5.7 (4.1)	0	15			
All patients	4.5 (3.9)	0	15	2.1 (1.5)	0 - 18	
Energy						
All patients	subscale not scored with sample 1			8.1 (1.9)	0 - 12	
Positive Well-being						
Men	13.5 (3.7)	6	18			
Women	12.6 (4.1)	2	18			
All patients	13.2 (3.8)	2	18	12.9 (2.7)	0 - 18	
General Well-being						
Men	43.1[1] (8.8)	18	54		0 - 54[1]	Sample 1
Women	39.0[1] (9.5)	13	54			
All patients	(1.4[1] (9.3)	13	54	51.7[2] (6.2)	0 - 66[2]	Sample 2

Sample 1 of people with Type 2 diabetes from Table 2 of Bradley and Lewis (1990)
Sample 2 of people with Type 1 diabetes from Tables 24a, b and c of Thibult (1990)

Associations of Well-being scales with complications of diabetes: It would be expected that those patients with complications of diabetes or other physical disorders such as arthritis, respiratory, gastro-intestinal, genito-urinary or central nervous system disorders, would be likely to report lower levels of well-being compared with patients who were free of disorders other than their diabetes. Bradley and Lewis (1990), in the study of patients with tablet-treated diabetes, compared those with one or more disorders on screening (N=140) with those patients without other disorders (N=44) and found significant differences on the total Well-being scores and on each of the three subscales, Depression, Anxiety and Positive Well-being, in the expected direction with p values of 0.05 or less.

Associations of Well-being scales with HbA$_1$ and other measures of diabetes control: Bradley and Lewis (1990) reported that tablet-treated patients with higher Depression and Anxiety scores were significantly more overweight [r = 0.14; p<0.05 (Depression), r = 0.24; p<0.001 (Anxiety)] and rated their diabetes to have been poorly controlled recently [r = 0.23; p<0.01 (Depression), r = 0.21; p<0.01 (Anxiety)]. However, no significant association was found between HbA$_1$ and depression, anxiety or positive well-being. As sex differences were found in Depression and Anxiety scores and women had poorer diabetes control, rated it as such, and were more overweight than the men, correlations between psychological Well-being and the metabolic variables were examined separately for each sex. The correlation between HbA$_1$ levels and the Well-being scales remained non-significant in each case. However, the correlation between Anxiety and percent ideal body weight was significant for women only (r = 0.43; p<0.001) whilst the association between depression and percent ideal body weight became non-significant for either sex separately, although for women, those who were more overweight tended to have higher Depression scores (r = 0.15; p=0.09). It was suggested tentatively that, for women, depression and anxiety may be causally associated with being overweight given that the correlation between these scales and percent ideal body weight was significant or approached significance for women. However, intervention studies would be needed to investigate whether weight loss would lead to improved well-being or vice versa.

Interrelationships between the scales: Bradley and Lewis (1990) reported that Depression and Anxiety scores were strongly correlated with each other (r = 0.64, p<0.001) and with the Positive Well-being scores (Depression; r = -0.68, p<0.001: Anxiety; r = -0.60, p<0.001), indicating some covariance between the measures. Although there was a high degree of intercorrelation there were instances where Positive Well-being was correlated with variables not related to Depression and Anxiety. For example, women who had experienced a stroke had significantly lower Positive Well-being scores than their counterparts not affected by strokes (r = -0.24, p<0.02) while there was no significant association with Depression (r = 0.09, n.s.) nor Anxiety scores (r = 0.00, n.s.). Thus absence of negative affect does not necessarily indicate a positive state of well-being and such findings support the inclusion of a separate Positive Well-being subscale.

Sensitivity to Change

Detection of treatment effects in people with Type 2 diabetes

Subsamples of Sample 1 patients with Type 2 diabetes were involved in two studies reported by Lewis (1994) and by Jennings *et al.* (1991). One subsample of patients was invited to take part in a trial of insulin therapy using either CSII pumps or injections. These patients were those who were classified as 'borderline poorly controlled' because their blood glucose levels were not well controlled by diet and oral agents and were close to the threshold where insulin would be routinely prescribed.

Patients who did not meet the selection criteria for the insulin study were invited to attend an education session. They were encouraged to bring a partner or friend if they wished. Of the 173 invited, 81 (47%) attended an education session. Comparisons of Well-being scores before and after education indicated a tendency towards reduced General Well-being following education. A mean score of 40.6 (s.d. 9.1) at baseline compared with a mean of 39.6 (10.0) post education. The difference which approached significance ($p < 0.062$) was mainly attributable to increased depression scores with a mean of 4.2 (2.7) at baseline and 4.6 (3.0) post education; $p < 0.052$. Changes in the Anxiety and Positive Well-being subscales (the Energy subscale was not scored for this sample) were in the direction of reduced well-being but nowhere near significance.

Changes in other variables measured in this study were more dramatic than changes in General Well-being or Depression scores. Notably, scores from the Satisfaction with Treatment scale, a forerunner of the Diabetes Treatment Satisfaction Questionnaire (DTSQ) described elsewhere in this book by the present author, showed highly significant increases in Satisfaction with Treatment following education. The Health Belief measures developed by Lewis *et al.* (1990) and described by Lewis and Bradley in a chapter of this *Handbook* were also included and showed Perceived Benefits of Treatment increased and Perceived Barriers to Treatment were significantly reduced following education. Thus the small increases in Depression scores associated with education sessions were offset by much larger increases in Satisfaction with Treatment.

The subsample of patients with poorly-controlled diabetes who took part in the insulin study was much smaller. Of the thirty two patients who fulfilled the selection criteria, twenty five agreed to participate. There was a three-month run-in period to maximise diet and sulphonylurea therapy. Twenty patients whose control did not improve sufficiently were randomised to CSII or CIT. Follow-up at four months showed no changes on the Depression, Anxiety or Positive Well-being subscales or on the General Well-being total score though Satisfaction with Treatment did improve significantly and so did diabetes control as indicated by HbA_1 levels (Jennings *et al.*, 1991; Lewis, 1994). Thus it can be concluded that introduction of insulin therapy in these patients led to a significant improvement in metabolic control without any deterioration in psychological aspects of well-being. Although psychological gains were observed on, for example, the Satisfaction with Treatment measure, they were not apparent on the Well-being scales used here. Had the Energy subscale been scored it is likely that it would have been the most sensitive to changes in this particular study where insulin therapy would be expected to impose quite an unwelcome burden on patients used to tablet treatment and the best that might be hoped for would be improved energy associated with improved metabolic control and that other aspects of psychological well-being would not be impaired. Clinical trials of CSII pump use in Sample 2 patients are described below and the Energy scale scored in that sample was indeed one of the most sensitive to change following CSII pump therapy in patients previously treated by injection therapy.

Detection of treatment effects in clinical trials involving people with Type 1 diabetes

The WHO study comparing CSII with injection treatment provides evidence of the value of the scales in detecting changes in well-being associated with the different treatments during the various periods of the study. In the French centre at Hotel Dieu where patients used the CSII pumps during the run-in phase of the study for at least two months, any improvement in well-being associated with CSII pumps would be expected to be most apparent in comparisons between baseline scores (when using conventional injection regimens) and scores taken at the time of randomisation (at the end of two months of CSII pump use). Patients who chose to take part in the study and who remained in the study at the end of the run-in period were likely to be patients who were initially less satisfied with their injection regimen and found that they preferred the pump. If they preferred the injection regimen they would be less likely to stay in the study. These issues of patients' preferences and randomised controlled trials have been discussed in detail elsewhere (e.g. Bradley, 1991; Bradley, 1993). Table 5 presents the analyses of changes in well-being scores from baseline, when the study was proposed to subjects, to the time of randomisation. Well-being was shown to be improved with CSII pumps compared with injections for three of the four subscales, Depression, Positive Well-being and Energy, but not for Anxiety. The improvement in General Well-being scores during the two months on the pump did not quite reach significance (see Table 5). During the crossover phase of the study, the four subscales showed patterns of change similar to those found in the run-in phase at Hotel Dieu. Significant period effects complicated the picture, with Well-being tending to be reduced during the first phase of the crossover compared with the second. However, the Energy subscale did show significant differences, with patients reporting more energy during pump treatment than during injection treatment (CSII - CIT: mean 0.29, s.d. 2.23, $p < 0.03$). Although all the subscales followed the expected pattern, with improved well-being during CSII treatment, the General Well-being scale did not reach significance (CSII - CIT: mean 1.52, s.d. 8.32, $p < 0.1$ n.s.).

Table 5 Insulin dependent patients from sample 2; changes in Well-being during the run-in on pumps in the French centre at Hotel Dieu

	Injections (Start of run-in) Mean (s.d.)		Pumps (End of run-in) Mean (s.d.)		Pumps-Injections (Δ during run-in) Mean (s.d.)		p
Depression (range 0-18)	4.1	(2.2)	3.4	(2.2)	-0.75	(2.2)	<0.04
Anxiety (range 0-18)	6.3	(3.6)	6.0	(3.7)	-0.34	(3.1)	<0.5 n.s.
Energy (range 0-12)	7.8	(2.6)	8.5	(2.2)	0.78	(2.2)	<0.04
Positive Well-being (range 0-18)	12.2	(3.4)	13.6	(3.0)	1.38	(3.5)	<0.02
General Well-being (range 0 - 66)	46.0	(9.7)	49.0	(9.2)	2.72	(7.9)	<0.06

Sample 2 of people with Type 1 diabetes from Tables 25a, b and c of Thibult (1990)

Table 6 Insulin dependent patients from sample 2; effects of CSII pump vs Injections in the German centre. Means (s.d.) scores on the well-being scales are shown for each of the treatment phases and for the differences between treatments

	Injections Mean (s.d.)		CSII Pump Mean (s.d.)		Pumps-Injections Mean (s.d.)		p
Depression (range 0-12)	1.7	(1.4)	1.0	(1.3)	-0.39	(1.3)	<0.08
Anxiety (range 0-18)	3.0	(2.8)	2.5	(2.0)	-0.54	(2.0)	<0.1 n.s.
Energy (range 0-12)	8.7	(2.4)	9.3	(2.1)	1.13	(2.6)	<0.01
Positive Well-being (range 0-18)	12.4	(2.8)	13.5	(2.8)	1.12	(2.5)	<0.01
General Well-being (range 0 - 66)	46.4	(8.0)	49.6	(6.9)	3.16	(6.5)	<0.005

n.b. There were no significant sequence or period effects, therefore the means are combined for the two groups in the crossover study and the pooled standard deviation reported.

Sample 2 of people with Type 1 diabetes from Tables 27a, b and c of Thibult (1990)

The German centre in the WHO study was the only one of the three centres on which psychometric analyses have been conducted, to follow the original protocol with a run-in period on injection treatment and no option to use pen-injectors instead of CSII or CIT during the study period. Whereas in Hotel Dieu with run-in on CSII pump there were no significant differences in Well-being or in HbA_1 levels during the crossover phases on CSII or CIT, in the German centre significant effects of treatment on Well-being and HbA_1 were apparent. Significant improvements in HbA_1 were associated with CSII use (mean 10.25, s.d. 0.93) compared with CIT (mean 9.70, s.d. 1.03; p<0.03) (Thibult, 1990, Table 19b). Table 6 shows that well-being was significantly improved with CSII compared with CIT. The most significant effect is seen in the total scale General Well-being score though significant effects are seen for the Positive Well-being and Energy subscales. There were no significant differences on the Anxiety subscale and the differences on the Depression subscale did not reach significance. Thus, as expected, the main benefits of CSII are to be seen in the implications for increased energy and improved positive well-being rather than in any improvements in anxiety or depression in this population which was not notably depressed or anxious to start with.

Norms

Means and standard deviations for each of the subscales and overall scale scores (and for men and women separately in the case of patients with tablet-treated diabetes) are presented in Table 4. Scores for the two samples of patients with Type 2 and Type 1 diabetes appear similar with the exception of the anxiety scores which appear higher in the Type 2 sample. The overall Well-being scores appear very similar if corrected for the number of items in the scale. A mean of 41.4 (for the tablet-treated patients responding to the 18-item scale) with a possible range of scores of 0 to 54 would be equivalent to a mean of 50.6 for a 22 item scale with scores from 0 to 66 and this is very similar to the mean of 51.7 obtained with the 22 item scale by the sample of patients with Type 1 diabetes.

Short Forms of the Measure

The Depression, Anxiety, Energy or Positive Well-being subscales may be selected from the twenty two-item scale and used separately though it should be noted that there are occasions when the total General Well-being score produces the most highly significant treatment effects as in the German centre of the WHO trial described above.

A short form of the measure was felt to be needed for a Royal College of Physicians/British Diabetic Association National UK study of audit of diabetes care (Williams *et al.*, 1992; Wilson *et al.* 1993). In order to reduce the scale for a single-page format and at the same time extend our knowledge about the nature of the measure, a scale was devised which included the six-item depression scale from the present Well-being scales together with six items to measure diabetes-specific depression with items such as "Because of my diabetes I cry or feel like crying". The diabetes-specific depression items were modifed from items used in The Diabetes Profile described in the Appendix (Meadows, 1989). Preliminary results show that, as expected, patients score higher on the Diabetes-specific Depression scale than on the General Depression scale and it is anticipated that the measure will be useful in identifying which cases of depressed mood are likely to be helped most effectively by the diabetes care team and which may require psychological or psychiatric referral. This scale may be useful in identifying problems with impaired psychological well-being in need of intervention though it would not be expected to be sensitive to change in clinical trials of new treatments in the way that the full Well-being scale has been shown to be.

DISCUSSION

The Well-being scales including each of the four subscales, Depression, Anxiety, Energy and Positive Well-being, have been shown to be useful as measures of psychological outcomes in clinical trials. The scales minimise the possibility of confusing symptoms of poor diabetes control with symptoms of depression. Data from Bradley and Lewis (1990) support the view that the measures of Depression, Anxiety and Positive Well-being are not related to HbA_1 measures of diabetes control. In addition, a major advantage offered by these scales compared with other existing measures (such as the HAD scale) that may well prove suitable for people with diabetes, is that the present scales measure positive aspects of well-being as well as negative states of anxiety and depression. Thus the Well-being scales are useful in determining the incremental benefits to well-being of new treatments designed with a view to improving patients' quality of life rather than just their blood glucose control. The Positive Well-being and Energy subscales were the subscales most sensitive to change in clinical trials of CSII use in patients with Type 1 diabetes. Although the Anxiety subscale has construct validity support, it has not shown itself to be sensitive to change in studies conducted to date though none of the interventions studied were expected to increase or decrease anxiety and the subscale may yet prove to be useful in the circumstances of other studies where effects on anxiety are anticipated. The Depression subscale has proved sensitive to change in the education intervention study as well as in the WHO clinical trial of CSII.

A problem with the Depression and Anxiety subscales is that scores are highly skewed with means lying between 3 and 4 on the 0 to 18 six-item scale. Thus it would be expected that the discriminatory power of these subscales would be less than that obtainable with the Positive Well-being and Energy subscales and this indeed has been found in the WHO study. The Depression and Anxiety subscales may prove to be more useful in detecting problems with psychological well-being in the course of auditing diabetes care and studies are now underway.

The factor structure of the Depression and Anxiety subscales was less clear cut than that observed for the Positive Well-being and Energy subscales. This seems in part to be attributable to the mixture of positively- and negatively-worded items in the Depression and Anxiety subscales. Future studies will examine the possibility of limiting the Anxiety subscale to the four negatively worded items and will add in additional negatively-worded items, including some concerned with low self-esteem, which may improve the coherence of the Depression subscale. Although there are clearly ways in which the scales might be improved, as they stand they have been shown to be useful measures and have at least adequate, and in the case of Positive Well-being and Energy, highly satisfactory levels of internal consistency.

Although the scales have not yet been used with people with diabetes treated with diet alone, there is every reason to believe that the scales will be equally appropriate for them but the psychometric properties of the scales have yet to be checked with such a sample. There is also every reason to believe that the scales may be useful with people who do not have diabetes as none of the items are specific to diabetes. The scales may be useful to those wishing to compare samples of people with diabetes with non-diabetic control samples or other patient groups though care is needed in interpreting such comparative data. The Depression and Anxiety subscales were originally developed with non-diabetic samples (Warr *et al.*, 1985) though the psychometric properties of these subscales should be examined if they are used with other samples not studied previously.

SUMMARY

The twenty two-item Well-being Questionnaire includes subscales to measure Depression, Anxiety, Energy and Positive Well-Being. It has been developed for use with insulin users and with people who have tablet-treated Type 2 diabetes, and is probably suitable for use with other populations including patients with other disorders and healthy people. The scales are designed for patient self completion, are quick to complete and can be scored (taking care to reverse-score items/subscales as specified in Table 1) to provide a total score of General Wellbeing as well as subscale scores to measure Depresison, Anxiety, Energy and Positive Well-being.

ACKNOWLEDGEMENTS

The author wishes to thank Nadine Thibult at INSERM for her detailed checking of the WHO data reported in this manuscript and for her valuable comments. The key role of Kirsten Staehr Johansen and the Quality of Care and Technologies programme at the WHO Regional Office for Europe in recognising the need for this measure and encouraging its design and development is appreciated and acknowledged.

REFERENCES

Beck, A.T., Ward, C.H., Mendelson, M., Mock, J. and Erbaugh, J. (1961). An inventory for measuring depression. *Archives of General Psychiatry*, **4**, 561-571

Bradley, C. (1987) WHO multicentre international study of CSII pumps. Report on translation problems in the Finnish version of the psychological scales. Report to the World Health Organisation, Regional Office for Europe, Copenhagen, May 1987

Bradley, C. (1991) Psychological issues in research design and measurement. In C. Bradley, P. Home and M. Christie (Eds.) *The Technology of Diabetes Care: Converging Medical and Psychosocial Perspectives.* Chur: Harwood Academic Press

Bradley, C. (1993) Designing medical and educational intervention studies: a review of some alternatives to conventional randomised controlled trials. *Diabetes Care*, **16**, 509-518

Bradley, C. and Lewis, K.S. (1990) Measures of Psychological Well-being and Treatment Satisfaction developed from the responses of people with tablet-treated diabetes. *Diabetic Medicine*, **7**, 445-451

Bradley, C., Meadows, K.A. and Sowden, A.J. (1992) General Well-being and Satisfaction with Treatment scales for use with people with insulin requiring diabetes. Part 1: Psychometric development and retranslation of the English, French and German versions. Report to the World Health Organisation, Regional Office for Europe, Copenhagen, June 1992

Bradley, C., Meadows, K.A. and Sowden, A.J. (1992a) General Well-being and Satisfaction with Treatment scales for use with people with insulin requiring diabetes. Part 2: Retranslation of the Albanian, Finnish, Hungarian, Serbo-Croat and Spanish versions. Report to the World Health Organisation, Regional Office for Europe, Copenhagen, August 1992

Bramley, P.N., Easton, A.M.E., Morley, S., Snaith, R.P. (1988) The differentiation of anxiety and depression by rating scales. *Acta Psychiatrica Scandinavica*, **77**, 133-138

Cronbach, L. J. (1951) Coefficient alpha and the internal structure of tests. *Psychometrika*, **16**, 297-334

Derogatis, L.R. (1986) Psychology in cancer medicine: a perspective and overview. *Journal of Consulting and Clinical Psychology*, **54**, 632-638

Friis, R. and Nanjundappa, G. (1986) Diabetes, depression and employment status. *Social Science and Medicine*, **23**, 471-475

Gamsu, D.S. and Bradley, C. (1987) Clinical staff's attributions about diabetes: scale development and staff versus patient comparisons. *Current Psychological Research and Reviews*, (Special Issue on Health Psychology), **6**, 69–78

Gillespie, C. R. and Bradley, C. (1988) Causal attributions of doctor and patients in a diabetes clinic. *British Journal of Clinical Psychology*, **27**, 67–76

Harman, H.H. (1967) *Modern Factor Analysis*, 2nd edn. Chicago: University of Chicago Press

Jennings, A.M., Lewis, K.S., Murdoch, S., Talbot, J.F., Bradley, C. and Ward, J.D. (1991) Randomised trial comparing continuous subcutaneous insulin infusion and conventional insulin therapy in Type II diabetic patients poorly controlled with sulphonylureas. *Diabetes Care*, **14**, 738–744

Jones, E.E. and Nisbett, R.E. (1971) The actor and the observer: divergent perceptions in the causes of behaviour. In E.E. Jones, D.E.Kanouse, H.H. Kelly, R.E. Nisbett, S. Valins and B.Weiner (ed.s) *Attribution: perceiving the causes of behaviour.* New Jersey: General Learning Press

Krans, H.M.J., Porta, M. and Keen, H. (1992) Diabetes Care and Research in Europe: the St Vincent Declaration Action Programme Implementation Document. World Health Organisation, Regional Office for Europe, Copenhagen

Lewis, K.S. (1994) An Examination of the Health Belief Model When Applied to Diabetes Mellitus. PhD thesis January 1994, University of Sheffield, Sheffield, UK

Lewis, K.S., Jennings, A.M., Ward, J.D. and Bradley, C. (1990) Health belief scales developed specifically for people with tablet-treated Type 2 diabetes. *Diabetic Medicine*, **7**, 148–155

Meadows, K.A., Brown, K.G., Thompson, C. and Wise, P.H. (1989) The diabetes health questionnaire (DHQ): preliminary validation of a new instrument (Abstract). *Diabetic Medicine*, **6** (Suppl. 2), P78

Plumb, M.M. and Holland, J. (1977) Comparative studies of psychological function in patients with advanced cancer - 1. Self-reported depressive symptoms *Psychosomatic Medicine*, 39, 264–276

Ross, L. (1977) The intuitive psychologist and his shortcomings: distortion of the attribution process. In L. Berkowitz (ed.) *Advances in Experimental Social Psychology*. New York: Academic Press

Staehr Johansen, K. (1989) World Health Organisation Multicentre Continuous Subcutaneous Insulin Infusion Pump Feasibility and Acceptability Study Experience. WHO Regional Office for Europe, Copenhagen

Thibult, N (1990) Tables: Clinical, biological and psychological analyses of the continuous subcutaneous insulin infusion (CSII) pump study. Report to the World Health Organisation, Regional Office for Europe. July 1990.

Warr, P.B., Banks, M.H. and Ullah, P. (1985) The experience of unemployment among black and white urban teenagers. *British Journal of Psychology*, **76**, 75–87

Wilkinson, G., Borsey, D.Q., Leslie, P., Newton, R.W., Lind, C. and Ballinger, C.B. (1988) Psychiatric morbidity and social problems in patients with insulin-dependent diabetes mellitus. *British Journal of Psychiatry*, **153**, 38–43

Williams, D.D.R., Home, P.D., Bishop, A., Bradley, C., and Members of a Working Group of the Research Unit of the Royal College of Physicians and British Diabetic Association (1992) A proposal for continuing audit of diabetes services. *Diabetic Medicine*, **9**, 759–764

Wilson, D.D.R., Home, P.D., Bishop, A., Bradley, C., Brown, K.J.E., Hargreaves, B. and Members of a Working Group of the Research Unit of the Royal College of Physicians and British Diabetic Association (1993) A dataset to allow exchange of information for monitoring continuing diabetes care. *Diabetic Medicine*, **10**, 378–390

Zigmond, A.S. and Snaith, R.P. (1983) The Hospital Anxiety and Depression Scale. *Acta Psychiatrica Scandinavica*, **67**, 361–370

DIABETES TREATMENT SATISFACTION QUESTIONNAIRE (DTSQ)

CLARE BRADLEY

Department of Psychology, Royal Holloway, University of London, Egham Hill, Egham, Surrey, TW20 0EX, UK

INTRODUCTION

The Diabetes Treatment Satisfaction Questionnaire (DTSQ) has been specifically designed to measure satisfaction with diabetes treatment regimens in people with diabetes. The version of the scales presented here is appropriate for patients with Type 1 or Type 2 diabetes. The scales were originally designed to evaluate changes in satisfaction with changes in treatment regimen and the present version of the scales is also appropriate for comparing satisfaction levels in patients using different treatment regimens. The scales have been shown to be useful in clinical trials evaluating new technologies for insulin delivery including continuous subcutaneous insulin infusion (CSII) pumps (Bradley *et al.*, 1992; Jennings *et al.*, 1991) and other devices (Menzel *et al.*, 1990), introduction of insulin for patients with tablet-treated diabetes (Bradley and Lewis, 1990; Jennings *et al.*, 1991), and the effects of a diabetes education programme (Lewis, 1994). More recently the scales have been widely used as one outcome indicator in routine audit of diabetes care.

A tendency of most measures of patient satisfaction to neglect measurement of patients' satisfaction with the outcome of medical care has been pointed out (Hall and Dorman, 1988; Fitzpatrick, 1991). The measurement of outcome perception is likely to be particularly problematic if a questionnaire is intended to be suitable for a wide variety of patients with a wide range of outcome goals and an even wider variety of unwanted side effects of treatment. In focusing on satisfaction with treatment of diabetes, the present satisfaction questionnaire is able to include items concerned with satisfaction with perceived frequency of hyper- and hypoglycaemia which are important aspects of the short-term outcomes of diabetes management.

The present questionnaire is intended only to measure satisfaction with treatment and is not designed to measure satisfaction with other aspects of the diabetes care service. Other measures have been designed to measure diabetic patients' satisfaction with the consultation (Gillespie and Bradley, 1988; Gillespie, 1989) and patients' satisfaction with a broad range of aspects of the diabetes care service (Wilson *et al.*, 1993). This last measure is described in the Appendix of this book.

Translations of the scales are available in French and German (Bradley *et al.*, 1992) and untested draft translations in Albanian, Finnish, Hungarian, Serbo-

Croat and Spanish (Bradley *et al.*, 1992a). Following a meeting organised by the World Health Organisation and the International Diabetes Federation in Oslo, June 1992, it was decided that scores from the scales are to be included in the basic information sheet designed for the multicentre European Diabcare project which aims to promote continuous quality improvement with a view to meeting and extending the targets of the St Vincent Declaration (Krans *et al.*, 1992).

The DTSQ has evolved through three stages. The earliest version of the measure was designed to evaluate changes in satisfaction after one year in a feasibility study of CSII pumps conducted in Sheffield (Lewis *et al.*, 1988). The Change in Treatment Satisfaction Questionnaire was used to evaluate improvements in satisfaction with treatment in that study where baseline reports of satisfaction were not available and a retrospective comparison was needed (Lewis *et al.*, 1988). Although the change measure proved valuable, interpretation of results is hampered by lack of information about baseline levels of satisfaction. With change scores only, a lack of improvement in satisfaction could be due to a ceiling effect if patients were highly satisfied to start with but could also occur with low levels of satisfaction on both occasions. A measure of absolute levels of satisfaction at a particular point in time is preferable where baseline measures can be taken and compared with post-intervention measures. In the second stage of development of satisfaction with treatment scales, the measures of absolute levels of satisfaction with treatment were developed first on a sample of patients with Type 2 tablet-treated diabetes and, subsequently, on a sample of Type 1 patients. One of the items that worked well in the Type 2 version of the scale was found to compromise the reliability of the scale when used with Type 1 patients and two slightly different versions of the Satisfaction with Treatment scales were developed, one for people with tablet-treated diabetes (which was probably equally suited to people treated with diet alone) (Bradley and Lewis, 1990), and one for insulin users (Bradley *et al.*, 1992). In the third and present stage of development, the two versions of the scales developed in stage 2 have been modifed slightly (changing one item in each scale) to produce a single version of the measure - The Diabetes Treatment Satisfaction Questionnaire (DTSQ) - which is designed to be appropriate for people with all types of diabetes regardless of the form of treatment used. This is the version of the questionnaire which is currently recommended for use, in preference to earlier versions.

THE SCALE

Design

Stage 1: Construction of items for the original Change in Treatment Satisfaction Questionnaire

Items were devised on the basis of qualitative data collected in the early stages of the Sheffield feasibility study of CSII pumps (Lewis *et al.*, 1988). The sample stud-

ied was all insulin users in a Sheffield diabetes outpatient clinic. After patients
had chosen one of three treatments, CSII pump therapy, intensified conventional
injection treatment (ICT) or conventional treatment (CT), they were given a
questionnaire asking why they had chosen their particular treatment regimen.
Both positive reasons for treatment choice and negative reasons for not choosing
other treatments were given. Items for the Change in Satisfaction Questionnaire
were derived by categorising the responses, e.g. "Pump too big and not practical
for a woman to wear" was classified as a response concerning convenience. Items
had to be sufficiently general to apply to each of the three treatments that
patients could be using. The questionnaire was intended to cover all those characteristics of treatments which were mentioned by the patients as important in
determining treatment preferences. Seven items were included which asked
respondents to compare their experience now with that of a year ago with respect
to general control of diabetes, hypoglycaemic episodes, hyperglycaemia, convenience of the treatment, flexibility, understanding of diabetes and the demands
of treatment.

Stage 2: Design of the questionnaire to measure absolute satisfaction with treatment

The version of the questionnaire designed to measure absolute levels of satisfaction with treatment, rather than change in satisfaction, was put together by the
present author following discussions with diabetologists and psychologists at a
meeting, organised by WHO Copenhagen, to plan a multicentre European study
evaluating the use of CSII pumps in the management of Type 1 diabetes. The initial, undeveloped questionnaire consisted of eleven items including modifed versions of the seven items from Lewis *et al.*'s (1988) change measure together with
five additional items designed during the course of discussions in Copenhagen.

*Stage 3: Modification of the questionnaire to produce a single measure of satisfaction with
treatment for diabetes - the DTSQ*

The eleven-item Satisfaction with Treatment Questionnaire was reduced to eight
items when psychometrically developed in a study of people with tablet-treated
diabetes. The version of the scales presented in Figure 1 has been modified to be
appropriate for people with Type 1 or Type 2 diabetes treated with insulin, tablets
and/or diet. Figure 1 differs from the previous developed versions of the scale in
the following ways:
    1) "How well controlled do you feel your diabetes has been recently?" has been
omitted as it only worked well for the tablet-treated sample, did not prove internally consistent with the other items when used with insulin-treated patients and
was dropped from the insulin-users' scale.
    2) "Would you recommend this form of treatment to someone else who needed
insulin treatment?" has been modified (item 7 Figure 1) to be suitable for people

who do not use insulin as well as for insulin users as it contributed usefully to the internal consistency of the measure for insulin users.

The modified scales presented in Figure 1 have now been used in a general pratice setting (Plowright, 1993) and the findings confirm the expected structure and high reliability of the scales.

Scoring

The numbers circled by respondents for six of the eight items in the questionnaire in Figure 1 are summed to produce a measure of Satisfaction with Treatment. Items to be summed are 1, 4, 5, 6, 7 and 8. Scores can range from 0 (very dissatisfied) to 36 (very satisfied). The remaining two items are treated individually. Item 2 provides an indication of Perceived Frequency of Hyperglycaemia on a scale ranging from 0 "none of the time" to 6 "most of the time". Item 3 provides an indication of Perceived Frequency of Hypoglycaemia ranging from 0 "none of the time" to 6 "most of the time"

SCALE DEVELOPMENT

Psychometric development work on the Change in Treatment Satisfaction Questionnaire is reported elsewhere (Lewis *et al.*, 1988) and will not be included here. Work on that scale was referred to in the introduction and design sections because the seven items from that measure formed the basis of the present questionnaire. The available psychometric analyses of relevance to the current version of the scales have been conducted on the questionnaires described in stage 2 of the design section. The version for Type 1 patients has had one item modified only trivially. The version for tablet-treated Type 2 patients has been modified by substitution of one item. Evidence is provided for the adequate reliability of the scales even if the modified/substitute item is excluded. Recent, unpublished data are now available confirming that the new substitute item adds usefully to the psychometric properties of the measure (Plowright, 1993).

Subject Samples and Procedures

The subject samples and procedures used in the two main scale development studies were the same as those fully described in the preceeding chapter concerned with development of the Well-being Questionnaire and are outlined only briefly here. A third sample studied by Plowright (1993) is also described.

Figure 1

The Diabetes Treatment Satisfaction Questionnaire: DTSQ

The following questions are concerned with the treatment for your diabetes (including insulin, tablets and/or diet) and your experience over the past few weeks. Please answer each question by circling a number on each of the scales.

1. How satisfied are you with your current treatment?
   very satisfied   6   5   4   3   2   1   0   very dissatisfied

2. How often have you felt that your blood sugars have been unacceptably high recently?
   most of the time   6   5   4   3   2   1   0   none of the time

3. How often have you felt that your blood sugars have been unacceptably low recently?
   most of the time   6   5   4   3   2   1   0   none of the time

4. How convenient have you been finding your treatment to be recently?
   very convenient   6   5   4   3   2   1   0   very in convenient

5. How flexible have you been finding your treatment to be recently?
   very flexible   6   5   4   3   2   1   0   very inflexible

6. How satisfied are you with your understanding of your diabetes?
   very satisfied   6   5   4   3   2   1   0   very dissatisfied

7. Would you recommend this form of treatment to someone else with your kind of diabetes?
   Yes, I would   6   5   4   3   2   1   0   No, I would
      definitely   definitely not
    recommend the   recommend the
      treatment   treatment

8. How satisfied would you be to continue with your present form of treatment?
   very satisfied   6   5   4   3   2   1   0   very dissatisfied

Please make sure that you have circled one number on each of the scales.

Study 1: Initial Sheffield scale development study: tablet -treated patients

Two hundred and nineteen patients (130 men and 89 women) agreed to take part in one or more of a series of studies and were screened to establish their health status. Participants (92% of those invited) did not differ from those declining to participate on any of the available measures including haemoglobin A_1 (HbA$_1$) levels. A booklet of questionnaires, including an eleven-item version of the Satisfaction with Treatment scales, was given to patients, at the screening appointment, for completion at home and return, in confidence, direct to the university psychology department. One hundred and eighty-seven (85%) patients (110 men, 77 women) returned completed questionnaires including 181 completed Satisfaction with Treatment questionnaires which provided data for the psychometric analyses reported in Bradley and Lewis (1990) and summarised here.

Study 2: WHO Multicentre European Study of CSII Pump Treatment vs Intensified Injection Therapy

The World Health Organisation multicentre European study used a crossover design where patients acted as their own controls and the order of the two treatments (CSII and ICT) was allocated at random (Staehr Johansen, 1989). A run-in period of at least two months preceded the two six-month treatment phases. During run-in, all centres except Hotel Dieu in Paris optimized injection therapy and introduced self monitoring of blood glucose levels. Previous experience at Hotel Dieu suggested that there would be a high drop-out rate among patients using CSII for the first time. In order to avoid high drop-out rates in the crossover phases of the study, experience of the CSII pump was provided during run-in at Hotel Dieu. Thus the Parisian patients who agreed to continue with the study after the run-in were likely to be more satisfied with the CSII pumps than patients who dropped out of the study. Eleven centres in nine countries participated in the study. The psychometric properties of the Satisfaction with Treatment Questionnaire were explored in three of the centres involved in the study: Paris, France; Karlsburg, Germany; Sheffield, UK. Psychometric analysis focused on these three centres because the numbers of patients participating in these centres were greater and/or translation problems with the questionnaires were absent or less apparent than was the case for other centres. Translation problems were first identified during preliminary analysis of the Finnish data (Bradley 1987), were subsequently found to be widespread, and are discussed in Chapter 3 of this volume. Back translation of the French and German translations of the Well-being scales revealed fewer and less substantial translation discrepancies than were apparent in other centres.

Psychometric analyses were conducted on data collected at the beginning of the run-in from N≤41 English, N≤69 French and N≤40 German patients who completed the questionnaire at the end of the run-in period, prior to randomisation. The effects of treatment on satisfaction scores are reported for N=19 English, N=41 French and N=39 German patients. The ratio of women/men who completed the run-in was 17/24 in the English sample, 34/35 in the French and 10/30 in the German. Mean ages (and standard deviations) were: English 35 years (10.0); French 37 (10.0); German 30 (9.0). Mean duration of diabetes (and standard deviations) were: English 12 years (8.0); French 12 (8.0); German 11.5 (7.0) (Thibult, 1990, Table 8a).

The make of pump used varied from centre to centre. Of greater impact on the findings was the fact that pen-injector devices (Novopen) became available in the Sheffield, UK, centre during the course of the study. Six patients used pen-injectors rather than conventional injections in the second treatment phase of the study following a first phase on pump treatment. Three patients used a pen-injector instead of a pump during the second phase following a first phase on conventional injections. Furthermore, five patients who used conventional injections during phase 1 continued with these injections instead of crossing over to pump treatment for phase 2. Thus interpretation of treatment effects in the English centre is especially problematic, though the pre-randomisation responses to the questionnaires used in psychometric analyses were unaffected by these problems.

Interpretation of pre-randomisation data for psychometric development purposes was generally less influenced by protocol differences between centres and deviations within centres than the analysis of treatment effects. However, the experience of pumps obtained in the French sample may well have influenced the data and the kind of patients willing to be recruited into the study may have varied from centre to centre as a result of the different protocols described to them when the study was proposed. Thus the samples need to be analysed and interpreted separately though similar psychometric characteristics in data from different samples will provide strong evidence of a pattern that is robust.

Study 3: General practice sample using the DTSQ (Plowright, 1993).

Fifty nine patients attending the diabetes clinic in a general practice with five partners in South-East England, UK participated in the study. The sample included thirty two women and twenty seven men aged between sixteen and eighty five and treated with insulin and diet, tablets and diet, or diet alone. The DTSQ was one of three short questionnaires patients were asked to complete and return in a sealed envelope to the researcher either before leaving the practice or subsequently by post. In addition to the fifty nine completed questionnaires, seven were distributed to patients but were not returned resulting in an 89% response rate.

Statistical Methods and Qualitative Judgements

Selection of items for inclusion in the Satisfaction with Treatment scales was guided by a series of forced and unforced factor analyses together with reliability analyses. Items 2 and 3, concerned with perceived frequency of hyper- and hypoglycaemia, did not load with the other high-loading items on Factor 1 in any of the samples studies. However, because these items were likely to be important in the assessment of treatment satisfaction in certain contexts, the items were recommended for inclusion in the questionnaire for scoring as single items in future. No further analyses were reported using the single-item scales with the tablet-treated Sheffield sample, though data on the use of these scales are available for the WHO sample patients and from additional studies.

In WHO sample analyses, one of the six items included in the British and German versions had to be excluded from the scoring of the French version due to problems with the translation. The French data from the WHO study were scored as a five item scale with the item "Would you recommend this form of treatment to someone else who needed insulin treatment?" excluded from the scoring. Items 2 and 3, relating to hyper- and hypoglycaemia, as for the Sheffield tablet-treated sample, did not load with the other high-loading items on Factor 1 in any of the three languages.

The distributions of scores on the scales were skewed, indicating the need for transformation or non-parametric statistical tests in subsequent analyses of these measures. The Sheffield data from study 1 were analysed using non-parametric tests on SPSSX while the WHO data from study 2 used non-parametric correlation methods but for the purposes of analysis of variance, transformed the data so that distributions were statistically normalised using an SAS procedure. Analysis of the WHO study data was conducted by Nadine Thibult at the Institut National de la Sante et de la Recherche Medicale (INSERM) near Paris.

For the purpose of analysing the results of the WHO study, the inaccurately translated item which adversely affected the reliability of the French translation was excluded for scoring purposes. This item has since been retranslated but the results described in this chapter refer to a five-item Satisfaction with Treatment French translation instead of the full six-item scale in English and German versions.

Structure of the Scale

Satisfaction with Treatment Scale for people with tablet-treated diabetes (developed with Sheffield tablet-treated sample)

Factor analyses and reliability analyses guided selection of six items for final inclusion in the Satisfaction with Treatment scale plus two items (Items 2 and 3 in Figure 1) to be considered as separate items in Sheffield tablet-treated patients. Items included in the six item scale were items 1, 4, 5, 6, and 8 from Figure 1 together with the additional item "How well controlled do you feel your diabetes has been recently?" which only loaded well for this sample of tablet-treated patients and failed to load for any of the centres in the WHO study.

Satisfaction with Treatment scale developed with WHO sample of insulin users

In WHO analyses of the UK and German centres, five of the six items included in the version of the scale developed with the Sheffield tablet-treated sample loaded highly on Factor 1 together with one additional item. The five items in common are recommended for future use and are numbered 1, 4, 5, 6, and 8 in Figure 1. The sixth item, " Would you recommend this form of treatment to someone else who needed insulin treatment?", which loaded highly on Factor 1 in the WHO sample analyses, has been modified for inclusion in Figure 1 (item 7) and for use in future studies.

DTSQ with general practice sample of insulin, tablet and/or diet-treated patients (Plowright, 1993).

Factor analysis confirmed the expected structure of the scale with the newly modified item 7 loading highly with the other five items on Factor 1 with factor loadings ranging from 0.67 to 0.90. Items 2 and 3 loaded separately on Factor 2. Thus the scale structure remains unchanged following the recent modifications which allow the questionnaire to be used by patients treated with insulin, tablets and/or diet.

Reliability

Internal consistency

Cronbach's alpha coefficient for the Satisfaction with Treatment scale for patients with tablet-treated diabetes (Sheffield sample) was 0.79 which is very satisfactory for a six-item scale. Alpha coefficients for the six-item English and German versions for insulin users (WHO sample) were better still at 0.82 and 0.86 respectively.

The five-item French version for insulin users had an alpha coefficient of 0.81, demonstrating that reliability can be retained without the item which specified insulin treatment, "Would you recommend this form of treatment to someone else who needed insulin treatment?" . This item was mistranslated and excluded from the French version of the scale but, by good fortune, it was the item which has now been modified in order to make the scales more generally appropriate for people with all kinds of diabetes rather than just insulin users. The French results show that, even if this modified item is excluded, the measure not only retains sufficient internal consistency but also performs well in terms of sensitivity to change, construct and discriminant validity. Reviewing printouts from the WHO sample analyses, the reliability analyses suggested that this item could be omitted without reduction of the alpha coefficient to unacceptable levels, partly because the alpha coefficients were excellent to start with (ranging from 0.81 to 0.85). Loss of this item would, however, cause a more substantial drop in alpha than would occur if almost any one of the other items was dropped and, in addition, this item was one of the highest loading items in the factor analyses. This item was therefore reworded slightly to be appropriate for tablet-treated as well as insulin-treated patients ("Would you recommend this form of treatment to someone else with your kind of diabetes?") and is included in the Figure 1 scales recommended for future use.

The item that had been included in the scale for tablet-treated patients but could not be included in the version for insulin users without seriously reducing the reliability of the scale was "How well controlled do you feel your diabetes has been recently?". With the tablet users, this item loaded on the same factor as the items which appear as items 1, 4, 5, 6 and 8 in the DTSQ shown in Figure 1. With the insulin users, however, this item loaded with item 2 or with items 2 and 3 in the English, French and German centres of the WHO study.

There was evidence to suggest that the item concerning diabetes control could be omitted from the version for tablet-treated patients without seriously affecting the reliability. Reviewing the printouts of the reliability analyses conducted for the Sheffield tablet-treated patients, it could be determined that the alpha coefficient would only have been reduced from 0.79 to 0.75 if the item "How well controlled do you feel your diabetes has been recently?" had been omitted and a five-item scale used.

Plowright (1993) examined the alpha coefficient for the DTSQ obtained with her heterogenous sample of general practice patients and, although the sample is rather small for such analyses, the alpha of 0.89 obtained for the latest version of the six-item scale suggests that reliability is highly satisfactory following the modifications.

Validity

Face and content validity

The source of the items in the scale (see Design) ensured that the core items chosen were salient to the preferences of insulin users for the different forms of treatment available, CSII and two different levels of intensity of injection regimen. These core items have since been shown to be useful in studies of people with tablet-treated diabetes and in mixed general practice samples including patients treated by diet alone.

The content is broad and while six of the items form a very reliable scale, researchers and clinicians wishing to intervene to improve patient satisfaction may also find it useful to look at scores for individual items with a view to identifying particular reasons for any dissatisfactions with treatment.

Concurrent validity

No concurrent validity information is presently available and there are no developed scales used widely with a diabetic population to offer themselves as obvious candidates for use in assessing concurrent validity. Scales are available to measure aspects of patient satisfaction, e.g. Wolf *et al.*'s (1978) medical interview satisfaction scale, and a modified version of this measure has been used with insulin using patients (Gillespie and Bradley, 1988; Gillespie, 1989). It would be expected that a patient who is satisfied with the consultation would also be likely to be satisfied with their treatment.

A single-page questionnaire, the Diabetes Clinic Satisfaction Questionnaire, asks patients to rate on a three-point scale their satisfaction with eighteen aspects of the diabetes care service (see Appendix for further details). This questionnaire has been designed for use in a British Diabetic Association/Royal College of Physicians national study of audit of diabetes care (Wilson *et al.*, 1993). One of the items is "The treatment recommended including diet, footcare and any medication for diabetes". This item in particular would be expected to relate to the present DTSQ. It is anticipated that this latter questionnaire might be used to identify problem areas which might then be explored in more detail using measures such as the current DTSQ in order to determine more precisely the nature of any dissatisfaction.

Construct validity and sensitivity to change

Construct validity was assessed by correlating the scales with other variables collected at the time of questionnaire completion in the Sheffield study of Type 2 diabetes. Support for scale validity was provided if associations were consistent, predicted and/or intuitively sensible. The WHO data were examined for expected changes in satisfaction levels.

Sheffield sample analyses; tablet-treated patients: Bradley and Lewis (1990) reported that greater treatment satisfaction in the Sheffield tablet-treated patients was associated with being less overweight (r = 0.19; p<0.05), better glycaemic control as indicated by lower HbA_1 levels (r = -0.28; p<0.001), and optimistic patient estimates of recent diabetes control (r = 0.56; p<0.001). Similar relationships between changes in treatment satisfaction and HbA_1 levels, and subjective estimates of diabetes control were found in earlier work with insulin treated patients using the change in satisfaction measure. The correlation with percent ideal body weight was in accordance with expectations and therefore provides further evidence of construct validity.

WHO sample analyses; insulin users: An opportunity to test construct validity and sensitivity to change was offered by the conventional randomised controlled crossover trial design employed in the WHO study which compared patients' experience of CSII with their experience of injection regimens. Prior to participating in the study, patients had no experience of using CSII pumps. Under these circumstances it was expected that patients who agreed to participate in the study (38% of those invited on average across centres) would prefer the idea of CSII pumps to injections. Those who continued in the study after experiencing CSII pump treatment would be likely to be more satisfied with CSII than with injection treatment. These issues of patients' preferences and randomised controlled trials have been discussed in detail elsewhere (e.g. Bradley, 1991, 1993). Forty seven of the sixty nine Hotel Dieu patients who agreed to participate (68%) continued beyond the run-in period on CSII pumps in the French centre where, exceptionally, CSII was used during run-in. Table 1 shows that there were highly significant improvements in satisfaction with treatment during the run-in period at Hotel Dieu, averaging more than seven points on the scale and significant at $p<0.001$. Similar differences in satisfaction with treatment were apparent during the crossover periods at Hotel Dieu, with patients reporting significantly greater levels of satisfaction during CSII pump therapy compared with injections (see Table 2). Changes in satisfaction levels during the run-in period in other centres where injections rather than pumps were used during the run-in indicated some improvement in satisfaction but, as expected, these were much smaller than the changes seen in Hotel Dieu (England mean 1.22 (s.d. 4.05) $p<0.22$; Germany mean 3.44, (6.18) $p<0.002$ (Thibult, 1990 Tables 24c and 27c)).

Table 3 reports data from the German centre which was the only one of the three centres contributing to the present psychometric analyses to follow the original protocol. The German centre was also the least effected by patients dropping out of the study: only one patient (from the injections followed by pump condition) dropped out. Results showed significant effects of treatment on HbA_1. Significant improvements in HbA_1 were associated with CSII use (mean 9.70, s.d. 1.03) compared with CIT (mean 10.25, s.d. 0.95; $p<0.03$) (Thibult, 1990, Table 19b). There were also significant effects of treatment used on satisfaction. However, as Table 3 shows, not only were there treatment effects, with patients reporting greater satisfaction with CSII than with injection treatment, but there were also significant sequence effects. Following run-in, the patients who continued with injections during the first phase of the study showed no change in their levels of satisfaction compared with satisfaction levels at the end of run-in. Patients who used CSII pumps during the first phase of the study, and then reverted to injections during the second phase, reported a marked decrease in satisfaction with injections. It is interesting to note that the most dramatic changes in satisfaction levels during injections treatment after pump treatment were seen in this German centre where only one of the patients dropped out of the study. The majority of patients stayed in the study but registered their new-found dissatisfaction with injection treatment via the Satisfaction with Treatment Questionnaire.

Thus the differences observed between satisfaction scores for CSII pump therapy and injection treatment were in the expected direction, providing support for the construct validity of the scale. Not only did the six-item scale demonstrate excellent sensitivity to change in the French and German centres, but the single item Perceived Frequency of Hyperglycaemia also changed significantly in the Hotel Dieu centre as shown in Tables 1 and 2. (Analyses of the single-item variables were not reported for the German centre.) In Hotel Dieu, patients reported fewer episodes of unacceptably high blood glucose levels while using CSII pumps than

Table 1 Type 1 patients from WHO sample; changes in satisfaction during the run-in on pumps in the French centre at Hotel Dieu

	Injections (Start of run-in) Mean (s.d.)	Pumps (End of run-in) Mean (s.d.)	Pumps-Injections (Δ during run-in) Mean (s.d.)	p
Satisfaction with Treatment (range 0-30)	17.8 (3.9)	24.8 (4.1)	7.05 (5.3)	<0.001
Perceived Frequency of Hyperglycaemia (range 0-6)	3.3 (1.5)	2.3 (1.0)	-1.0 (1.5)	<0.001
Perceived Frequency of Hypoglycaemia (range 0-6)	2.6 (1.4)	2.5 (1.3)	0.1 (1.8)	n.s.

WHO sample of people with Type 1 diabetes from Tables 25c and 25d of Thibult (1990)

Table 2 Type 1 patients from WHO sample; changes in satisfaction during the crossover periods in the French centre at Hotel Dieu

	Injections Mean (s.d.)	Pumps Mean (s.d.)	Pumps-Injections (Δ during crossover) Mean (s.d.)	p
Satisfaction with Treatment (range 0-30)	18.2 (5.1)	25.2 (4.0)	7.00 (6.8)	<0.0001
Perceived Frequency of Hyperglycaemia (range 0-6)	3.0 (1.2)	2.4 (1.2)	-0.54 (1.5)	<0.02
Perceived Frequency of Hypoglycaemia (range 0-6)	2.5 (1.4)	2.1 (1.2)	0.24 (1.49)	n.s.

WHO sample of people with Type 1 diabetes from Tables 25c and 25d of Thibult (1990)
n.b. There were no significant sequence or period effects, therefore the means are combined for the two groups in the crossover study and the pooled standard deviations reported.

Table 3 Type 1 patients from WHO sample; effects of CSII pump vs Injections in the German centre. Means (s.d.) for the Satisfaction with Treatment scale are shown for each of the 2 groups of patients 1) Injections followed by Pump and 2) Pump followed by Injections

	1) Injections>Pumps N=19 Mean (s.d.)	2) Pumps>Injections N=20 Mean (s.d.)	p
Baseline	25.0 (5.4)	23.3 (7.9)	<0.45
At time of randomisation	28.1 (4.6)	27.0 (6.5)	<0.54
Randomisation - Baseline	3.44 (6.18)		<0.002
The Cross-over			
Sequence effect			<0.0001
Injection treatment	27.6 (4.3)	19.1 (6.8)	<0.0001
Pump treatment	33.6 (1.8)	33.4 (2.9)	<0.88
First Period	**Injections**	**Pumps**	**p**
Treatment effect 1*	27.6 (4.3)	33.4 (2.9)	<0.0001
Second Period	**Pumps**	**Injections**	**p**
Treatment effect 2**	33.6 (1.8)	19.1 (6.8)	<0.0001

* Comparison of satisfaction with CSII treatment vs satisfaction with injection treatment in patients with no prior experience of CSII use.

** Comparison of satisfaction with CSII treatment vs satisfaction with injection treatment in patients where injection treatment followed CSII use.

WHO sample of people with Type 1 diabetes from Table 27c of Thibult (1990) modified by Thibult (1993, personal communication).

when using injection treatment. There was no change in the Perceived Frequency of Hypoglycaemia.

Detection of treatment effects in studies involving subsamples of Sheffield, UK, sample with Type 2 diabetes: Subsamples of Sheffield patients with Type 2 diabetes were involved in studies reported by Lewis (1994) and by Jennings *et al.*(1991). One subsample of thirty two patients was invited to take part in a trial of insulin therapy using either CSII pumps or conventional injection treatment. These patients were those who were classified as "borderline poorly controlled" because their blood glucose levels were not well controlled by diet and oral agents and were close to the threshold where insulin would be routinely prescribed. Twenty five patients agreed to participate having been informed of their poor diabetes control and the increased risk of complications associated with poor control. There was a three-month run-in period to maximise diet and sulphonylurea therapy. Twenty patients whose control did not improve sufficiently were randomised to CSII or injections. Follow-up at four months showed that glycosylated haemoglobin levels had improved significantly in both groups of patients studied whether using CSII or injections. Despite small sample sizes and incomplete questionnaire data on 25% of the sample, leaving seven injection-treated and eight CSII-treated patients contributing data on Satisfaction with Treatment, patients' reported satisfaction improved significantly with insulin treatment (p<0.02) compared to previous levels of satisfaction with sulphonylurea tablets. Analysis of the two treatment groups separately showed only the injection therapy group to have significantly improved satisfaction levels (p<0.05). Medians and ranges of satisfaction scores before insulin treatment and at four months were as follows for the injection-treated groups: pretreatment 28 (9–34) and post treatment 33 (25–35). Comparable data for the CSII-treated group were pretreatment 24 (13–33) and post treatment 32 (15–35). Although treatment satisfaction increased in five of eight CSII-treated patients, two patients reported no significant change and one patient was markedly less satisfied with CSII than they had been with sulphonylurea therapy. Individuals differed more in their perceptions of CSII than in their perceptions of injection treatment, leading to no significant overall change in satisfaction scores for the CSII group when analysed separately.

Patients who did not meet the selection criteria for the insulin study were invited to attend an education session. Of the 173 invited, 81 (47%) attended one of the thirteen sessions. Satisfaction with Treatment scores increased significantly after education (baseline mean 29.1 (s.d. 5.1), post education 30.8 (4.9), p< 0.003; Lewis, 1994 p. 143). However, greater improvements in knowledge were associated with lower Treatment Satisfaction (r = -0.21, p<0.05) and a range of other negative states including lower Well-being scores. Although these negative effects of education were not predicted, Lewis suggested that these findings indicate that prior lack of knowledge may have been associated with an unrealistic view of diabetes and thus large increases in knowledge would have been very disconcerting (Lewis, 1994, p. 172).

Table 4 Scale means (s.d.), minimum and maximum scores for tablet-treated patients in the Sheffield, UK, sample and for the UK centre insulin dependent patients in the WHO sample

	Sheffield, UK: Type 2 (N=219)			WHO : Type 1(N=19)	
	Mean (s.d.)	Minimum found	Maximum found	Mean (s.d.) (at baseline)	Range
Satisfaction with Treatment scales (range 0 - 36)	29.4 (5.9)	6	36	26.2 (4.9)	0-36
Perceived Frequency of Hyperglycaemia (range 0 - 6)				2.4 (1.5)	0-6
Perceived Frequency of Hypoglycaemia (range 0 - 6)				2.0 (1.4)	0-6

Sheffield, UK, sample of people with Type 2 diabetes from Table 2 of Bradley and Lewis (1990)
WHO sample people with Type 1 diabetes, UK subsample from Table 24c and 24d of Thibult (1990)

The Health Belief measures described by Lewis and Bradley and the Perceived Control scales described by Bradley in this *Handbook* were also measured pre and post education and related sensibly and significantly with the Satisfaction with Treatment scale, providing further evidence for construct validity. Higher Treatment Satisfaction scores were significantly related to fewer perceived Barriers to Treatment (r = -0.23, p<0.05), more perceived Benefits of Treatment (r = 0.31, p<0.01), lower perceived personal Vulnerability to Complications (r = -0.22, p<0.05) with comparable results for other measures of perceived vulnerability, and greater perceived Personal Control over diabetes (r = 0.33, p<0.01) (Lewis, 1994 pp.150–152).

Norms

Means and standard deviations for each of the subscales and overall scale scores for UK samples of patients are presented in Table 4. To date, the measure has not been used for case finding of patients who are dissatisfied and would benefit from intervention to modify their treatment regimen in some way, though studies are planned.

Alternative Versions of the Measure

The Change in Satisfaction with Treatment scale reported by Lewis *et al.* (1988), though for most purposes superceded by the more readily interpretable scales reported here, may nevertheless have a place in studies where baseline measures of satisfaction cannot be obtained. Under such circumstances, a measure of change in satisfaction may be desirable. The items included in the scales in Figure 1 could be modified to form a change version of the measure similar to that employed by Lewis *et al.* (1988).

Additional Studies

"Catheter-pen" study (Menzel et al., 1990)

Menzel and colleagues, in a study evaluating "catheter-pen" devices for insulin delivery, included what appears to be the German translation of the full undeveloped version of the Satisfaction with Treatment Questionnaire used in the WHO study of CSII pumps. The "catheter-pens" were described as hand-driven insulin pumps which are more easily concealed under clothes than CSII pumps. However, they do not provide continuous insulin but merely provide the means for delivering frequent insulin doses through a needle which remains in place subcutaneously allowing more convenient insulin delivery without the need for multiple skin punctures. Thirty patients with Type 1 diabetes used the pens for one year. HbA_1 levels did not improve significantly over the year but significant improvements were reported with the satisfaction scales. Menzel and colleagues reported the pre- and post-treatment ratings for each of the items separately. Of the fifteen items in the undeveloped questionnaire, significant changes in a positive direction were shown for ten items (eight at $p<0.01$ and 2 at $p<0.05$). Of the six items that were subsequently selected to form the Satisfaction with Treatment scale (Bradley *et al.*,1992), five showed significant effects of treatment. The item that did not show significant effects of treatment was "How satisfied are you with your understanding of your diabetes?" which would perhaps not be expected to change in the circumstances of this study as the patients had been on multiple injection regimens for a long time prior to the study. The item "Would you recommend this form of treatment to someone else who needed insulin treatment?" was one of the two items showing the largest differences in ratings of any of the six scale items (with pre-treatment means of less than three and post-treatment means close to the maximum of six) adding further support to the view that it was important to modify this item in order to retain it in the present questionnaire suitable for people with Type 2 as well as for people with Type 1 diabetes. The item concerning Perceived Frequency of Hyperglycaemia indicated significant improvements following treatment with the pen ($P<0.05$) but there was no significant improvement in ratings of Perceived Frequency of Hypoglycaemia. Thus the Menzel *et al.* (1990) study demonstrated the value of exploring changes in ratings of individual items as well as in investigating changes in summed scale scores.

DISCUSSION

The Satisfaction scales have been shown to be useful measures of psychological outcomes in clinical trials which allow measurement of benefits of new treatments designed with a view to improving patients' quality of life rather than just their blood glucose control. They have also proved useful in studies evaluating treatment aimed primarily at improving blood glucose control (Jennings *et al.*, 1991). Increased Satisfaction with Treatment accompanied intensification and allayed any fears that the advantages of improved diabetes control may be offset by psychological disadvantages for these patients.

The DTSQ presented here and recommended for use in future studies provides a minimum of three or maximum of eight scores. Summing items 1,4,5,6,7 and 8 provides a highly reliable scale ranging from 0 to 36 which will offer the greatest discriminatory power. Most of the single items have also proved to be sensitive to change despite their limited range of scores (0 to 6). However, it should be noted that in the Menzel *et al.* (1990) study, where significant changes in single-item scores were found, there was considerable room for improvement in satisfaction levels to start with. With a sample of patients who were less dissatisfied at baseline, greater discriminatory power would be offered by the six-item scale score than by single-item scores.

Patients' satisfaction scores are often higher than their physicians expect (e.g. Rashid *et al.*, 1990; Sowden, 1992). The data from the German centre in the WHO study showed that satisfaction with injection regimens reduced significantly following experience with CSII pumps, suggesting that the patients may have expressed satisfaction with their injection regimens thinking that the treatment they were using was the best that was available. When they tried and preferred CSII pumps they became dissatisfied with the injection treatment with which they were previously satisfied. There are several statistical and design implications of this phenomenon. Satisfaction scores are usually skewed and will require the use of non-parametric statistical tests or transformation to reduce the skew to an acceptable level for parametric tests to be used. Sequence effects such as those found in the German centre, where satisfaction with injection regimens depended on whether this regimen preceded or followed CSII pump treatment, may undermine the main advantages of a randomised controlled crossover design. Crossover designs are typically used to reduce the sample size required for a study, but any advantage is lost if dissatisfied patients drop out at a high rate or where sequence effects occur and the two subgroups cannot be combined. However, use of the randomised crossover design in the German centre, where only one patient dropped out, allowed us to see the effects that prior experience of CSII pumps had on satisfaction with injection treatment. An independent-groups design where patients used one or other treatment but not both would have underestimated the impact of CSII pumps on satisfaction levels and would have underestimated the disenchantment with injection regimens that patients would be likely to experience if their CSII pumps were withdrawn following the study. Thus the sequence effect seen in the pump study can be understood as a significant finding of interest and importance. Measurement of psychological outcomes may help in interpreting and understanding sequence effects for metabolic and other clinical outcomes that might otherwise be inappropriately dismissed as bewildering and inconvenient quirks in the data.

Although the scales have been little used with people with diabetes treated with diet alone, there is every reason to believe that the scales will be equally appropriate for them but the psychometric properties of the scales have as yet only been checked with a mixed sample of general practice patients which included some patients treated with diet alone. The DTSQ, as it stands, is only appropriate for people with diabetes though it would be easily modified for use with other chronic disorders such as asthma or epilepsy. However, the breadth and salience of the content would need to be examined with such samples and the psychometric properties of the adapted scales examined.

Unlike most patient satisfaction measures, the present measure has included items to measure patient satisfaction with treatment outcomes (aspects of diabetes control) as well as satisfaction with the experience of following the treatment regimen. However, it was only with the tablet-treated patients in the Sheffield sample that any of the three items concerned with diabetes control loaded on the same factor as the other five items which were used in the Satisfaction with Treatment scale. This item, "How well controlled do you feel your diabetes has been recently?" had to be excluded from the scale developed with the Type 1 patients in the WHO sample. Type 1 patients would have had more accurate knowledge of their degree of metabolic control because they tended to have more feedback about their blood glucose levels at the start of the study whereas feedback for tablet-treated patients was very much more limited. It is therefore likely that tablet-treated patients' views of their diabetes control, being less informed by data, are more influenced by their general feelings about the demands of their treatment than by any objective evidence of blood glucose control. The Type 1 patients, on the other hand, having more accurate data on blood glucose control, gave ratings that were less likely to be influenced by other feelings about treatment. Indeed, patients on a demanding multiple-injection regimen with frequent blood glucose monitoring, might well have excellent metabolic control while at the same time being dissatisfied with the demands of the treatment regimen. Patients who are on minimal treatment with a single injection and occasional blood glucose monitoring might, on the other hand, be very satisfied with their less demanding regimen but have poor diabetes control. Thus it is unsurprising that the item concerned with diabetes control did not load highly with the items concerned with the nature of treatment demands.

Patients' satisfaction with treatment scores, obtained by summing six items from the DTSQ, will not necessarily correlate with their HbA_1 level. Improvements in satisfaction may be accompanied by improved HbA_1 (as, for example, in the German centre of the WHO study) or they may not (as in Menzel et al.'s, 1990 study). It is quite possible that in future studies of new treatments, metabolic control improves while patients become more dissatisfied with treatment. Indeed, this has been the case for some individuals in studies reported here, with some patients having improved metabolic control but reduced satisfaction with treatment. Even if tight metabolic control can be gained in the short term, in a clinical trial lasting only a few months it is unlikely to be maintained in the longer term if the patient is dissatisfied with the treatment.

DTSQ scores should be interpreted and conclusions reached only in the light of other important outcome measures such as metabolic control and well-being. Ideally the aim would be to have a satisfied patient with low HbA_1 levels and high Well-being scores. High HbA_1 levels or evidence of poor well-being would indicate that the treatment regimen should be reconsidered, even if the patient reports being satisfied, with a view to improving control or well-being without undue reduction in satisfaction levels. The identifying of strategies of intervention to optimize outcome profiles provides a challenge for clinicians and researchers that is more likely to move us closer to meeting the needs and wishes of people with diabetes than is the single-track pursuit of tight metabolic control.

SUMMARY

The eight-item DTSQ has been developed for use by people with Type 1 and tablet-treated Type 2 diabetes and, more recently with a mixed general practice sample including those who treat their diabetes with diet alone. The questionnaire is designed for self administration, is quick to complete and can be scored to provide a total score of Satisfaction with Treatment and two separate item scores to indicate perceived frequency of hyper- and hypoglycaemia. The DTSQ is most useful when used as one of a profile of important outcome measures including metabolic control. Used in this manner the DTSQ can help to identify instances where patient satisfaction is achieved at the expense of metabolic control or where metabolic control is only achieved at the expense of patient satisfaction (a danger when medical audit focuses only on traditional medical outcomes). The DTSQ has proved to be highly reliable with good construct validity, sensitivity to change and discriminatory power. It has proved particularly useful in identifying advantages of new treatments such as CSII pumps that may not be reflected in measures of diabetes control but may be demonstrated clearly in treatment satisfaction scores.

ACKNOWLEDGEMENTS

The author wishes to thank Nadine Thibult at INSERM for her detailed checking of and valuable comments on the WHO data reported in this manuscript.

REFERENCES

Bradley, C. (1987) WHO multicentre international study of CSII pumps. Report on translation problems in the Finnish version of the psychological scales. Report to the World Health Organisation, Regional Office for Europe, Copenhagen, May 1987

Bradley, C. (1991) Psychological issues in research design and measurement. In C. Bradley, P. Home and M. Christie (eds) *The Technology of Diabetes Care: Converging Medical and Psychosocial Perspectives*. Chur: Harwood Academic Press

Bradley, C. (1993) Designing medical and educational intervention studies: a review of some alternatives to conventional randomised controlled trials. *Diabetes Care*, **16**, 509–518

Bradley, C. and Lewis, K.S. (1990) Measures of Psychological Well-being and Treatment Satisfaction developed from the responses of people with tablet-treated diabetes. *Diabetic Medicine*, **7**, 445–451.

Bradley, C., Meadows, K.A. and Sowden, A.J. (1992) General Well-being and Satisfaction with Treatment scales for use with people with insulin requiring diabetes. Part 1: Psychometric development and retranslation of the English, French and German versions. Report to the World Health Organisation, Copenhagen, June 1992

Bradley, C., Meadows, K.A. and Sowden, A.J. (1992a) General Well-being and Satisfaction with Treatment scales for use with people with insulin requiring diabetes. Part 2: Retranslation of the Albanian, Finnish, Hungarian, Serbo-Croat and Spanish versions. Report to the World Health Organisation, Copenhagen, August 1992

Fitzpatrick, R. (1991) Surveys of patient satisfaction: 1 - Important general considerations. *British Medical Journal*, **302**, 887–889

Gillespie, C. R. and Bradley, C. (1988) Causal attributions of doctor and patients in a diabetes clinic. *British Journal of Clinical Psychology*, **27**, 67–76

Gillespie, C. R. (1989) Psychological variables in the self-regulation of diabetes mellitus. PhD Thesis, University of Sheffield, Sheffield, UK

Hall, J. and Dorman, M. (1988) What patients like about their medical care and how often they are asked: a meta-analysis of the satisfaction literature. *Social Science and Medicine*, **27**, 935–940

Jennings, A.M., Lewis, K.S., Murdoch, S., Talbot, J.F., Bradley, C. and Ward, J.D. (1991) Randomised trial comparing continuous subcutaneous insulin infusion and conventional insulin therapy in Type II diabetic patients poorly controlled with sulphonylureas. *Diabetes Care*, **14**, 738–744

Krans, H.M.J., Porta, M. and Keen, H. (1992) Diabetes Care and Research in Europe: the St Vincent Declaration Action Programme Implementation Document. World Health Organisation, Regional Office for Europe, Copenhagen

Lewis, K.S. (1994) An Examination of the Health Belief Model When Applied to Diabetes Mellitus. PhD thesis, University of Sheffield, Sheffield, UK

Lewis, K.S., Bradley, C., Knight, G., Boulton, A.J.M. and Ward, J.D. (1988) A measure of treatment satisfaction designed specifically for people with insulin-dependent diabetes. *Diabetic Medicine*, **5**, 235–242

Lewis, K.S., Jennings, A.M., Ward, J.D. and Bradley, C. (1990) Health belief scales developed specifically for people with tablet-treated Type 2 diabetes. *Diabetic Medicine*, **7**, 148–155

Menzel, R., Chlup, R., Jutzi, E. and Hildman, W. (1990) "Catheter-Pens" - an alternative to insulin pump treatment? *Experimental Clinical Endocrinology*, **95**,157–164

Plowright, R. (1993) Patient well-being and satisfaction with diabetes care: similarities and differences between patients' and doctors'/nurses' perceptions. Unpublished undergraduate research project report, Department of Psychology, Royal Holloway, University of London, UK

Rashid, A., Forman, W., Jagger, C. and Mann, R. (1990) Consultations in general practice: a comparison of patients' and doctors' satisfaction. *British Medical Journal*, **299**, 1015–1016

Sowden, A.J. (1992) Beliefs, Policies and Health Outcomes in Diabetes Management: The Effects of Patients' Age and Mode of Treatment. PhD thesis, University of London, UK

Staehr Johansen, K. (1989) World Health Organisation Multicentre Continuous Subcutaneous Insulin Infusion Pump Feasibility and Acceptability Study Experience. WHO Regional Office for Europe, Copenhagen

Thibult, N. (1990) Tables: Clinical, biological and psychological analyses of the continuous subcutaneous insulin infusion (CSII) pump study. Report to the World Health Organisation, Regional Office for Europe, July 1990

Wilson, D.D.R., Home, P.D., Bishop, A., Bradley, C., Brown, K.J.E. and Hargreaves, B. and Members of a Working Group of the Research Unit of the Royal College of Physicians and British Diabetic Association (1993) A dataset to allow exchange of information for monitoring continuing diabetes care. *Diabetic Medicine*, **10**, 378–390

Wolf, M.H., Putnam, S.M., James, S.A. and Stiles, W.B. (1978) The medical interview satisfaction scale: development of a scale to measure physician behaviour. *Journal of Behavioral Medicine*, **1**, 391–401.

CHAPTER 8

THE FEAR OF HYPOGLYCAEMIA SCALE

AUDREY IRVINE, DANIEL COX, and LINDA GONDER-FREDERICK

University of Virginia, Department of Behavioral Medicine, Charlottesville, Virginia, USA

INTRODUCTION

The therapeutic objective of normalizing blood glucose (BG) levels in diabetic patients minimises the chances of acute ketoacidosis and ensuing coma, while increasing the chances of hypoglycaemic episodes (Lorenz *et al.*, 1988). While hypoglycaemia is a risk for all IDDM patients, tight control increases this risk and episodes can be easily precipitated by insufficient food (a missed meal or snack), physical activity, or too large a dose of insulin.

The consequences of hypoglycaemia can be quite aversive and potentially life threatening. The physical sequelae, in themselves, provide ample reason for patients to fear hypoglycaemia and avoid episodes. These may include: dizziness, slurred speech, confused thinking, visual impairment, lack of coordination, emotional lability, trembling, palpitations, seizures, coma, and, in about four percent of cases, death (Cryer *et al.*, 1989; Boyle *et al.*, 1985; Pennebaker *et al.*, 1981). Symptoms can also place the individual at risk for compromising situations in daily living. Social consequences of hypoglycaemia may run the gamut from embarrassment to loss of a job or physical injury to self or others.

PURPOSE OF SCALE AND RANGE OF USES

The Hypoglycemic Fear Survey (HFS) was developed (Cox *et al.*, 1987) as a research and clinical tool measuring the degree of fear experienced with respect to hypoglycaemia. This instrument allows the exploration of a variety of aspects of fear of hypoglycaemia (FH). These include: events precipitating fear, the phenomenological experience of the fear response, behavioural reactions to hypoglycaemia (both adaptive and maladaptive), and physiological outcomes.

The HFS may also be used as a clinical tool identifying individuals at risk for inadequately controlled levels of BG (hyper and hypoglycaemia). The HFS was initially targeted to individuals manifesting chronically high BG levels due to high fear of hypoglycaemia (phobic). Subsequent research suggests that the HFS may also identify individuals who are at high risk of hypoglycaemia but evidence low levels of fear (denial). In the following pages, the preliminary studies validating the HFS and exploring the nature of hypoglycaemic fear will be examined.

THE SCALE

Scale Design

Scale items were derived from interviews with diabetes health professionals and twenty insulin-requiring diabetic patients using an open-ended questionnaire format. The investigators then compiled the responses from both sources into two clusters reflecting behavioural and affective (fear) aspects. This resulted in thirty four items that were placed in a five point Likert form scaled from Never (1) to Always (5). This scale was administered to twelve patients and twelve diabetes health providers. Redundant items (inter-item correlations > .80) were deleted or rewritten leaving twenty seven items.

The scale was then administered to thirty-five IDDM patients. This pilot of the scale yielded a high level of internal consistency for the scale (Cronbach's alpha of .87). All twenty-seven items were positively correlated with the total scale. This original version of the HFS was later revised (see Study IV below) yielding a twenty-three item scale. See Figure 1 for the scale.

Figure 1: The Hypoglycaemic Fear Survey (HFS)

Name _____

Date _____

LOW BLOOD SUGAR SURVEY

I. Behaviour: Below is a list of things people with diabetes do in order to avoid low blood sugar. Read each item carefully. Circle one of the numbers to the right that best describes what you do during your daily routine to AVOID low blood sugar.

	Never	Rarely	Sometimes	Often	Always
1. Eat large snacks at bedtime	0	1	2	3	4
2. Avoid being alone when my sugar is likely to be low	0	1	2	3	4
3. If test blood glucose, run a little high to be on the safe side	0	1	2	3	4
4. Keep my sugar high when I will be alone for awhile	0	1	2	3	4
5. Eat something as soon as I feel the first sign of low blood sugar	0	1	2	3	4
6. Reduce my insulin when I think my sugar is low	0	1	2	3	4
7. Keep my sugar high when I plan to be in a long meeting or at a party	0	1	2	3	4
8. Carry fast-acting sugar with me	0	1	2	3	4
9. Avoid exercise when I think my sugar is low	0	1	2	3	4
10. Check my sugar often when I plan to be in a long meeting or out to a party	0	1	2	3	4

II. <u>Worry</u>: Below is a list of concerns people with diabetes sometimes have. Please read each item carefully (do not skip any). Circle one of the numbers to the right that best describes how often you WORRY about each item because of low blood sugar.

I worry about...	Never	Rarely	Sometimes	Often	Always
11. Not recognising/realising I am having low blood sugar.	0	1	2	3	4
12. Not having food, fruit, or juice with me	0	1	2	3	4
13. Passing out in public	0	1	2	3	4
14. Embarrassing myself or my friends in a social situation	0	1	2	3	4
15. Having a reaction while alone	0	1	2	3	4
16. Appearing stupid or drunk.	0	1	2	3	4
17. Losing control	0	1	2	3	4
18. No one being around to help me during a reaction.	0	1	2	3	4
19. Having a reaction while driving	0	1	2	3	4
20. Making a mistake or having an accident	0	1	2	3	4
21. Getting a bad evaluation or being criticised	0	1	2	3	4
22. Difficulty thinking clearly when responsible for others	0	1	2	3	4
23. Feeling lightheaded or dizzy	0	1	2	3	4

Scoring

The revised HFS (HFS-II) consists of ten behaviour or avoidance items and thirteen Worry or Fear items. Subscale scores are determined by adding item responses. Total HFS scores can also be calculated by adding all Behaviour and Worry subscale items.

SCALE DEVELOPMENT

To date, seven studies have contributed data regarding the reliability and validity of the FH concept and the HFS scale in particular. In the following pages, these studies will be reviewed for their contributions to the development of the scale. We will begin by examining the subject samples and procedures used in each study and will follow this with a discussion of the scale reliability and validity.

Subject Samples and Procedures

Study I

The primary objective of this study was to determine the scaling properties of the HFS. Specific attention was paid to the internal consistency of the scale and the relationship of the HFS to metabolic control. It was hypothesised that the HFS would be:

1) positively correlated with glycosylated haemoglobin (HbA_1) and
2) able to discriminate levels of HbA_1 that were clinically diffferent.

Subjects: A total sample of 158 insulin-dependent (IDDM) patients from four locations in the United States [Kaiser Permanante in San Diego (n=38), International Diabetes Center in Minneapolis, Minnesota (n=32), University of Virginia, Virginia (n=70), and Lewis Gale Clinic in Salem, Virginia (n=16)] participated in the study (Cox *et al.*, 1987). Sample ages ranged from 15 to 80 years (mean=38.1, s.d.=16.7). Education levels ranged from 4th grade to graduate school (mean=13.5 years, s.d.=2.8). Duration of disease ranged from 1 to 48 years (mean=12, s.d.=8.6). Data on age at diagnosis yielded a bimodal distribution separated at age 35, with 108 subjects diagnosed before age 35 (young diagnosis) and 50 after age 35 (older diagnosis).

Mean score for the total HFS was 64 (s.d.=17). The respective means for the younger and older diagnosed subjects were 66 (s.d.=15) and 61 (s.d.=21) respectively for the total score, 28 (s.d.=5) and 25 (s.d.=8) for the Behaviour subscale and 38 (s.d.=12) and 37 (s.d.=16) for the Worry subscale. There was no significant difference in HFS score between the younger and older samples. Duration of diabetes was also unrelated to the HFS.

Procedure: Questionnaires were mailed to the various clinics where they were distributed to patients as they arrived for routine clinic appointments. Glycosylated Haemoglobin (HbA_1: Herold *et al.*, 1986) was measured in 152 of the subjects within twenty-four hours of completing the HFS. Because the HbA_1 tests were analyzed at different laboratories, the HbA_1 results were transformed to Z scores.

Study II

This study used a convenient data set to examine the test-retest reliability of the HFS (Cox *et al.*, 1989).

Subjects: The twenty-two subjects participating in this study averaged 32.4 years of age and had a mean length of diagnosis of 7.8 years.

Procedure: Subjects responded to advertisements soliciting volunteers for an ongoing diabetes research programme at the University of Virginia Health Sciences Center. Subjects were given $300.00 and a free medical examination for participating in the entire project. Only individuals with IDDM of at least one year duration and who had used insulin since diagnosis were eligible. A subset of twenty-two subjects from the total sample (Cox *et al.*, 1987) completed the HFS just before entering the primary introductory session and again, just before entering the primary experimental manipulation. Average inter-trial interval was three months.

Study III

Study III attempted to demonstrate the external validity of the HFS by using it with a different medical "culture" (i.e., in the United Kingdom). It was expected that the HFS would be a valid and reliable measure when used with this population.

Subjects: Twenty-two subjects from Cambridge, UK, took part in the study. Mean age for the group was 44.3 years (s.d.=7.9) and mean duration of illness was 25.7 (s.d.=8.5). The means and standard deviations for the total scale and Behaviour and Worry subscales were 60.0 (s.d.=13.8), 26.4 (s.d.=4.5) and 33.4 (s.d.=10.9) at the first testing and 62.3 (s.d.=7.9), 26.4 (s.d.=5.2), and 35.6 (s.d.=14.8) at the retest.

Procedure: To assess the test-retest reliability of the HFS, subjects participating in a drug trial were asked to complete the HFS twice: at the initial screening and, again, at home. This second testing was returned to the research team by mail. Mean inter-trial interval was six weeks.

Study IV

This study compared Type 1 and Type 2 diabetic patients for differences in FH. Due to differences in insulin regimen and the nature of hypoglycaemic episodes in Type 1 and Type 2 patients, it was expected that Type 1 subjects would:

1) show more fear,
2) have more frequent and distressing hypoglycaemic episodes,
3) have more anxiety but fewer other psychological symptoms

Subjects: To investigate these proposed differences, Irvine *et al.* (1990) sampled 133 insulin-requiring patients from a diabetes outpatient clinic. Thirty seven were diagnosed before age thirty and weighed less than 120% of their ideal body weight (Type 1). Ninety six were diagnosed after age thirty and weighed over 120% of their ideal body weight (Type 2). The average age for the entire group was 48.7 (s.d.=14.1). The average length of time with diabetes was 10.1 years (s.d.=9.8). Mean Behaviour subscale scores for Type 1 and Type 2 patients were 27.3 (s.d.=5.29) and 26.54 (s.d.=6.6). Worry subscale scores averaged 28.9 (s.d.=9.8) and 28.25 (s.d.=9.88) for Type 1 and Type 2 patients, respectively.

Procedure: Subjects were mailed questionnaire packets containing the HFS-II and the Hopkins Symptom Checklist (SCL-90: Derogatis, *et al.*, 1974). Patients then went to the laboratory for HbA_1 testing. Subjects were paid for their participation. Six weeks later all subjects were sent a follow-up questionnaire containing the HFS-II and questions concerning the number and severity of hypoglycaemic experiences over the previous year.

The HFS-II is a twenty-three item revised version of the HFS. Four items were deleted from the original scale due to low response variance. These items included "having a reaction while asleep", "developing long-term complications from frequent low blood sugar", "having an insulin reaction" and "having seizures and convulsions". Four additional items in the original scale were rewritten slightly to clarify their meaning.

Study V

Polonsky et al. (1992) examined whether FH in Type 1 and Type 2 insulin-requiring patients was associated with:

1) higher levels of anxiety and general fearfulness,
2) difficulty in differentiating symptoms and hypoglycaemia,
3) past experience with hypoglycaemia.

They hypothesised that FH was most likely to occur in those patients with preexisting generalized anxiety. Frequent experience with hypoglycaemia and an inability to distinguish between symptoms of anxiety and early hypoglycaemia was expected to predict fear in Type patients.

Subjects: Subjects included 232 Type 1 (n=169) and Type 2 (n=61) patients. Subjects were all insulin-requiring and between the ages of 13 and 85 (Mean=45.0, s.d.=16.6). Type 1 subjects averaged 39.2 (s.d.=15.1) years of age, whereas Type 2 subjects averaged 60.5 (s.d.=8.7). Duration of illness was 26.7 years for the total sample, 19.2 (s.d.=12.2) for Type 1 and 14.0 (s.d.=8.3) for Type 2 Mean Worry subscale scores were 34.4 (s.d.=12.0), 36.2 (s.d.=12.3), and 29.3 (s.d.=9.5) for the total sample, Type 1 and Type 2 subjects, respectively. The sample averaged 5.9 (s.d.=6.9) hypoglycaemic events over the previous month with Type 1 reporting 6.6 (s.d.=7.0) and Type 2 reporting 3.9 (s.d.=6.3).

Procedure: Eligible subjects were identified through medical records and completed questionnaires at their routine clinic visit. Questionnaires included the HFS, the Bendig, a short form of the Taylor Manifest Anxiety Scale (Bendig, 1956), a fear survey schedule (Greer, 1965) and a scale reporting frequency and quality of mild and major hypoglycaemic episodes over the previous month.

Study VI

Previous studies have found elevated distress, somatic complications, depression, anxiety, and fear among visually impaired individuals. Kiernan et al., (1992) hypothesized that visually impaired diabetic subjects in general and blind patients in particular would demonstrate:

1) elevations in fear of hypoglycaemia,
2) increased levels of perceived stress,
3) increased levels of Somatisation, Depression, Anxiety, Phobic anxiety, and total psychological symptoms on the SCL-90.

Subjects: Of the 112 IDDM subjects recruited for the study, forty nine were visually impaired and sixty two had no visual impairment. The visually impaired group was divided into two groups: totally blind (n=21) and partially sighted (n=29). Visually impaired subjects were older (partially sighted, mean=49 years, totally blind, mean=46 years, and normally sighted, mean=34 years) and had had diabetes longer (partially sighted: mean=21.5 years, blind: mean=21 years, and normally sighted: mean=11 years). Mean Worry subscale scores for the normally sighted, partially sighted and blind groups were 36 (s.d.=10), 32 (s.d.=9.8) and 40 (s.d.=18), respectively.

Procedure: The forty nine subjects with diabetes-related visual impairment were recruited through advertisements from the Ophthalmology Clinic at the University of Virginia and from the mailing list of the Virginia Department of Visually Handicapped. IDDM patients with no visual impairment (n=62) were recruited through advertisements as part of an unrelated behavioural diabetes research programme. The normally-sighted group completed the measures by hand as part of a larger assessment battery; whereas, the visually-impaired groups were assessed through telephone interviews.

Study VII

Irvine *et al.* (1992) examined the relationship of FH to psychological symptoms, perceived stress, risk of hypoglycaemia, and HbA_1 in a Type 1 sample. They hypothesised that greater levels of FH would be associated with:

1) increased levels of phobic anxiety and total psychological symptoms,
2) more perceived stress, and
3) increased risk of hypoglycaemia.

Subjects: Subjects included forty one women and twenty eight men, who were diagnosed with IDDM before age thirty. Average duration of diabetes was 11.9 years (s.d.=7.86). Average age was 33.4 years (s.d.=9.4). Subjects used reflectance metres to monitor their blood glucose (BG) levels. Average insulin use per day ranged from .25 units/kg to 1.54 units/kg (mean=.65, s.d. =.24). Mean HbA_1 was 12.2 (s.d.=3.53).

Scores on the HFS Behaviour subscale ranged from 15 to 37 with a mean of 26.1 (s.d.=8.1). The Worry subscale scores ranged from 19 to 76 (mean=37.4, s.d.=2.0). The subscale scores were unrelated to age or gender. Duration of disease was significantly related to the Worry (r=.23, p<.01) and the Behaviour (r=.25, p<.01) subscales.

Procedure: Subjects responded to advertisements soliciting volunteers for an ongoing diabetes research programme at the University of Virginia Health Sciences Center. Subjects were given $300.00 and a free medical examination for participating in the entire project. Only individuals with IDDM of at least one year duration and who had used insulin since diagnosis were eligible.

Data collection began at an orientation meeting where subjects completed the HFS (Cox *et al.*, 1987), the Hopkins Symptom Checklist (Derogatis *et al.*, 1974), the Perceived Stress Scale (Cohen *et al.*, 1983), and the Hypoglycaemic Experiences Questionnaire (Cox and Gonder-Frederick, 1989). Blood samples were drawn for HbA_1 analysis.

The Perceived Stress scale is a fourteen-item scale measuring the degree of control the individual is experiencing over daily events. The Hypoglycaemic Experiences Questionnaire is a self-report measure of the number of hypoglycaemic experiences in the previous twelve months, the number of events at work, home, in social situations, or while alone, and the degree of distress caused by these episodes.

After orientation, subjects were given a beeper that was randomly activated four times a day (morning, early afternoon, late afternoon, and evening) for ten consecutive days. At the beep, subjects recorded the time, performed SMBG, and recorded the results. Blood glucose measures ranged from 30 to 400+ mg/dl with a mean of 189.2 mg/dl (s.d.=51.3).

Structure of Scale

As a part of Study I, a factor analysis was conducted including all the items of the HFS. This analysis used Image factor with Varimax factor rotation. One primary factor was generated, with high loading items exclusively from the Worry subscale. Items included "losing control", "feeling light headed or faint","difficulty thinking clearly when responsible for others", developing long-term complications from frequent low blood sugar", and "having an insulin reaction". The factor had an eigen value 6.6, and accounted for 40 percent of the variance.

Reliability

Internal consistency

Internal consistency of the scale was measured in three studies. Reliability was high for the Worry subscale in Study I (alpha=.89), Study IV (alpha=.90), and Study VII (alpha=.96). Reliability of the Behaviour subscale was high in Study VII (alpha=.84) but was moderate in Studies I (alpha=.60) and IV (alpha=.69). No negative item-to-total-scale correlations were found in these studies.

Test-retest

Test-retest reliability was measured in two studies: Study II and III. Both studies found moderate to high levels of test-retest reliability for both subscales. For the Behaviour subscale correlations were .68 (Study II) and .59 (Study III). For the Worry subscale, the correlations were .64 (Study II) and .76 (Study III).

Validity

Face and content validity

To assure adequate content and face validity, items for the scale were solicited from both diabetic patients and health-care professionals. This allowed us to take advantage of the unique perspectives of both these groups and permitted as wide a sampling of the universe of items concerning FH as possible.

Concurrent validity

If, as expected, the HFS measures psychological fear, it should be moderately related to other measures of anxiety or fearfulness administered concurrently. Four studies, Study IV, V, VI, and VII, provide information demonstrating this expected relationship.

Study IV (Irvine *et al.*, 1989) compared Type 1 and Type 2 patients on their responses to the HFS-II and the SCL-90. Although there was no mean difference in HFS scores for Type 1 and Type 2 subjects, correlations between the SCL-90 and the HFS-II yielded different relationships for the two groups. Type 1 patients showed a negative relationship between the Behaviour subscale and Phobic Anxiety (r=-.36, p<.05) such that high levels on the SCL-90 were related to fewer behaviours to avoid hypoglycaemia. The Behaviour subscale was unrelated to anxiety for Type 2 subjects.

However, Type 2 subjects showed a strong positive relationship between the SCL-90 and the Worry subscale. The Anxiety (r=.43, p<.05) and Phobic Anxiety (r=.29, p<.05) subscales were both significantly associated with the HFS-II. Anxiety was unrelated to the Worry subscale for Type 1 subjects.

Polonsky *et al.* (1992) (Study V) used Type 1 and Type 2 subjects to examine the relationship between FH, using the Worry subscale, and both trait anxiety and general fearfulness. For both groups, FH was positively correlated with trait anxiety (Type 1: r=.42, p<.0005; Type 2: r=.34, p<.05) and general fearfulness (Type 1: r=.39, p<.0005; Type 2: r=.44, p<.005). For Type 1, but not Type 2 subjects, FH was associated with self-reported difficulty distinguishing between anxiety and initial hypoglycaemic symptoms (r= -.33, p<.0005).

Hierarchical regressions were conducted predicting FH for Type 1 and Type 2 subjects. Trait and general fear measures were entered first into the models as a block accounting for 24% of the variance in FH for Type 1 subjects and 20% of the variance for Type 2 subjects. For the Type 1 subjects, but not Type 2 subjects, prediction of HFS was significantly enhanced by the addition of frequency of recent hypoglycaemic events and symptom discrimination.

Kiernan *et al.* (1992) (Study VI) found that blind patients had significant elevations in Anxiety and Phobic Anxiety subscale scores of the SCL-90 and the HFS relative to partially-sighted and normally-sighted subjects. The investigators suggest that this is consistent with previous findings which report an increased sense of vulnerability among the blind which seems to heighten their anxiety in general and FH in particular.

Irvine *et al.* (1992) (Study VII) associated the Behaviour and Worry subscales to the SCL-90 for a strictly Type 1 sample. As expected, the Behaviour and Worry subscales significantly correlated with the Anxiety and Phobic Anxiety subscales of the SCL-90. Post hoc analysis (at the p<.01 level) also found that the Worry subscale was also related to the Interpersonal Sensitivity, Paranoia, and Psychoticism subscales. The Behaviour subscale was associated only with the Somatization subscale. Table 1 presents these correlations.

The significant associations between the HFS and measures of anxiety and fear suggest common variance in these constructs. The correlations have, however, not been as strong as one might initially expect. On reflection, this may not be surprising. The HFS is a diabetes-specific measure of fear/worry regarding a specific diabetes-related phenomenon (i.e., hypoglycaemia). The other anxiety measures are general measures of anxiety. Therefore, it might be expected that beyond the variance commonly accounted for by measuring anxiety, the HFS should be accounting for context dependent variance related to the management of diabetes.

Table 1 Study VII: Pearson correlations among HFS subscales and dependent variables

			HFS subscales	
	Mean	SD	Behaviour	Worry
SCL-90				
Somatisation	7.5	5.9	.37**	.20
Obsessive-compulsive	10.2	7.1	.13	.29*
Interpersonal sensitivity	8.8	6.3	.13	.36**
Depression	11.2	8.5	.06	.29*
Anxiety	6.1	4.8	.22*	.31*
Anger/Hostility	1.4	3.0	-.09	.10
Phobic Anxiety	3.9	3.7	.13	.26*
Paranoia	3.9	3.7	.15	.30**
Psychoticism	3.7	4.1	.15	.37**
Total SCL-90	5.3	3.8	.18	.29*
Perceived Stress	23.4	8.3	-.10	-.30**
Frequency of episodes[1]	.7	1.6	.39*	.23
# while asleep	2.3	12.6	.04	-.13
# at work	.3	.7	.12	-.13
# in social situations	.4	1.4	.13	-.03
# while alone	1.0	3.5	.16	-.02
HbA$_1$	12.2	3.5	.06	.02
Mean BG	189.5	51.5	-.13	.32**
BG variability	5,940.3	3,041.3	.04	-.05
# episodes < 50[2]	.9	1.6	.16	.27**
# episodes > 250[3]	7.6	8.8	-.14	-.29**
Duration[4]	5.3	6.9	.25**	.23**
Age	33.4	9.4	-.04	.13

*p<.05 ** p<.01

1 Episodes refer to number of self-reported hypoglycaemic episodes over the previous 12 months.
2 Hypoglycaemic episodes are defined by BGs below 50 mg/dl.
3 Hyperglycaemic episodes are defined by BGs above 250 mg/dl.
4 Duration is length of time since diagnosis with diabetes.

Postdictive validity

Fear of hypoglycaemia has been theoretically related to previous experience with hypoglycaemia. Studies have explored this relationship in several ways, using HbA$_1$, frequency and degree of distress caused by the episodes, and risk of having future episodes as measures of the likelihood of previous experience with hypoglycaemia.

In the initial validation of the HFS (Study 1: Cox *et al.*, 1987), no correlation was found between the HFS and HbA$_1$. Subsequently, HbA$_1$ values were categorised into clinically meaningful categories: average (± 1 s.d. around the mean), high (> 1 s.d. around the mean), low (< 1 s.d. below the mean). All twenty seven items of the HFS were then used in a discriminant function analysis. The resulting discriminant function (Wilks =.57, F=2.95, df=30, p=.001) was able to classify correctly 70.3% of the HbA_1 cases, with six Behaviour items and nine Worry items. Table 2 presents the loadings for the two functions identified in the discriminant analysis. As seen in Table 3, these discriminant functions were unlikely to categorize incorrectly a subject who was low or average as high (.7% chance of a false positive error). Nor was it likely to categorise a subject who was high as low (5.8% false negative error). Taken together, these discriminant analyses suggest that the HFS can meaningfully differentiate clinically different levels of HbA_1.

Table 2 Study I: Discriminant analysis of HFS items predicting low, average, and high HbA_1

Items	Function 1	Function 2
1	+.63	+.24
4	-.62	+.09
5	-.46	-.14
7	-.12	-.44
8	-.32	-.16
9	+.16	+.35
11	+.42	+.11
15	+.07	-.68
16	+.68	-.36
18	-.26	+.48
19	-.94	+.21
21	-.07	+.41
22	+.16	+.55
24	+.51	+.00
26	+.28	-.49
26	+.28	-.49

Table 3 Study I: Discriminant function classification of low, average, and high HbA_1

	Predicted Groups		
	Low	Average	High
Actual groups			
Low	30 (60)	20 (40)	0 (0)
Average	14 (16.5)	70 (82.4)	1 (1.2)
High	1 (5.9)	9 (52.9)	7 (41.2)

Absoloute values (n) with percentages in parentheses

Irvine and colleagues (1989) (Study IV) hypothesised that FH would be related to the number of previous hypoglycaemic episodes and the distress of these episodes. Predictive validity of the HFS-II was examined by correlating the HFS-II scale with the number of hypoglycaemic episodes in the past year and level of distress generated by these episodes. For Type 1 subjects, the Worry subscale of the HFS-II was associated with degree of distress experienced while having an episode alone (r=.69, p<.05), in social situations (r=.52, p<.05) or when unable to treat the episode (r=.59, p<.05). The HFS-II was unrelated to numbers of self-reported hypoglycaemic episodes.

For Type 2 subjects, the Behaviour subscale was significantly related to the number of episodes while alone (r=.22, p<.05) and degree of reported severity of the episodes (r=.32, p<.05), and distress when the individual was unable to treat the episode (r=.26, p<.05). The Worry subscale was associated with the number of episodes while asleep (r=.22, p<.05) and in public (r=28, p<.05). It was also associated with the degree of distress the episodes caused when experienced at work (r=.26,p<.05) or when unable to treat the episode (r=.34, p<.05).

No significant correlation was found between the HFS-II and HbA_1 for either the Type 1 or Type 2 subjects. However, discriminant function analyses showed that the HFS-II discriminated between three levels of HbA_1: high ($HbA_1 \geq 12$), medium ($8 < HbA_1 \leq 12$), and low ($HbA_1 < 8$). The discriminant model generated for the Type 1 sample was a one function model (Wilks=.04, p=.0001). Sixty-two percent of the items included in the model were in the discriminant model in the first validation study (Cox *et al.*, 1987). In addition, this model was able to classify correctly 97% of the Type 1 subjects. The discriminant model for Type 2 sample yielded a two function model (Wilks=.61, p=.0002). The classification procedure was able to place correctly 61.7% of the Type 2 subjects by level of HbA_1. Seventy-one percent of the items included were in the model from the initial validation study (Cox *et al.*, 1987). Although different for Type 1 and Type 2 patients, these results suggest a high level of predictive validity for the revised HFS.

Using the original version of the HFS Worry scale, Polonsky *et al.* (1992) also demonstrated a relationship between FH and previous episodes. Comparison of the Type 1 and Type 2 subjects showed that Type 2 subjects were less prone to severe glycemic fluctuations and less likely to have experienced hypoglycaemia than the Type 1 group. Type 1 subjects reported significantly more occurrences of both hypoglycaemia and ketoacidosis during the previous month and significantly more fear on the Worry subscale (mean=36.2, s.d.=12.3) than Type 2 subjects (mean=29.3, s.d.=9.5). For Type 1 subjects, but not Type 2 subjects, FH was positively associated with frequency of hypoglycaemic episodes over the previous month (r=.25, p<.005)

In Study VII, Irvine *et al.* (1992) corroborated earlier work showing the relationship between previous hypoglycaemic experiences and FH while using as measures of glycaemic control both HbA_1 and a measure of hypoglycaemic risk (i.e. how 'at risk' for hypoglycaemia were individuals based on the previous frequency of hypoglycaemia) derived from actual reported BGs.

Self-reported (i.e., paper and pencil) frequency of hypoglycaemic experiences over the previous year was significantly associated with the Behaviour subscale (r=.39, p<.05), but not the Worry subscale. The Behaviour and Worry subscale scores were unrelated to the frequency of hypoglycaemia in specific situations (e.g. having experiences while asleep, alone, at work or in social situations). The inability to find these relationships may have been due to the small number of hypoglycaemic episodes reported (n=33).

To examine the relationship between risk of having hypoglycaemia and fear, two measures of glycaemic control were used: HbA_1 and BG variability. Neither HbA_1 nor variability in daily BG correlated significantly with the HFS subscales.

Subjects were categorised according to risk of hypoglycaemia using mean splits for BG mean and variability. This was based on the assumption that individuals exhibiting high variability of BG and a low mean BG would be at highest risk (in the past and future) for hypoglycaemia whereas individuals with a high mean BG and low variability would be at lowest risk for hypoglycaemia. Analysis of variance was used to compare HFS subscale scores across these different levels of hypoglycaemic risk. Analysis of variance models for the Behaviour subscale scores did not differ across the risk groups. However, a significant Main Effect for mean BG ($F(1,50)=6.29$, p=.01) and a two-way mean-by-variability interaction ($F(1,50)=3.84$, df=1, p=.056) was found for the Worry subscale. Table 4 presents the Worry subscale scores across the four risk groups. These data show that while fear is significantly lower for individuals with high mean BG (low risk of hypoglycaemia), variability of BG is also a significant factor. For example, when BG is variable and mean BG is low (i.e. high risk), fear is highest.

Table 4 Study V: Mean (and standard deviation) for Worry subscale, number[1] of hypo and hyperglycaemic episodes by mean and variability of BG

	N	Worry	# Hypo[2] episodes	# Hyper[3] episodes
High mean BG				
Low variability	8	36.0	.25	19.38
		(19.8)	(.46)	(12.5)
High mean BG				
High variability	13	23.7	.54	16.69
		(17.8)	(.96)	(6.0)
Low mean BG				
Low variability	17	37.2	.71	1.88
		(18.7)	(1.1)	(2.3)
Low mean BG				
High variability	16	43.8	2.69	7.06
		(12.8)	(2.3)	(2.3)

1 Hypo and hyperglycaemic episodes represent the number identified during the 10 days of daily BG reporting.
2 Hypoglycaemic episodes are defined as BGs below 50 mg/dl.
3 Hyperglycaemic episodes are defined as BGs above 250 mg/dl.

The two high-mean groups did not differ significantly on level of Worry ($F(1,50)=1.6$, p=.11); however, the high-mean, high-variability group evidenced significantly lower Worry subscale scores (fear) than the low-mean low-variability ($F(1,50)=2.16$, p=.036) and the low-mean high-variability ($F(1,50)=3.18$, p=.003) groups. A model testing for the equivalence of the two high-mean groups and a linear increase in fear over the low-mean, low-variability and low-mean, high-variability groups was significant ($F(1,50)=2.38$, p=.04) suggesting a possible floor effect for mean BG. That is, risk for hypoglycaemia may continue to decline, but beyond a certain point fear will not correspondingly decrease.

To validate the reliability of the risk groups as defined above, frequencies of hypo and hyperglycaemic episodes were examined. (see Table 4). This included both self-reports of episodes occurring over the previous twelve months and episodes occurring during the daily BG testing phase. No significant difference in self-reported frequency of hypoglycaemic episodes over the previous year was found ($F(3,50)=.67$, p>.10). Significant differences were found for number of daily hypoglycaemic (BG<50) ($F(3,50)=7.83$, p=.001) and hyperglycaemic (BG> 250) ($F(3,50)=24.9$, p=.0001) episodes. As expected, the highest number of hypoglycaemic episodes was found for subjects with low-mean BG and high-variability. One way ANOVA contrasts supported the significantly greater number of episodes found in this group when compared to the other three groups ($F(1,50)=3.85$, p=.001; $F(1,50)=3.76$, p=.001; $F(1,50)=3.80$, p=.001). The lowest number of hypoglycaemic episodes were found for subjects with high-mean and low-variability of BG. Frequency of hypoglycaemia was significantly related to the Worry subscale but not to the Behaviour subscale. Hyperglycaemia was most frequent for subjects with high-mean BG irrespective of variability in BG and was least frequent for those with low-mean and low-variability ($F(3,25)=24.8$, df=3, p=.02). These data suggested that mean and variability of BG may reflect increased risk of hypoglycaemia (i.e. increased frequency) and that FH increases with risk as expected.

Predictive validity

To date, no attempt has been made to use the HFS to predict future BG levels or behaviours relevant to FH.

Discriminant validity

A relationship has been postulated between the HFS and the Anxiety and Phobic Anxiety subscales of the SCL-90. As a measure of discriminant validity, the relationship of the HFS to the other subscales of the SCL-90 can be examined. In Study IV (Irvine *et al.*, 1989) post hoc analyses at the p< .01 level did not yield any significant relationships between the SCL-90 subscales and the HFS. Study VII (Irvine *et al.*, 1992) found a significant post hoc association between the HFS and the Interpersonal-Sensitivity (r=.36), Paranoia (r=.30), and Psychoticism (r=.37) subscales of the SCL-90. These correlations were of moderate strength accounting for a maximum of 15% of the variance. These results suggest that some variance is held in common between the HFS and the aforementioned subscales of the SCL-90. However, the majority of the variance seems to be unique to each construct, suggesting adequate discriminate validity.

Study VII also postulated an association between the HFS and Perceived Stress. The correlation was significant (r=-.30, p<.05) with the Worry subscale. This correlation again suggested considerable unique variance in the two constructs (i.e. stress and HFS).

External validity

The generalizability of the HFS was demonstrated in its validity across a variety of types of diabetic populations including Type 1 and Type 2 subjects (Studies I, IV, and V) and the visually impaired (Study VI). Generalisabilty across different geographic samples was demonstrated in Study III with the sample from Cambridge, UK.

Sensitivity to Change

Currently, the sensitivity of the HFS to changes in fear level has not been experimentally determined. A case study conducted by Cox *et al.* (1990), however, does suggest an adequate level of sensitivity in the scale. Cox and his colleagues followed a patient for several months before and after a severe hypoglycaemic episode involving personal injury to the patient. In an interview after the episode, the patient reported feeling extremely frightened by the episode and having a difficult time returning to his previous pattern of intensive treatment. Results from the HFS showed a marked increase in the Worry score. Group trials examining sensitivity of the HFS to changes in fear resulting from Blood Glucose Awareness Training are currently under way.

DISCUSSION

The results of the studies described above support the validity and reliability of the HFS. See Table 5 for a summary of the demographic and reliability data for these studies. Internal consistency for the subscales was high and test-retest was moderate to high. Adequate construct validity was suggested by the subscales' association with several measures of anxiety or fear, risk of hypoglycaemia, and number of hypo- and hyperglycaemic episodes. Correlations between the HFS and other theoretically unrelated constructs suggests adequate discriminant validity. The HFS is generalisable to a variety of diabetic subject populations and seems to be sensitive to changes in fear over time.

Table 5 Summary of demographic and reliability data for Behaviour and Worry subscales of the Hypoglycaemic Fear Survey

	N	Age	Duration	Mean	Alpha	retest
Study I	158	38.1 (16.7)	12.0 (8.6)			
Behaviour					.60	
Type 1				28 (5)		
Type 2				25 (8)		
Worry					.89	
Type 1				38 (12)		
Type 2				37 (16)		
Study II	22	32.4	7.8			
Behaviour						.68**
Worry						.64*
Study III	22	44.3 (7.9)	25.7 (8.5)			
Behaviour				26.4 (4.5)		.59*
Worry				33.4 (10.9)		.76**
Study IV	133	48.7 (14.1)	10.1 (9.8)			
Behaviour					.69	
Type 1				27.3 (5.3)		
Type 2				26.5 (6.6)		
Worry					.90	
Type 1				28.9 (9.8)		
Type 2				28.3 (9.9)		
Study V	232	45.0 (16.6)	18.2 (12.0)			
Worry						
Type 1				36.2 (12.3)		
Type 2				29.3 (9.5)		
Study VI	112					
Total scale						
Blind		45.9 (12.6)	21.0 (9.4)			
P.S.		48.8 (15.1)	21.5 (11.3)			
Sighted		34.0 (9.8)	10.7 (8.9)			
Behaviour						
Blind				25.2 (5.8)		
P.S.				26.0 (6.1)		
Sighted				27.6 (5.3)		
Worry						
Blind				32 (9.9)		
P.S.				36 (10.0)		
Sighted				40 (18.0)		
Study VII	69	33.4 (9.4)	11.9 (7.9)			
Behaviour				26.1 (8.1)	.84	
Worry				37.4 (2.0)	.96	

N - Sample size
Duration - Duration of illness
Alpha - Cronbach's alpha, test for internal consistency
Retest- test/retest correlation
P.S. - Partially sighted
*p<.01   ** p<.001
All samples are Type I (IDDM) unless otherwise noted.

In the process of validating the HFS, we have learned much about the anteced-ents to FH. As a result of this work, we have also identified limitations in the initial FH model, measurement design, and outcome measures. In the following para-graphs, we would like to examine the theoretical underpinning of FH and make some suggestions for future research using the HFS.

Initial models explaining the role of FH in diabetes management suggested that FH could motivate maladaptive self-care behaviour in the avoidance of hypogly-caemia, resulting in poor glycaemic control (Irvine *et al.*, 1990). The relationships were outlined as follows:

$$\text{Hypoglycaemia} \rightarrow \text{Fear (Worry)} \rightarrow \overset{\text{Avoidance}}{\text{Behaviour}} \rightarrow \overset{\text{Elevated}}{\text{BG level}}$$

While this linear model was straightforward and easily testable, research sug-gests that it is too simplistic, ignoring a variety of factors related to FH and glycae-mic control. These include: factors related to the experience of hypoglycaemia such as risk and degree of distress caused by the episodes, psychological predispo-sition toward anxiety, and adequacy of the self-care response.

Recent studies suggest that risk of hypoglycaemia is an important determinant of the level of FH. This is significant in two ways:

1) level of risk implies what is appropriate FH in the present and
2) suggests appropriate self-care behaviour in the future.

Deviations from the expected FH responses would suggest that an individual is at risk for maladaptive self-care behaviours to hypoglycaemia and poorly con-trolled BG levels. Risk of hypoglycaemia, itself, is influenced by a number of vari-ables including degree of metabolic control (Lorenz *et al.*, 1988), variability of BG, and the individual's ability to perceive (i.e. hypoglycaemic awareness) and then treat hypoglycaemic symptoms.

The quality of hypoglycaemic episodes may also affect FH. Characteristics of ep-isodes of particular interest include severity, predictability of episodes, distress ex-perienced, and the consequences of these episodes. Consequences may be either physical, social or emotional. The presence of seizures, coma, injury, or severe symptoms would logically increase FH, as would the social and emotional conse-quences of mistakes, accidents at work, or having an episode in public or other so-cially important situation.

While psychological factors were not a part of the initial model, a variety have been related to FH in subsequent research including anxiety, total number of psy-chological symptoms, and perceived stress. A wide range of other predisposing psychological characteristics have yet to be examined. A potentially important ex-ample may be Health Beliefs. It is likely that when an individual believes that he/ she is susceptible to hypoglycaemia, outcomes of episodes are likely to be serious, adequate help is unavailable, and the cost of help or treatment is high, the indi-vidual may experience high fear.

Initially, FH was believed to be unidimensional, adaptive when low and maladaptive when high. Research now suggests (Irvine *et al.*, 1992) that the appropriateness of the coping behaviour is unrelated to the strength of the fear but is instead a function of the risk of future hypoglycaemic episodes. High fear when risk is high is appropriate and can motivate adaptive changes in self care. High fear when risk is low is inappropriate (i.e. phobic) and potentially maladaptive when it motivates avoidance behaviour that results in unwarranted elevation of BG. Maladaptive responses may also be seen in individuals at high risk but with low fear (denial). In this case, the individual is unlikely to take the adequate measures to avoid hypoglycaemia. Figure 2 presents a revised model of FH showing both adaptive and maladaptive responses.

Study VII identified sixteen percent of their sample at risk for maladaptive fear responses. Four subjects were found to be at high risk for hypoglycaemia (i.e: high variability and low mean BG) but reported fear levels below the group Worry mean (i.e. potential deniers). This is twenty-five percent of subjects at risk for hypoglycaemia. Seven patients were at low risk (i.e. high mean BG) but above the group mean for fear (i.e. phobic), representing thirty-three percent of subjects at low risk for hypoglycaemia. These data are suggestive; however, further research is needed to verify the role of adaptive and maladaptive responses to hypoglycaemia.

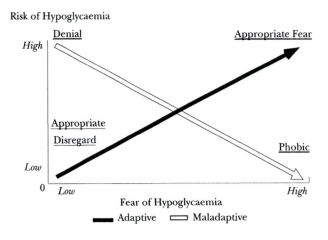

Figure 2 Maladaptive/adaptive hypoglycaemic fear at extremes of risk

In the original model, FH was assumed to be a relatively enduring, trait-like phenomenon. FH measured in the present was assumed to remain constant over months. Indeed, the relationship of FH to such relatively enduring variables as anxiety, and psychological symptomatology suggest that this may be the case. However, other research suggests that FH may vary (Cox *et al.*, 1990). Cox and colleagues followed a patient for several months after a severe hypoglycaemic episode and found that FH and HbA_1 increased immediately after the episode but decreased over time. This suggests that FH may follow a behavioural model. Such a model would predict that current FH is a function of the frequency and quality of recent hypoglycaemic experiences and, that, when no further episodes occur, FH would decrease until it reached pre-episode levels (i.e. was extinguished). This question can only be examined through prospective research designs.

Researchers were originally interested in FH because of its supposed impact on glycaemic control. Metabolic control, and HbA_1 in particular, was, therefore, the outcome variable of choice. It came as some surprise when no correlational relationship was found between HbA_1 and FH. In retrospect, as a measure of glycaemic control averaged over six to eight weeks, HbA_1 may be an inappropriate outcome measure. First, HbA_1 can also be conceptualized as a risk factor for hypoglycaemia. Low HbA_1 suggests a person at greater risk for hypoglycaemia. This problem is compounded by the fact that it is impossible in a cross-sectional study to separate the role of BG as a predictor variable in the etiology of the fear of hypoglycaemia from its role as a dependent variable.

Secondly, HbA_1 obscures the role of BG as a risk factor for hypoglycaemia by failing to reflect variability in BG. By using HbA_1 exclusively as an outcome measure, individuals with stable BG levels are grouped with individuals with labile (high risk) BG at the same level of HbA_1. To assess adequately the role of BG in manifestation of FH, daily measures of BG will be needed.

In addition to BG levels, a variety of other outcome variables could be examined including: specific self-care behaviours, number of subsequent hypoglycaemic episodes, accidents, hospitalisations, or days lost at work. Such measures may be more sensitive to FH and could give us a better understanding of the phenomenology of FH.

An additional problem in the study of FH concerns the use of cross-sectional research designs. To date, research has relied exclusively on these designs making it difficult to tease apart the predictors of FH from outcome variables. Cross-sectional designs also limit researchers to self-reports of episodes and their consequences as remembered over weeks or months. Self reports under these conditions are notoriously susceptible to memory distortion and self-presentation biases. Examination of hypoglycaemic events is also limited by cross-sectional designs to global characteristics such as number of episodes and overall distress. Prospective examination of hypoglycaemia would allow the expansion of the models of FH to include information on the nature and consequences of hypoglycaemic episodes.

Finally, the usefulness of the Behaviour subscale has been a focus of some discussion. The subscale has a lower level of internal consistency and, in the factor analysis, its items failed to load on the major factor. On reflection, the subscale may be measuring multiple dimensions including both appropriate and inappropriate behaviours to avoid hypoglycaemia. To make matters more complicated, the appropriateness of a behaviour may change according to the level of risk for hypoglycaemia. For example if "Keep my sugar high if I'm going to be alone for a while" is endorsed by an individual at high risk, the behaviour may be appropriate.

If it is endorsed by an individual who is at low risk, the behaviour is likely to be inappropriate. In addition, the items reflect behaviours undertaken in a variety of situations both public and private.

Alternatives to the use of the behaviour subscale may include reconstructing the subscale to reflect either appropriate or inappropriate behaviours or to simply drop the behaviour subscale in favour of measuring self-care behaviour directly.

While the work on FH has only recently begun, our understanding of this phenomenon has increased markedly. The results have been both unexpected and rewarding. Our model describing the factors predicting FH has expanded, as has our appreciation of adaptive and maladaptive responses to FH. Future research holds promise for understanding how FH is related to self-care, quality of life, and glycaemic control and for the development of interventions to enhance appropriate response to hypoglycaemia.

SUMMARY

In summary, the HFS was developed as a research and clinical tool to measure fear of hypoglycaemia. As a research tool, it allows examination of the role of FH in diabetes self-care and subsequent metabolic control. The HFS will also permit examination of antecedents to fear and the nature of the fear experience. Clinically, the HFS allows identification of individuals at risk for inadequately controlled BG levels (both hypo and hyperglycaemia). It is suitable for use with any group of individuals with diabetes that requires insulin.

An advantage of the HFS is the ease with which it can be administered. Because it is a relatively short paper and pencil measure, it can be administered in a variety of settings, both clinical and research. Scoring requires only a summation of the scale items for the subscales and total scale score.

REFERENCES

Bendig, A. (1956) The development of a short form of the Manifest Anxiety Scale. *Journal of Consulting Psychology*, **5**, 384–386

Boyle, P., Swartz, N., Suresh, D., Shah, M, Clutter, W. and Cryer, P. (1985) Plasma glucose concentrations at the onset of hypoglycaemic symptoms in patients with poorly controlled diabetes and in nondiabetics. *New England Journal of Medicine*, **318(23)**, 1487-1492

Cohen, S., Camarck, T. and Mermelstein, R. (1983) A global measure of perceived stress. *Journal of Health and Social Behaviour*, **24**(December), 385–396

Cox, D. and Gonder-Frederick, L. (1989) *Hypoglycaemic Experiences Questionnaire*, (unpublished questionnaire)

Cox, D, Gonder-Frederick, L., Antoun, B., Cryer, P. and Clarke, W. (1990) Psycho-behavioral metabolic parameters of severe hypoglycaemic episodes. *Diabetes Care*, **9(11)**, 81–86

Cox, D., Gonder-Fredrick, L., Lee, J., Julian, D., Carter, W. and Clarke, W. (1989) Effects and correlates of blood glucose awareness training among patients with IDDM. *Diabetes Care*, **12**, 313–318

Cox, D., Irvine, A., Gonder-Frederick, L., Nowacek, G., and Butterfield, J. (1987) Fear of Hypoglycaemia: Quantification, validation, and utilization, *Diabetes Care*, **10(5)**, 617–621

Cryer, P., Binder, C., Bolli, G., Cherrington, A., Gale, E. Gerich, J. and Sherwin, R. (1989) Hypoglycaemia in IDDM. *Diabetes*, **38**, 1193–1199

Derogatis, L., Lipman, R., Rickels, K., Uhlenhuth, E. and Covi, L. (1974) The Hopkins Symptom Checklist (HSCL): A self report symptom inventory. *Behaviour Science*, **19**, 1–15

Greer, J. (1965) The development of a scale to measure fear. *Behavioral Research and Therapy*, **3**, 45–53

Herold, D., Mifflin, J., Boyd, J., Savory, J. and Burns, D. (1986) Measurement of glycosylated hemoglobin by bornate affinity chromatography. In W. Clarke, J. Larner, S. Pohl, (eds.), *Methods in Diabetes Research, (vol II, pp. 505-520)*, New York: Wiley

Irvine, A., Cox, D. and Gonder-Frederick, L. (1990) Methodological issues in the examination of fear of hypoglycaemia. *Diabetes Care*, **14(1)**, 76

Irvine A., Cox, D. and Gonder-Frederick, L. (1992) Fear of hypoglycaemia: Relationship to physical and psychological symptoms in patients with insulin-dependent diabetes mellitus. *Health Psychology*, **11(2)**, 135–138

Irvine, A., Saunders, T., Cox, D. and Gonder-Frederick, L. (1989) Fear of hypoglycaemia: Replication and extension, paper presented at the American Diabetes Association Meeting, Detroit USA

Kiernan, B., Cox, D., Schroeder, D. and Crowley, M. (1992). Psychosocial sequelae of visual loss in diabetes. (manuscript under review)

Lorenz, R., Siebert, C., Cleary, P., Santiago, J. and Heyse, S. for the DCCT Research Group (1988) Epidemiology of severe hypoglycaemia in the DCCT. *Diabetes*, **37**, (Supplement 1)

Pennebaker, J., Cox, D., Gonder-Frederick, L., Wunsh, M., Evans, W. and Pohl, S. (1981) Physical symptoms related to blood glucose in insulin-dependent diabetics. *Psychosomatic Medicine*, **43(6)**, 489–500

Polonsky, W, Davis, C., Jacobson, A. and Anderson, B. (1992) The context of hypoglycaemic fear in diabetes mellitus, (unpublished manuscript)

SECTION 3

KNOWLEDGE AND
COGNITIVE FUNCTION

CHAPTER 9

MEASUREMENT OF DIABETES KNOWLEDGE – THE DEVELOPMENT OF THE DKN SCALES

LINDA J. BEENEY[1], STEWART M. DUNN[2] AND GARRY WELCH[3]

[1]Medical Psychology Unit, Department of Medicine, University of Sydney, NSW 2006, Australia; [2]Medical Psychology Unit, Royal Prince Alfred Hospital and Department of Medicine, University of Sydney, NSW 2006, Australia; [3]Mental Health Unit, Joslin Diabetes Centre, One Joslin Place, Boston, Massachusetts, MA 02215, USA.

INTRODUCTION

The past twenty-five years have seen great advances in our understanding of the underlying aetiology and pathophysiology of diabetes mellitus with consequent technological improvements in our ability to treat the disease and to prevent or delay the onset of complications (Centers for Disease Control, 1991). There has been a corresponding increase in the complexity of recommendations given to patients, and increased emphasis on self-management. In the late 1970s, diabetes education programmes (DEPs) were initiated to ensure patients had sufficient knowledge and understanding of their disease and its treatment to manage their diabetes. The need to evaluate these DEPs led to the development of tests of diabetes knowledge. Early questionnaires were inconsistent in content, and no attempts were made to assess reliability and validity (Williams *et al.*, 1967; Collier and Etzwiler, 1971; Simon and Stewart, 1976). Many were lengthy and time-consuming as the authors attempted to measure comprehensively all aspects of an individual's knowledge of diabetes and scores were often confounded by differences in intelligence, educational level and test sophistication.

Lengthy or complex assessment of knowledge is frequently unnecessary in research and clinical evaluation. Consequently the assessment of knowledge, as only one of a variety of important psychosocial factors, demanded shorter, more efficient tests retaining the vital characteristics of high reliability, validity and patient acceptability. The DKN scales were developed for use with IDDM and NIDDM patients, particularly in situations where knowledge needed to be assessed quickly, reliably, and repeatedly in programme evaluation and research.

This chapter describes the early development of the DKN scales, modifications to the original forms and their rationale, and published and unpublished data using the scales in the wider context of diabetes education research.

The original published versions of the three scales were used in all analyses presented in this chapter unless otherwise specified. Updated versions of the scales, modified to take into account changes in management and outdated terminology, are presented in Figures 1–3.

DKN SCALE FORM A

NAME: _____ AGE: _____ SEX: _____ (M or F)

HOW LONG HAVE YOU HAD DIABETES? _____

HOW IS IT TREATED? (tick one) DIET ____ DIET & TABLETS ____ DIET & INSULIN ____

INSTRUCTIONS: This is a short quiz to find out how much you know about diabetes. There are 15 questions and each one has several possible answers. For questions 1 to 12 only one answer is correct. If you know the right answer, circle the letter in front of it. If you don't know the answer, circle the letter in front of "I don't know". Notice that Questions 13, 14 and 15 have more than one correct answer, so you should circle all the answers you think are right.

---

1. **In uncontrolled diabetes the blood sugar is:**
   A. Normal
   B. Increased
   C. Decreased
   D. I don't know

2. **Which one of the following is true?**
   A. It does not matter if your diabetes is not fully controlled, as long as you do not have a coma
   B. It is best to show some sugar in the urine in order to avoid hypoglycaemia
   C. Poor control of diabetes could result in a greater chance of complications later
   D. I don't know

3. **The NORMAL range for blood glucose is:**
   A. 4 - 8 mmol/l
   B. 7 - 15 mmol/l
   C. 2 - 10 mmol/l
   D. I don't know

4. **Butter is mainly:**
   A. Protein
   B. Carbohydrate
   C. Fat
   D. Mineral and vitamin
   E. I don't know

5. **Rice is mainly:**
   A. Protein
   B. Carbohydrate
   C. Fat
   D. Mineral and vitamin
   E. I don't know

6. **The presence of ketones in the urine is:**
   A. A good sign
   B. A bad sign
   C. A usual finding in diabetes
   D. I don't know

7. **Which of the following possible complications is usually not associated with diabetes?**
   A. Changes in vision
   B. Changes in the kidney
   C. Changes in the lung
   D. I don't know

8. **If a person on insulin has a high blood or urine sugar level and ketones were present they should:**
   A. Increase insulin
   B. Decrease insulin
   C. Keep insulin and diet the same, and test blood/urine later
   D. I don't know

PLEASE TURN OVER TO CONTINUE

9.   **When people wih diabetes on insulin become ill and unable to eat the prescribed diet:**

A.   They should immediately stop taking insulin

B.   They must continue to take insulin

C.   They should use diabetic tablets instead of insulin

D.   I don't know

10. **If you feel the beginnings of hypoglycaemia you should:**

A.   Immediately take some insulin or tablets.

B.   Immediately lie down and rest

C.   Immediately eat or drink something sweet

D.   I don't know

11. **You can eat as much as you like of which of the following foods:**

A.   Apples

B.   Celery

C.   Meat

D.   Honey

E.   I don't know

12. **Hypoglycaemia is caused by:**

A.   Too much insulin

B.   Too little insulin

C.   Too little exercise

D.   I don't know

IN THESE LAST THREE QUESTIONS, THERE WILL BE MORE THAN ONE CORRECT ANSWER. PLEASE CIRCLE THE LETTERS IN FRONT OF ALL THE ANSWERS YOU THINK ARE CORRECT

13. **A kilogram is:**

A.   A metric unit of weight

B.   Equal to 10 pounds

C.   A metric unit of energy

D.   A little more than two pounds

E.   I don't know

14. **Two of the following substitutions are right:**

A.   One portion (1oz) bread = 4 cracker biscuits (e.g. Sao biscuits)

B.   One egg = one portion of mince

C.   5 oz milk = 5 oz orange juice

D.   3/4 cup cornflakes = 3/4 cup cooked porridge

E.   I don't know

15. **If I don't feel like the egg allowed on my diet for breakfast I can:**

A.   Have extra toast

B.   Substitute one small lamb cutlet

C.   Have an ounce of cheese instead

D.   Forget about it

E.   I don't know

DKN SCALE FORM B

NAME: _____ AGE: _____ SEX: _____ (M or F)

HOW LONG HAVE YOU HAD DIABETES? _____

HOW IS IT TREATED? (tick one) DIET ____ DIET & TABLETS ____ DIET & INSULIN ____

INSTRUCTIONS: This is a short quiz to find out how much you know about diabetes. There are 15 questions and each one has several possible answers. For questions 1 to 12 only one answer is correct. If you know the right answer, circle the letter in front of it. If you don't know the answer, circle the letter in front of "I don't know". Notice that Questions 13, 14 and 15 have more than one correct answer, so you should circle all the answers you think are right.

1.   **The key to the control of diabetes is:**

A.   The balance between regular amounts of insulin/tablets, food and exercise

B.   The maintenance of a low level of sugar in the urine in order to prevent hypoglycaemia

C.   A high-protein, high-fibre diet

D.   I don't know

2.   **The NORMAL range for blood glucose is:**

A.   4 - 8 mmol/l

B.   7 - 15 mmol/l

C.   2 - 10 mmol/l

D.   I don't know

3.   **Margarine is mainly:**

A.   Protein

B.   Carbohydrate

C.   Fat

D.   Mineral and vitamin

E.   I don't know

4.   **Rice is mainly:**

A.   Protein

B.   Carbohydrate

C.   Fat

D.   Mineral and vitamin

E.   I don't know

5.   **Glucose is detected in the urine when:**

A.   The build-up of ketones in the urine prevents insulin from working properly

B.   The kidney threshold is passed and glucose spills over into the urine

C.   The dose of insulin or diabetic tablets is too large

D.   I don't know

6.   **One egg can be substituted for:**

A.   One ounce of cheese

B.   Half a cup of mushrooms

C.   One slice of bread

D.   Two ounces of cream

E.   I don't know

7.   **A person with diabetes on insulin who becomes ill, often needs:**

A.   More insulin

B.   Less insulin

C.   No insulin

D.   I don't know

8.   **The best food for someone with diabetes to eat before prolonged exercise or sport would be:**

A.   A protein-rich food, like meat

B.   A carbohydrate, like bread or a plain biscuit

C.   Nothing until afterwards

D.   Honey

E.   I don't know

PLEASE TURN OVER TO CONTINUE

9. **People with diabetes should take good care of their feet because:**

A. After a long period of time, injecting insulin into the legs may cause swelling of the feet

B. Flat feet are commonly associated with diabetes

C. Older people with diabetes may have poor circulation of the blood in this area

D. I don't know

10. **When people wih diabetes on insulin become ill and unable to eat the prescribed diet:**

A. They should immediately stop taking insulin

B. They must continue to take insulin

C. They should use diabetic tablets instead of insulin

D. I don't know

11. **When a person on insulin has a high blood or urine sugar level and ketones were present they should:**

A. Increase insulin

B. Decrease insulin

C. Keep insulin and diet the same, and test blood/urine later

D. I don't know

12. **Hypoglycaemia is caused by:**

A. Too much insulin

B. Too little insulin

C. Too little exercise

D. I don't know

IN THESE LAST THREE QUESTIONS, THERE WILL BE MORE THAN ONE CORRECT ANSWER. PLEASE CIRCLE THE LETTERS IN FRONT OF ALL THE ANSWERS YOU THINK ARE CORRECT

---

13. **On a diabetic diet which of the following can be taken freely?**

A. Lettuce, celery, cucumber

B. Herbs and spices

C. Marmite, Vegemite, soup cubes

D. Fresh fruit

E. I don't know

14. **"Empty calories" is a term used to describe foods which supply calories and no other nutrients. Which of the following are sources of "Empty Calories"?**

A. Fruit juices

B. Margarine

C. Soft drinks

D. Sugar

E. I don't know

15. **Hypoglycaemia is likely to occur if:**

A. Blood sugar drops too low

B. You miss your normal dose of insulin or tablets

C. You miss your normal meal

D. Blood sugars exceed 2+

E. I don't know

DKN SCALE FORM C

NAME: _____ AGE: _____ SEX: _____ (M or F)

HOW LONG HAVE YOU HAD DIABETES? _____

HOW IS IT TREATED? (tick one) DIET ____ DIET & TABLETS ____ DIET & INSULIN ____

INSTRUCTIONS: This is a short quiz to find out how much you know about diabetes. There are 15 questions and each one has several possible answers. For questions 1 to 12 only one answer is correct. If you know the right answer, circle the letter in front of it. If you don't know the answer, circle the letter in front of "I don't know". Notice that Questions 13, 14 and 15 have more than one correct answer, so you should circle all the answers you think are right.

1. **When a person with diabetes on insulin undertakes unusually heavy exercise, they should have:**
   A. More insulin before the exercise
   B. Extra carbohydrate beforehand
   C. Less food just beforehand
   D. I don't know

2. **People with diabetes should:**
   A. Have their food cooked separately from that of the family
   B. Eat the same foods at the same time each day
   C. Vary their diet by substituting different foods correctly from the diet exchange list
   D. I don't know

3. **The NORMAL range for blood glucose is:**
   A. 4 - 8 mmol/l
   B. 7 - 15 mmol/l
   C. 2 - 10 mmol/l
   D. I don't know

4. **Rice is mainly:**
   A. Protein
   B. Carbohydrate
   C. Fat
   D. Mineral and vitamin
   E. I don't know

5. **Insulin causes blood sugar to:**
   A. Decrease
   B. Increase
   C. Neither A nor B above
   D. I don't know

6. **Which of the following is rich in carbohydrate?**
   A. Meat
   B. Eggs
   C. Butter
   D. Corn
   E. I don't know

7. **Which one of the following symptoms is not usually associated with hypoglycaemia?**
   A. Weakness
   B. Hunger
   C. Chest pain
   D. I don't know

8. **If a person on insulin has a high blood or urine sugar level and ketones were present they should:**
   A. Increase insulin
   B. Decrease insulin
   C. Keep insulin and diet the same and test blood/urine later
   D. I don't know

PLEASE TURN OVER TO CONTINUE

9. When a person with diabetes on insulin becomes ill and unable to eat the prescribed diet:

A. They should immediately stop taking insulin

B. They must continue to take insulin

C. They should use tablets instead of insulin

D. I don't know

10. You can eat as much as you like of which one of the following foods?

A. Fruit

B. Lettuce

C. Steak

D. Honey

E. I don't know

11. You must avoid becoming overweight if you have diabetes because:

A. Insulin can be harmful to overweight people

B. Being overweight makes diabetes worse

C. Hypo attacks occur more frequently in overweight people

D. I don't know

12. Hypoglycaemia is caused by:

A. Too much insulin

B. Too little insulin

C. Too little exercise

D. I don't know

IN THESE LAST THREE QUESTIONS, THERE WILL BE MORE THAN ONE CORRECT ANSWER. PLEASE CIRCLE THE LETTERS IN FRONT OF ALL THE ANSWERS YOU THINK ARE CORRECT

13. Which of the following so-called "DIABETIC" food items are APPROVED by the Diabetic Clinic?

A. Diabetic jam

B. Diabetic jellies

C. Sorbitol-sweetened, sugar free canned fruit

D. "Low Calorie" soft drinks

E. I don't know

14. If someone with diabetes becomes sick and has vomiting and diarrhoea s/he should:

A. Stop all food and drink

B. Take their usual insulin/tablets

C. Take sugar sweetened drinks every two hours

D. Call the doctor if vomiting persists

E. I don't know

15. Special "DIABETIC" foods are:

A. Forbidden in a diabetic diet

B. Essential in a diabetic diet

C. Acceptable if used selectively and correctly

D. Usually more expensive than the non-diabetic equivalent

E. I don't know

    ISBN 0 9598171 8 2 C

THE DKN SCALES

Applications

The Diabetes Knowledge (DKN) scales were developed during the late 1970s and early 1980s in response to the need for a short theoretically-based knowledge test which met psychometric criteria of reliability and validity, and had practical advantages in being short and easily-administered. They were designed to be applicable to individuals with either IDDM or NIDDM, principally for applications in empirical research and programme evaluation. A primary aim was to develop a test of diabetes knowledge using a subset of items of high internal consistency selected from the full domain of diabetes knowledge.

Research

The scales were designed to allow rapid and reliable measurement of knowledge for research studies investigating the relationships between knowledge, psychological and social factors, and health status and metabolic control (e.g. Dunn *et al.*, 1984, 1990; Dougherty *et al.*, 1992). They have been used to explore the range of factors that influence changes in diabetes knowledge among diabetes patients.

Evaluation

An important focus of programme evaluation in diabetes education is the assessment of changes in knowledge over the course of an intervention. The specific focus may be a change in group knowledge scores (e.g. treatment versus control in randomised designs), or change in individual scores in longitudinal follow-up studies. Typically the design of such evaluation studies will involve repeated measurement of knowledge scores over a short period of time. For this reason, three parallel forms of the DKN scales were developed to ensure that recall of previous responses did not bias subsequent test scores.

Clinically the scales have been used with groups ranging in age from teenagers to the elderly, with individuals from a variety of ethnic backgrounds (including Greek, French, Italian, German), and with both IDDM and NIDDM populations.

Design

The latest versions of the DKN scales are presented in Figures 1-3. The scales were designed as a practical alternative to lengthy comprehensive tests and their content reflects the kind of information that was presented to patients attending DEPs at the time the scales were developed. In the late 1970s, the prevailing educational philosophy was that patients required an understanding of the theoretical aspects of diabetes (e.g. underlying physiology and the rationale for treatment) in order to manage their diabetes adequately. The authors did not make a distinction between theoretical and practical knowledge and therefore the scale contains a mix of the two item types. Since the initial development of the scales, understanding of different types of knowledge and their relationship to behaviour and outcomes has become more sophisticated, and distinctions between theoretical and practical knowledge have become an issue.

The DKN scales (DKNA, DKNB, DKNC) are three parallel tests containing fifteen multiple-choice items each. The fifteen questions on each form were designed to sample knowledge in five broad categories:

1) basic physiology of diabetes including insulin action
2) hypoglycaemia
3) food groups and food substitutions
4) sick day management
5) general diabetes care.

DKN items were designed to cover the general principles of diabetes management so that overall performance on the questionnaire would be minimally affected by treatment modality or prior experience. Patients with previous formal diabetes education who are not treated with exogenous insulin should still understand the physiological action of endogenous insulin secretion and its role in diabetes. Therefore, items related to insulin action were selected so as to minimise the effects of personal experience with insulin treatment. The alternative of developing separate scales designed specifically for subgroups would only complicate the task of using these questionnaires. It was expected, based on previous findings and our hypotheses in developing the item pool, that IDDM patients would obtain higher scores on the scales compared with NIDDM patients, and this constituted one aspects of the scales' validation.

Multiple-choice item format was selected for the final version of the scales. The true/false format trialed was not retained as it allowed a 50% probability of correctly guessing answers, and as a consequence generated a wide range of item difficulties compared to the more restricted range of the multiple-choice format. Open-ended format items were trialed and rejected as they introduced a bias against people with limited verbal ability who constituted a substantial proportion of the hospital population in which the instrument was to be used. The forty-five items included a subset of thirteen items from Collier and Etzwiler (1971).

Scoring

Each item is assigned a score of 1 for a correct response and 0 for an incorrect response. Items 1 to 12 on each form require a single correct answer. For items 13 to 15 several answers are correct and all must be checked to obtain a score of 1. The scale includes instructions for these different items, although clinical experience showed that a small number of patients did not follow the instructions. A wrong answer for any of the options for an item leads to a score of zero for the item. Thus, if a person circles all the alternatives including the correct ones, this will lead to a score of 0. Only scores of 0 or 1 are used, partially correct answers are scored as 0. The correct answers to the items from the three DKN scales are listed below:

Item	Version A Correct option	Version B Correct option	Version C Correct option
1	B	A	B
2	C	A	C
3	A	C	A
4	C	B	B
5	B	B	A
6	B	A	D
7	C	A	C
8	A	B	A
9	B	C	B
10	C	B	B
11	B	A	B
12	A	A	A
13	A D	A B C	A B D
14	A B	C D	B C D
15	B C	A C	C D

The total score for each form is calculated by summing the scores on each of the fifteen items, to give a potential score range of 0 to 15, with higher scores indicating better diabetes knowledge. DKN scores are typically expressed as raw scores out of fifteen, or as a percentage of correct answers (Beeney *et al.*, 1988; Beeney and Dunn, 1990; Dougherty *et al.*, 1992). For example, a raw score of 12 out of 15 corresponds to 80% correct. Scores can also be converted to a standardised normal distribution with a mean of zero and a standard deviation of 1, as used by Dunn *et al.* (1990), who demonstrated mean knowledge increases of almost 1 SD, corresponding to a raw score improvement from 48% correct to 74% correct at post-test. Any of these presentations of DKN scores is acceptable, though standardised scores may have an advantage in making comparisons between individuals and across time intervals.

SCALE DEVELOPMENT

Subject Samples

The original scales were developed during 1976-80, using samples of patients drawn from diabetes outpatient clinics at Royal Prince Alfred Hospital (RPAH). The clinic population is characterised by a high proportion of people with poor English literacy due to the multiplicity of ethnic backgrounds in the community served by the hospital. The RPAH area serves a predominantly working class adult population, with 69% of the population at the three lowest levels of the Congalton Occupational Status Scales (Congalton, 1963). Characteristics of the RPAH diabetic clinic population at that time were: 60% female, mean age 44 yrs, mean diabetes duration 10 yrs, 61% insulin-treated, mean HbA_{1c} of 10.0% for insulin-treated, and 9.7% for non-insulin-treated patients, and 46% had previously attended education programmes. It is important to note that the DKN scales were developed within this distinctive population, and therefore may not be directly applicable in different populations.

Five samples of patients were used in the early development of the scales and summary characteristics of these samples are detailed in Table 1. Additional published and unpublished data have contributed to supporting the psychometric credentials of the DKN scales. Available details are provided for these samples in Table 1. Samples 1-4 were randomly selected from, and representative of, the general RPAH clinic population in all characteristics described above, with the exception of English literacy, as patients were required to be literate in English to complete the questionnaires. Sample 3 was comparable to Samples 1 and 2 in all respects except that patients who had formal diabetes education were underrepresented (33% vs 46% respectively). Sample 5 patients completed the DKN scales as part of a study comparing the effectiveness of several DEPs. The study and sample characteristics have been described in detail elsewhere (Beeney & Dunn, 1990). The sample was drawn from a similar population pool to Samples 1 to 5. The mean HbA_{1c} was significantly higher in IDDM and insulin-treated groups compared with NIDDM and non-insulin-treated groups.

Table 1 Summary characteristics of diabetes patient samples used in the early development of the DKN scales

Sample	Purpose	n	Source
1	initial face validity & item format	3 x 30	RPAH outpatient clinics
2	formal face & content validity & final item format	205	RPAH Outpatient Clinics
3	initial reliability testing	56	RPAH Outpatient Clinics
4	clinical trial of scales	219	RPAH Diabetes Centre DEPs - 1981
5	reliability & validity testing	558	Attending DEPs at 3 Sydney hospital diabetes centres
Maxwell et al. (1992)	reliability of 14-item DKN version	203	IDDM & NIDDM; 20-81 yrs; 46% male; 45% insulin-treated
Tu et al. (1993)	reliability testing	27	NIDDM; 60+ yrs; 89% insulin-treated
Campbell (1991)	validity testing	150	NIDDM; duration 1-10+ yrs; 50% 61-70 yrs
		229	NIDDM; mean age 59 yrs; 48% male; mean duration 5 months
Dougherty et al. (1992)	normative data	(1) 27	(1) IDDM; teenagers duration 5 months
		(2) 65	(2) parents of IDDM teenagers
White (1992)	normative data duration < 1 year	(1) 66	(1) IDDM teenagers
		(2) 60	(2) mothers of IDDM teenagers

STATISTICAL METHODS AND QUALITATIVE JUDGEMENTS

This section details the steps involved in developing the DKN scales, using the samples described in the previous section, and the methods and criteria for determining the item selection for inclusion in the final versions.

1) The initial item pool was generated from an extensive literature review, published questionnaires, and consultation with a range of experienced diabetes professionals including physicians, nurses, dietitians, psychologists and patients.

2) The initial pool of 89 DKN items was pilot tested for face validity and acceptability in 6 different presentation formats including multiple choice, true/false and open-ended items using 3 randomly selected samples of 30 patients from the RPAH Diabetes Clinic (Sample 1). Duplicated and redundant items were deleted to leave a total of 45 items.

3) These 45 mixed-format items included a subset of 13 items from Collier and Etzwiler (1971). These items were given to 205 patients during 1976-177 (Sample 2) for face validity testing. The final choice of item format was determined by examination of the response patterns for the 3 formats. The open-ended questions were found to introduce a bias against a majority of the subjects who were limited in their ability to express verbally abstract concepts such as 'renal threshold'. Subjects were frequently able to identify the correct answer among a list of multiple-choice alternatives although they were unable to answer the same question in open-ended format. The true/false format, by virtue of its 50% probability of a correct response by guessing alone, produced ambiguous item difficulties when compared with the multiple-choice format. Other studies employing the true/false format report similar variation in item difficulties (Windsor *et al.*, 1981). In this sample, only the multiple-choice items remained stable in terms of item difficulty. The mean score of 72% on these items was consistent with the mean of 77% from Collier and Etzwiler's earlier study (1971).

4) All items were translated into multiple-choice format for inclusion in a self-administered questionnaire. Five items with outmoded content were deleted leaving 40 items. The new set of 40 items consisted of 18 dietary and 9 general questions, 5 questions on hyperglycaemia and illness, 4 on hypoglycaemia, and 4 on urine testing. Sample 3 completed this scale in early 1980 for initial reliability testing. The mean DKN score was 34.1 ± 6.8 or 76% correct. Five items were deleted from the scale owing to unacceptably low item difficulty or item discrimination coefficients (<0.20).

5) These 35 items were distributed to form parallel scales (see section on parallel scales for details).

PROCEDURES

Instructions for completion of the test are provided at the top of each scale form and the DKN scales are designed to be self-administered by respondents, though individuals unfamiliar with questionnaire completion may require assistance. Campbell (1991) reported that some elderly patients required explanation of the multiple choice format, and did not understand that items about insulin should be answered even if they were not on insulin treatment themselves.

Samples 1-4 involved in the initial scale development were recruited from the waiting rooms of the outpatient clinic and asked to assist in developing a diabetes knowledge questionnaire by completing the current version and making comments on the wording and format. Informed consent was obtained from each patient and no patient refused to complete the scales. A research assistant helped individual subjects to ensure all items were completed and to note difficulties with instructions and item wording for the further refinement of the scale. In Sample 5, subjects attending DEPs completed the scale at the first education session in a supervised group. Follow-up questionnaires were sent by mail to subjects who completed them at home.

STRUCTURE OF SCALE

Parallel Scales

The repeated measurement of diabetes knowledge using the same test over a limited time span risks artificially inflating the correlations between measurements as subjects may recall previous responses and reproduce them. Parallel forms of a scale allow repeat testing using equivalent but different forms of the same test and present a solution to this problem. Psychometric criteria are set for parallel tests (Gulliksen, 1950): the different test forms should (1) be similar in content and item type; (2) have near-equal mean and standard deviation, and (3) show similar intercorrelations.

Data analysed from several patient samples confirm that the DKN scales satisfactorily meet these criteria. To ensure the different forms were similar in content, the set of items was assigned to three forms so that each scale contained representative items from the broad areas of diabetes management - insulin action, sick day management, food groups, general information and hypoglycaemia. All items were in multiple-choice format with a choice of four or five possible responses.

Four items consistently displayed the highest item-total correlations across different subsets of the total sample. These four items were considered by the clinical staff to represent basic information for all patients and were repeated in each of the three forms of the DKN scales. These assessed knowledge of:

1) the normal range for blood glucose
2) the causes of hypoglycaemia

3) insulin requirements during illness
4) carbohydrate food.

Items were assigned to DKNA, DKNB and DKNC according to the following criteria:

1) the minimum number of items for reliable knowledge should be used,
2) basic information should be represented in each form, and
3) items should be matched across forms for item content, item difficulty, item variance, and discrimination coefficient. Two items were repeated in modified form in two of the scales.

Responses to the three forms were normally distributed, based on analysis of Sample 3 data. Analysis of variance showed that the means and variances of the three scale forms were comparable (F=1.03, d.f.=2,165). A clinical trial of the three forms in 219 patients demonstrated that pre-test scores were normally distributed and ANOVA was not significant (F=0.67, d.f.=2,216). Correlations between the three forms were 0.90 to 0.91 (p<0.001), though this high correlation is partly due to replication of the four basic information items.

Data from Sample 5 were analysed using ANOVA to test for equivalence of mean scores on the three parallel forms at baseline and post-DEP. At baseline the mean scores (±s.d.) for DKNA, DKNB and DKNC were: 9.0 (3.5); 7.6 (3.3), and 8.0 (3.5) respectively. Analysis by planned comparisons indicated a significant main effect across the three means (F=10.85, df=2,664). Pair-wise t-test comparisons showed that the mean score for DKNA was higher in comparison with mean scores for DKNB and DKNC [A vs B: t_{664}=4.51; p<0.0001; A vs B: t_{664}=3.16; p<0.01; B vs C: t_{664}=-1.28; p>0.1]. The scale means were statistically different in these very large samples, however differences among the mean scores for the three parallel forms are not likely to translate to clinically significant differences. Intercorrelations among the forms for this larger sample were 0.66 to 0.74.

Additional and Modified Items

Other users of the DKN scales have modified the original scales or created additional items to suit their particular situation or population. We present several of these new items verbatim and discuss their psychometric characteristics below.

Dougherty *et al.* (1992) reported a ceiling effect in samples of adolescents with IDDM and their parents during pre-testing with the original DKN scales. They created five additional items shown below intended to improve the discriminatory power of the measure. The authors also modified the scale instructions to make them suitable for administration with parents of children with diabetes.

16. Exercise:
a. Can decrease insulin needs
b. Can increase insulin needs
c. Increases the sugar in the blood
d. I don't know

17. A fruit exchange can be:
a. 1/2 cup of milk
b. 1/2 cup sweetened orange juice
c. 4 plain sweet biscuits
d. I don't know

18. A diabetic who is hyperglycaemic must:
a. Stop taking his/her insulin
b. Increase his/her insulin dose
c. Decrease his/her insulin dose
d. I don't know

19. A diabetic who feels sick and has no appetite:
a. Should take more insulin
b. Consult the doctor or diabetes nurse to have insulin adjusted
c. Is a sign that I am sick or could be getting sick. I should call the doctor or diabetes nurse
d. I don't know

20. The presence of ketones in the urine:
a. Only happens when my blood sugar is high
b. Means my control is good
c. Is a sign that I am sick or could be getting sick. I should call the doctor or diabetes nurse
d. I don't know

The authors reported that subjects found item sixteen difficult, but no data are yet available concerning individual item means, standard deviations, ranges, or changes in scale reliability or validity as a result of these additional items. Inspection of the face validity of these items indicates that the question content is appropriate for IDDM patients, consistent with the target population, however an evaluation of the items by a group of expert diabetes health professionals indicated that items nineteen and twenty in particular suffer from poor English expression, are poorly designed, have ambiguous answers and distractors and their relevance to successful self-management is not clear.

Some of the original DKN items are outdated now: the scales included items on urinalysis and none on blood glucose measurement, they used sexist language and used the term 'diabetic' as a noun. We have responded to this problem by recently updating the versions, modifying sexist and 'diabetic' terminology, and adding an additional item on SMBG on all three versions. We have substituted the following item, taken from Lennon *et al.* (1990), for previous items on ketones and insulin in all three DKN parallel scale versions:

If a person on insulin has a high blood or urine
sugar level and ketones are present, they should :

(a) increase insulin
(b) decrease insulin
(c) keep insulin and diet the same and test blood/urine later
(d) I don't know

In using the modified scales, it is advisable to obtain a sufficiently large sample size in order to confirm reliability, and if possible, to compare the parallelism of the modified versions. It is likely that these modifications will result in enhanced internal consistency and validity.

Reliability

Internal consistency

Samples 3 and 5 and other studies (Maxwell *et al.*, 1992; Tu *et al.*, 1993) have provided data to evaluate the internal consistency of the DKN scales.

Sample 3 completed the revised forty-item multiple choice DKN scale prior to construction of the parallel forms. Homogeneity analysis supported the belief that the scale items measure a unitary concept (Cronbach alpha = 0.92). For tests of ability it is usually preferable to exclude items which have very low or very high item difficulty (i.e. very low or very high mean scores). Items which are too easy or too hard are not useful in discriminating between individuals. Item difficulties ranged from 0.14 to 0.93, with thirty-five items in the "acceptable" range of 0.30-0.90 (Windsor *et al.*, 1981). Thirty-eight items exceeded the minimum coefficient of 0.20. Corrected item-total correlations were positive and ranged from 0.15 to 0.73. Five items with unacceptable item difficulties or low corrected item-total correlations (<0.20) were deleted. The remaining thirty-five items had item difficulties ranging from 0.35 to 0.93, and item-total correlations from 0.24 to 0.73. The reliability analysis was replicated in a sample of IDDM and NIDDM patients with long duration (n=43: Cronbach alpha = 0.91) and in the subset of IDDM patients from that sample (n=25: Cronbach alpha = 0.86).

Cronbach alphas were computed for DKNA - 0.83, DKNB - 0.83, and DKNC - 0.85. Kuder-Richardson reliability coefficients were also computed to allow comparisons with reliability of another published diabetes knowlege scale (Windsor *et al.*, 1981). KR21 coefficients were 0.80 (DKNA), 0.77 (DKNB) and 0.81 (DKNC). In order to compare reliabilities of the separate tests, Ferguson's (1976) modification of the Spearman-Brown formula was used for estimating the increase in reliability with increased test length. The standardised coefficients were DKNA - 0.96, DKNB - 0.96, and DKNC - 0.97 in comparison with Windsor's results of 0.96 and 0.97. The three parallel forms of the DKN scales, therefore, retained high relative reliability when contrasted with a test which was 2.3 times longer.

The internal consistency of the fifteen-item versions considered together was 0.76 using Sample 5 data. Item difficulties ranged from 0.26 to 0.74. All item-total correlations were above 0.20, and the removal of items did not significantly inflate the reliability coefficient. The more heterogeneous nature of the latter sample compared to the original development sample is likely to have contributed to the lowered reliability.

Reliability of parallel forms: DKNA, DKNB, DKNC

Internal reliability coefficients of 0.84, 0.83 and 0.85 respectively were reported for the parallel forms in Sample 3 (Dunn, 1984). Initial data appeared promising and these analyses were repeated with the larger Sample 5. The coefficient alphas for DKNA (n=237), DKNB (n=217), and DKNC (n=208) for the mixed sample of IDDM and NIDDM patients were 0.80, 0.74 and 0.79 respectively. Item difficulties ranged from 0.17 to 0.85, and item-total correlations ranged from 0.17 to 0.55.

Maxwell *et al.* (1992) provided reliability data from a sample of 203 patients in their study of the effect of social support and diabetes education on metabolic control, knowledge and psychosocial outcomes. They reported Cronbach alphas for fourteen-item modified versions of the DKN scales as 0.75, 0.83 and 0.78 in mixed samples of IDD and NIDD patients.

Reliability for sample subsets

We examined internal consistency of the DKN scales separately for IDDM and NIDDM samples (Sample 5). Patients were diagnosed according to the criteria of Welborn *et al.* (1983). Patients wih IDDM were forty years or younger at diagnosis and on permanent insulin therapy within two years of diagnosis. Patients defined as NIDDM had an age of onset of diabetes after forty years. Published data showed differences between these groups in knowledge and in psychological adjustment (Beeney and Dunn, 1990; Welch *et al.*, in press), and thus it was considered necessary to demonstrate reliability in these more homogeneous subgroups in addition to the reliability for the scale in large heterogeneous samples. The results shown in Table 2 are data from Sample 5.

Table 2   A comparison of reliability coefficients for the 3 parallel DKN scales for diabetes type and treatment subgroups based on data from Sample 5

Subgroup		Cronbach alpha	
	DKNA (n)	DKNB (n)	DKNC (n)
NIDDM	0.79 (183)	0.72 (175)	0.76 (166)
IDDM	0.74 (53)	0.61 (42)	0.62 (42)
Non-insulin-treated	0.79 (128)	0.71 (123)	0.72 (119)
Insulin-treated	0.72 (109)	0.66 (93)	0.78 (89)

Additional reliability data were provided by Tu *et al.*(1993) who used Kuder-Richardson 20 to obtain a reliability estimate for one of the parallel DKN forms (which form was not stated). They reported a Cronbach alpha of 0.76 in a sample of twenty-seven healthy individuals over sixty years with NIDDM, of whom 89% were insulin-treated.

The pattern of coefficients for the parallel scales suggests that DKNA is more consistently reliable across different subgroups than the other two versions. The recommended minimum sample size for analysis of Cronbach alpha is 200 according to Nunnally *et al.* (1975) and thus it is difficult to draw firm conclusions regarding scale reliability for IDDM patients. The internal reliability of the DKN scales is moderate and acceptable for use with NIDDM samples, and with insulin-treated samples. These analyses were conducted using the original scale versions and may be expected to improve with modifications.

Test-retest reliability

Test-retest data have not been published on the DKN scales although alternate forms reliability has been estimated with Sample 5. Pearson product-moment correlations between the parallel forms used longitudinally at follow-up intervals of three to twelve months varied from $r=0.64$ for an interval of three months ($n=343$), to 0.59 for an interval of 11 months ($n=138$) (both $p<.001$) in Sample 5 subjects. Clinic attendance, intervening educational input and other vicarious learning between the first and second administrations of the DKN scales are likely to suppress correlations between scores in these samples.

Validity

Face/content validity

The sources of the initial pool of eighty-nine DKN items included an extensive search of the diabetes education literature, published questionnaires developed by Etzwiler and associates (e.g. Etzwiler and Robb, 1972; Collier and Etzwiler, 1971) and consultation with a range of diabetes health professionals including dietitians, nurses, physicians, diabetes educators and psychologists involved in all aspects of diabetes patient management at the Diabetes Centre at RPAH. Items to be included in the final form were selected on the basis of coverage of "basic diabetes information" as assessed by the expert panel, including dietary and general information, hyperglycaemia and illness, hypoglycaemia and urine glucose testing. All items were pilot-tested with patient samples to confirm face validity and acceptability in terms of content and item format (Samples 1 to 4 as detailed above).

The assessment of test validity is an evolving process. It is important to note here that although the scales satisfied content validity criteria when developed in the late 1970s and early 1980s, diabetes management has changed significantly since then. The approach to dietary advice is now more flexible, self monitoring of blood glucose has largely replaced urine testing, and many other advances have occurred that are relevant to the items included in a patient diabetes knowledge assessment. The modified DKN scales are presented in Figures 1-3. Several items containing references to units of measurement require rewording to suit different local contexts, for example weight (kg or pound) and blood glucose (mmol/l or mg/dl).

Some concerns have been raised by users of the scales regarding items assessing knowledge of insulin action and their relevance to individuals with NIDDM. The DKN items were designed to cover the general principles of diabetes management so that overall performance on the questionnaire would be minimally affected by treatment modality or prior experience. The scales were intended for use with all patients on the basis that individuals who are not treated with exogenous insulin should still understand the physiological action of endogenous insulin secretion and its role in diabetes. Therefore, items related to insulin action were selected so as to minimise personal experience with insulin treatment as a relevant factor in ability to respond correctly.

Some problems have been generated in attempting to develop scales suitable for all diabetes patients. Thus NIDDM patients on tablets and/or diet do not need to know about insulin requirements during illness for their own self-management, though it is important for tablet-treated patients to know that continuing medication is critical during illness. Although NIDDM patients do experience hypoglyceamia, those treated by tablets and/or diet are not at risk of hypoglycaemia "because of too much exogenous insulin" as the DKN item implies. The normal range for blood glucose is even more important information now that self-monitoring and feedback of blood glucose is available.

Concurrent validity

There are no reports on the correlation of the DKN scales with other tests of diabetes knowledge. However, thirteen items were common to both the DKN scales and the questionnaire of Collier and Etzwiler (1971), and the mean scores for these two scales were similar: 72% for the DKN scale in Sample 2 compared with 77% from the earlier Collier and Etzwiler (1971) study.

Predictive validity

An increase of 25% in DKN scores in a sample of 309 patients reported by Dunn *et al.* (1990) did not predict HbA_{1c} improvement over a fifteen month follow-up. Beeney and Dunn (1990) tested the hypothesis that improvement in scores in specific knowledge areas would predict changes in specific measures of diabetes control - HbA_{1c} and hypoglycaemic episodes. Patients (n=558) attending one of five DEPs completed the DKN scales at baseline and post-DEP. Diabetes knowledge improvement did not correlate significantly with baseline or post-DEP HbA_{1c}, or with changes in HbA_{1c} (r=0.03), and improvement in nine specific content areas failed to predict changes in HbA_{1c}. This study also found that improvement in knowledge of the causes of hypoglycaemia did not predict prospective changes in the frequency of reported hypoglycaemic episodes at follow-up. However, we cannot confidently conclude that an improvement in knowledge of the causes of hypoglycaemia would not predict a decline in the frequency of hypoglycaemia in patients for whom this issue is most relevant. The sample included a mix of patients with non-insulin-treated NIDDM, IDDM and insulin-treated NIDDM and was too small for valid statistical analysis of sub-groups. Non-insulin-treated patients on tablets are less prone to hypoglycaemic episodes generally, and when they do occur they will be due to missing or late mealtimes or extra exercise, not to too much insulin which is the correct response to the DKN item. If the sample is restricted to insulin users, the analysis would need to be further restricted to the subgroup who were having hypoglycaemic events before the DEP. Those people who improved their knowledge of hypoglycaemia might also improve their knowledge of the reasons for controlling their diabetes at lower blood glucose levels; if they implement this in practice they may well be at greater risk of hypoglycaemia than prior to the DEP. Larger sample sizes are needed for these sophisticated subgroup analyses to consider all the complexities of the relationship.

Construct validity

Research reports on diabetes knowledge present a confusing and often contradictory picture. Variables which might be expected to show a simple linear correlation with knowledge do not. Age is inconsistently related to knowledge in juvenile diabetic patients, and only appears to show a reliable negative correlation in adulthood (Etzwiler & Robb, 1972; Simon & Stewart, 1976; Karlander *et al.*, 1980). DKN scores correlated negatively (-0.31) with age in the first published samples (Dunn *et al.*, 1984) but were correlated positively in the study reported by Maxwell *et al.* (1992) (+0.38). IDDM patients did not differ in DKN scores according to age at diagnosis ($p>0.01$), although NIDDM patients who were diagnosed before fifty years had significantly higher scores than those diagnosed after sixty years of age ($p<0.01$; Sample 5 data).

Data are also inconsistent regarding the relationship between knowledge and diabetes duration (Simon & Stewart, 1976). Patients from Sample 3 with diabetes of long duration scored significantly higher than newly-diagnosed patients (76% vs 50%, respectively).

Significantly higher scores were reported for patients with lower occupational status ($r=-0.33$; $p<0.01$) (Dunn, 1984), consistent with previously published data (Collier and Etzwiler, 1971; Miller *et al.*, 1978). Higher DKN scores were associated ($p<0.001$) with reading more diabetes literature ($r=0.52$), regular urinalysis ($r=0.41$), and motivation to exercise frequently ($r=0.48$). In the clinical trial using Sample 4, baseline DKN scores were moderately correlated ($r=0.33$) with the 'B' scale on Cattell's 16PF personality questionnaire (Cattell, 1966), a measure of intelligence. The pattern of correlations between the DKN scores and other variables in Samples 2 and 3 supports the DKN scale construct validity. One third of the individuals in Sample 3 had attended DEPs compared to 46% in Samples 1 and 2. The mean score of 24.4 (60%) ± 8.7 for Sample 3 was lower than for Sample 2 (76%) and patients with more diabetes education tended to have higher DKN scores ($r=0.21$).

Maxwell *et al.* (1992) also reported a positive correlation between education and DKN scores (r=0.41). These relationships were consistent with previously published data (Collier and Etzwiler, 1971; Miller *et al.*, 1978).

Significantly higher DKN scores in insulin-treated or IDDM patient samples compared with non-insulin-treated NIDDM patients are consistently reported (Dunn, 1984; Dunn *et al.*, 1984; Beeney and Dunn, 1990; Maxwell *et al.*, 1992). Higher DKN scores were reported (r=0.34, p<0.01) for those patients treated with insulin in Samples 2-3. The summary data from Sample 5 in Table 3 compares the mean DKN scores for diabetes type and treatment subgroups.

We would expect IDDM or insulin-treated samples to score significantly higher overall on the total scales and on specific items related to insulin treatment or hypoglycaemia because of their greater experience and exposure to insulin, thus providing support for construct validity of the scale. Data from Sample 5 above confirms that IDDM and insulin-treated groups consistently score higher both at baseline and after educational intervention. IDDM patients also consistently score higher on individual DKN items related to the causes of hypoglycaemia. Differences at baseline between IDDM and NIDDM on sick day medication DKN items (91% vs 39%, p<0.0001) were eliminated following education (94% vs 88%, n.s.).

Table 3 Normative scores on the DKN scales according to subgroups: diabetes type and treatment, before and after a diabetes education programme (DEP)

SUBGROUP	source	n	DKN score	
			pre-DEP	post-DEP
IDDM	Sample 5	113	10.7 (2.4)	12.1 (2.1) [1]
	Dougherty *et al.*	(1) 27	75%	
	(1992)	(2) 65	83% [2]	
	White (1992)	(1) 66	86%	
		(2) 60	88% [2]	
NIDDM	Sample 5	460	7.6 (3.3)	10.5 (2.9) [1]
	Campbell (1991)	229	range: 4.8-5.9	7.5-9.2 [1]
			(32-39%)	(50-61%) [2]
Insulin-treated	Sample 5	252	9.9 (2.9)	11.6 (2.3) [1]
Diet/tablet-treated	Sample 5	321	6.9 (3.2)	10.2 (3.0) [1]
MIXED	Maxwell *et al.*	(1) 203	62%	75% [2]
	(1992)	(2) 100	55%	71% [2]

[1] DKN score expressed as mean (± sd)
[2] DKN score expressed a percentage
[All pre-post- DEP comparisons significant p<0.001]

The additional studies using the DKN scales in Table 3 provide data on various samples from a low of 32% correct in 229 older NIDDM patients prior to diabetes education (Campbell, 1991), through to 86% correct in a sample of sixty-six adolescents with IDDM diagnosed under one year (White, 1992, personal communication).

What can we conclude about the construct validity of the DKN scales from these data? The kind of knowledge the scales measure could best be described as predominantly theoretical as distinguished from practical or behavioural. The relationships between DKN scores and occupational status and intelligence supports this concept. The variables most useful in evaluating construct validity of the DKN scales will be diabetes type and treatment, education level, and other variables associated with knowledge in general.

It is important to recognise that there are more complex relationships among the variables relating to knowledge than simple correlations will reveal. For example, the relationship between knowledge and duration of diabetes is unlikely to be linear. We may expect an increase in knowledge in the first year after diagnosis, with a steep learning curve in the early stages as information and experience are integrated into daily routines, leading on to a learning plateau. Thus it is not surprising that few papers report clear relationships between duration and DKN scores, as most analyses have been confined to correlations.

It is difficult to predict clear links between patients' age and their level of diabetes knowledge - age is confounded with diabetes type and may have a relatively minimal contribution to predicting knowledge in comparison with other factors. The general trend to higher scores in younger patients may be partially due to the fact that most of them have IDDM and IDDM patients score higher on the DKN scales. In addition, anecdotal observations have suggested that younger patients with IDDM are more likely to be offered education than older NIDDM patients, perhaps because of the widespread perception that IDDM is a more serious disease than NIDDM, and it is believed that educational input is more effective in terms of outcomes with younger individuals. These questions can be answered using more sophisticated statistical analyses which control for the confounding effects of diabetes type and we offer this as a suggestion to researchers interested in pursuing this further.

Variables that are likely to have a stronger association with DKN scores are diabetes education and treatment type. If scores are responsive to interventions designed to affect knowledge, this is strong support for construct validity. The data presented here clearly support the sensitivity of DKN scores to the impact of interventions.

The DKN scales are designed to be a representative sample of the larger domain of diabetes knowledge. Insulin-treated and IDDM patients are exposed to a greater proportion of that domain of knowledge than tablet/diet treated NIDDM patients. Therefore if the scale is intended to assess patient knowledge of this large domain, it is logical that IDDM and insulin-treated NIDDM patients will obtain higher DKN scores. Our data and those of other groups confirm a consistent distinction among these groups in DKN scores.

Several published randomised trials of diabetes education programmes have failed to provide substantial evidence for a significant impact of increased knowledge on subsequent metabolic control (Bloomgarten *et al.*, 1987; Mazzuca *et al.*,

1986). Logically it would seem that more knowledge enables a patient to put into practice those self-care behaviours which will contribute to improvement in metabolic control, though it does not necessarily follow that a statistically significant relationship between these variables will be found. The strength of the association between knowledge and control will be diluted by the effect of intervening variables such as motivation and attitudes, and because measurement tools address many aspects of management, only some of which would be expected to relate to diabetes control in some of the patients studied. Some aspects of management are only relevant to control under certain special circumstances. Thus items on sick day rules would not be expected generally to relate to HbA_{1c} levels, but in a subset of people hospitalised with diabetic ketoacidosis (DKA) we might expect a much higher proportion of people who do not know the guidelines than would be expected in a group who have not been hospitalised with DKA. Subgroup analyses separating out those patients who are not prone to DKA are appropriate to test these hypotheses, and individual items must be tested separately.

The relationships between DKN scores and HbA_{1c} were tested in subgroups of Sample 5 patients: IDDM vs NIDDM, and insulin-treated vs non-insulin-treated. No correlations were significant between DKN scores at baseline or post-DEP and HbA_{1c} at baseline and at three months follow-up. However, linear correlations are likely to oversimplify real and important relationships between knowledge and control. More detailed analyses are required to unravel the complex associations among knowledge and metabolic parameters. Lockington et al. (1988), using a different knowledge questionnaire, grouped knowledge scores into quintiles, and found a higher mean HbA_{1c} in patients in the lowest scoring quintile compared with the pooled mean of the remaining knowledge quintiles. Beeney and Dunn (1990) did not replicate these findings in a similar analysis of DKN scale scores in Sample 5 subjects. Quintile groupings of DKN post-DEP scores showed no significant associations with HbA_{1c} at follow-up; the lowest quintile grouping was not different significantly from the pooled mean of the remaining quintiles. Of the other studies testing the relationship between DKN scales and metabolic control (Dougherty et al., 1992; Dunn, 1984; Campbell, 1991; Maxwell et al., 1992), only one reported a significant relationship between diabetes knowledge and measures of glycosylated haemoglobin (Maxwell et al., 1992). It is not clear what factors might account for this latter result. Campbell (1991) found DKN scores did not relate significantly to HbA_{1c}, body mass index, fasting blood glucose, or cholesterol.

Sensitivity to Change

The DKN scales are consistently reported to be sensitive to change in response to educational interventions with both the total scores and the percentage of correct individual items increasing significantly from pre-DEP to post-DEP (Dunn, 1984; Dunn et al., 1990; Beeney and Dunn, 1990). Dunn et al. (1990) reported mean DKN score increases of almost one standard deviation (i.e. 25%) from baseline to post-test after a two-day group education programme for a sample of 309 IDDM and NIDDM patients. These increases have been maintained for up to twelve months of follow-up. In comparison, scores of individuals who have not attended formal DEPs remained stable over the equivalent time frame (Beeney and Dunn, 1990). Results in Table 3 show the consistent statistically significant improvements in DKN scores that result from educational interventions.

Campbell (1991) in a randomised trial of four educational interventions reported significant mean improvements of 18% to 22% in DKN scores between groups at three and six months follow-up (p<0.001). Differences in the magnitude of these increases indicated that the DKN scales are sensitive to differences in programme presentation and intensity. Pair-wise comparisons among the four intervention groups showed that both the Behavioural and Group education interventions were associated with significantly greater improvement than the Minimal programme at three and six months follow-up.

Henderson (1992, personal communication) used the DKN scales to assess diabetes knowledge change among twenty-eight school staff attending a one-day diabetes education workshop. The workshop aimed to increase teachers' knowledge about diabetes thereby ensuring greater safety of children with diabetes under their care. A set of eleven items were selected from the DKN scales based on four content areas: hypoglycaemia, blood glucose control, exercise, and complications. Baseline median scores were high (73% correct) with wide variability. Scores increased to 91% correct immediately after the intervention and were 82% at two months follow-up.

Discriminatory Power

Data from Beeney and Dunn (1990) for 558 patients attending DEPs showed that total DKN scores at baseline and post-intervention were not normally distributed, being significantly skewed to the higher end of the distribution: 70% of the 558 patients scored ≥ 7/15 at baseline, and 21% scored ≤ 5/15. Dougherty *et al.* (1992) noted a ceiling effect in a sample of adolescent IDDM subjects and added five extra items to the original fifteen. The authors reported that the addition of these items improved the discriminatory power of the measure; however no evidence was provided to support this claim.

Standardisation and Norms

Table 3 includes a summary of normative scores for published and unpublished studies using the DKN scales. Mean scores range from a low of 32% in a sample of 229 older NIDDM patients with no previous diabetes education (Campbell, 1991) to a high of 86% in a sample of sixty six IDDM adolescents who had been diagnosed for at least one year (White, 1992, personal communication). Mean scores for adults after formal group diabetes education varied from 60% to 75% (Table 3). The average improvement in mean scores ranged from 13% to 25% following attendance at DEPs which varied in duration, health professional input and intensity.

DISCUSSION

The measurement of diabetes knowledge cannot be considered in isolation from the wider context of diabetes management and education. Our discussion of data accumulated over ten years of research with the DKN scales raises larger issues: the appropriateness of study designs and the underlying assumptions behind published research; the need for greater precision in definition, measurement and understanding of the construct of knowledge; and increasing psychometric rigour in developing such instruments.

As our understanding of the processes of behaviour change and their implementation in diabetes management becomes more sophisticated, so it becomes more important to distinguish the components of diabetes knowledge - theory, practice, and skills. Researchers seeking to develop measures of diabetes knowledge must specify a clear theoretical rationale for the type of measure of knowledge and give careful consideration to issues of practical application and skills performance which are expressions of true understanding.

The quality of studies in diabetes education research has improved (Padgett *et al.*, 1988) but the psychometric standards of scales used to measure knowledge and other psychosocial variables, are often inadequate. Sufficient psychometric information must be published to enable the reader to evaluate the quality and characteristics of the currently available instruments. It is difficult to be confident of any results using scales which do not have a strong track record or other supporting evidence.

According to one school of thought, the measurement of diabetes knowledge is inextricably linked with outcomes: knowledge is only important if improving knowledge means improved control. Another view is that measuring knowledge is critical, independent of the association with diabetes control, because people have the right to be fully informed of the principles of self-management.

While there has been a growing awareness that psychosocial factors such as motivation, health beliefs, and self-efficacy, contribute significantly to behaviour and health outcomes, knowledge remains the most frequently assessed outcome in research and evaluation of diabetes education interventions.

In practice, diabetes education has often operated along the lines of the school classroom with the primary object being to transmit facts about diabetes. This process was based on the assumption that increasing a patient's knowledge of the 'facts' of diabetes would lead to improved blood glucose control, and, in turn, reduce the incidence and severity of complications. This assumption is wrong. Several studies have confirmed improvements in diabetes knowledge following DEPs (e.g. Wise *et al.*, 1986; Beeney and Dunn, 1990); far fewer have reported improvements in metabolic control as a consequence.

The rationale behind the development of the DKN scales was primarily one of pragmatism: to produce short scales suitable for rapid and reliable assessment of diabetes knowledge in mixed samples of patients to avoid the necessity for separate questionnaires for IDDM and NIDDM groups. The data presented in this chapter generally supports the ability of the DKN scales to meet these objectives. However, others have argued that the content of some DKN items related to insulin action is not relevant to non-insulin requiring patients, and therefore the scales have poor content validity for NIDDM and should be used for IDDM patients only. We disagree. The items were designed to tap knowledge of the underlying theoretical principles of diabetes and its management which involve the action of insulin, regardless of therapy type. It is a simple fact that personal experience with insulin will enable IDDM and insulin-treated NIDDM patients to gain this knowledge more easily and quickly. However, our data demonstrate that NIDDM patients improve significantly on DKN items related to insulin as a result of DEP attendance and perform equally as well as IDDM subjects on those items. Thus personal experience is neither necessary nor sufficient (Beeney and Dunn, 1990). Some users of the DKN scales believe that patients not treated with insulin do not need to have information about insulin, and there should be separate scales for IDDM and NIDDM. We believe this is a narrow view of diabetes education and self-management and that every patient should be provided with full and accurate information about the underlying pathophysiology of diabetes as a rationale for its treatment. Nevertheless we acknowledge that there are no data to test the hypothesis that non-insulin-treated patients with a better understanding of diabetes, including insulin action, are better off in terms of metabolic control or other outcomes. While personal experience with insulin may contribute to some patients achieving higher scores, it does not therefore follow that there should be two separate questionnaires.

Clinical Utility of the DKN scales

The measurement of knowledge remains important to diabetes management. Scales such as the DKN have their use in diabetes education and in research, as diagnostic tools and as a general measure of patients' general understanding of diabetes. In considering the value and potential usefulness of DKN scales, it is important to consider the purpose for which knowledge is being measured. In their updated format, as reproduced in this chapter, the scales appear to have value for continued use in settings where it is desirable to measure knowledge quickly and reliably - (i.e. theoretical knowledge). The DKN scales were designed and used primarily with older patients and are therefore most appropriate for use with an older population. Data from other researchers using the DKN scales with IDDM patients suggests that the scales in their present format have item difficulties too low for younger samples such as adolescents. This limitation may be overcome by the addition of suitable items. The usefulness of the DKN is not only in its total score, but also in an examination of performance on individual items as demonstrated by Beeney and Dunn (1990). The DKN is not intended to be a comprehensive diagnostic instrument, however the scale has been used success-fully for this purpose with patients attending the RPAH Diabetes Centre and other researchers have indicated that the DKN scales are useful in quickly identi-fying areas of misunderstanding in diabetes management.

Limitations

The scale may easily be used in its self-administered form, although individuals unfamiliar with questionnaire completion may be given assistance. Campbell (1991) has cautioned that some elderly patients required explanation of the mul-tiple-choice format, and did not understand that items about insulin should be answered even if they were not on insulin treatment themselves. This is a peren-nial problem with any written questionnaire, viz. that those unfamiliar with forms of any sort will be at a disadvantage. The DKN scales were developed in a mostly older NIDDM population. Dougherty *et al.* (1992) reported ceiling effects using the scales with samples of young IDDM patients and their parents. The DKN scores of younger, better educated patients tend to be skewed to the high end of the distribution, and thus the test currently does not have good discriminatory power with that population.

The scales were originally developed in the early 1980s and some of the content and terminology are now outdated. For example, there are no items on blood glu-cose measurement, they include sexist language and use the term 'diabetic' as a noun. In response to this, we have recently updated the parallel versions by mod-ifying terminology where necessary, and substituting an item on blood glucose monitoring in all three versions. These changes may have effects on scale reliabil-ity and validity and for future use we recommend that a sufficiently large sample be used to check reliability and confirm the parallelism of the three scales. It is likely that these modifications will result in enhanced internal consistency and va-lidity.

It is important to note that items concerning ketostix and SMBG are only appro-priate for patients who are performing these particular tests. It is possible that other groups have designed and used substitute items that do not depend on ex-perience with these specific tests.

The data reported in this chapter support the construct validity of the DKN scales. However a more appropriate criterion for the DKN scales than metabolic outcomes may be the application of knowledge in performance of self-care skills. Such analyses have not been reported with the DKN scales.

The comprehensive assessment of diabetes knowledge is a desirable clinical objective, but there are many contexts in which it is not feasible. In assessing the variety of educational needs of individual patients, and in evaluative research applied to DEPs, we would argue that it is more important to assess knowledge rapidly and efficiently than it is to catalogue exhaustively the entire range of po-tential knowledge items. Our research has shown that it is possible to sample from this larger domain and to produce a brief instrument of high reliability. The DKN scales offer rapid and efficient assessment of diabetes knowledge without sacrificing reliability. The scales have shown good patient and health professional acceptability. Parallel forms of the scale help to overcome many of the difficulties in motivating patients to complete lengthy and complicated self-report questionnaires. As a result of their brevity, factors such as boredom and fatigue are minimised as confounding variables. Longer tests than the DKN may be suitable when sufficient time is available to assess comprehensively all areas of diabetes knowledge (Hess and Davis, 1983). However, there is little justification on theoretical and empirical evidence to date that knowledge can account for more than minimal variance in predicting patient outcomes, and therefore time spent on assessing diabetes knowledge will compete with the assessment of other important medical and psychosocial factors (Dunn *et al.* 1990).

SUMMARY

The DKN scales have helped to generate a great deal of research and we believe there is still an important use for scales such as these, as evidenced by the continued demand for them in clinical applications, and by the evaluation methods used in published research.

When the scales were first designed it was felt that knowledge was important in diabetes management, but knowledge is often considered to be of far less importance now, especially for diabetes control. Measurement of the sort of knowledge the DKN scales assess remains important - individuals still need the facts about their disease. However, there is a need for additional measures of the different concepts of knowledge - including more direct assessment of skills and behaviours, so that the extent to which patients are able to generalise what they learn in an educational setting to real life situations can be assessed. We would argue that though the accurate and reliable measurement of knowledge remains an important task particularly for clinical management, it requires reliable and valid instruments that are theoretically and empirically supported. Future attention must be directed to the assessment of largely neglected factors such as patient and health professional attitudes and behaviours which contribute significantly to the prediction of improved outcomes, and are amenable to modification.

The DKN scales have been used to evaluate a variety of diabetes educational interventions, and to screen groups and individuals for their level of understanding of diabetes. The scales are sensitive to interventions designed to improve patient understanding of diabetes and its management. The multiple choice item format allows the DKN scales to be used with individuals possessing a wide range of language abilities and literacy levels.

In summary, the three parallel DKN scales are intended to be reliable and valid measures of knowledge of information considered important for patients with diabetes. The DKN scales sample knowledge in the major areas of basic physiology of diabetes and insulin action, hypoglycaemia, food groups and food substitutions, diabetes management during intercurrent illness, and general principles of diabetes care. The scales have their principal application in research and the evaluation of educational interventions where clinic time and resources are at a premium.

ACKNOWLEDGEMENTS

We wish to acknowledge our indebtedness to the pioneering work in the assessment of diabetes knowledge of Donnell Etzwiler and associates in Minneapolis. Thanks are due to the staff of the RPAH Diabetes Centre for their assistance in updating and suggesting modifications for the DKN scales, and to Dr Clare Bradley for her insightful comments, many of which have been incorporated into the text of this chapter.

REFERENCES

Beeney, L.J., Dunn, S.M. and Turtle, J.R. (1988) Alternative approaches to formal diabetes education: A one-year follow-up. *Diabetes Research and Clinical Practice*, 5 (Suppl.1), S44

Beeney, L.J., and Dunn, S.M. (1990) Knowledge improvement and metabolic control in diabetes education: Approaching the limits? *Patient Education and Counselling*, 16, 217–229

Bloomgarten, Z.T., Karmally, W., Metzger, M.J., Brothers, M., Nechemias, C., Bookman, J., Faierman, D., Ginsberg-Fellner, F., Rayfield, E. and Brown, W.V. (1987) Randomized, controlled trial of diabetic patient education: improved knowledge without improved metabolic status. *Diabetes Care* 10, 263

Campbell, E. (1991) Behaviour change in the prevention and treatment of non-insulin-dependent diabetes mellitus. Unpublished doctoral dissertation, University of Newcastle, NSW, Australia

Cattell, R.B. (1966) *Handbook of Multivariate Experimental Psychology.* Chicago: Rand McNally

Centers for Disease Control (1991) *The Prevention and Treatment of Complications of Diabetes: A Guide for Primary Care Practitioners.* Atlanta, USA

Collier, B.N. and Etzwiler, D.D. (1971) Comparative study of diabetes knowledge among juvenile diabetics and their parents. *Diabetes* , 20, 51–57

Congalton, A.A. (1963) *Occupational Status in Australia.* Kensington, University of NSW School of Sociology

Dougherty, G., Schiffrin, A., White, D., and Ball, L. (1992) Predictors of initial glycaemic control in newly diagnosed diabetic children: A randomised trial. *American Journal of Diseases of Children*, 146, 468

Dunn, S.M. (1984) The Psychological Impact of Diabetes Education. Unpublished doctoral dissertation, University of Sydney, NSW, Australia

Dunn, S.M., Bryson, J.M., Hoskins, P.L., Alford, J.B., Handelsman, D.J. and Turtle J.R. (1984) Development of the Diabetes Knowledge (DKN) Scales: Forms DKNA, DKNB, and DKNC. *Diabetes Care* , 7 (1), 36–41

Dunn, S.M., Beeney, L.J., Hoskins, P.L. and Turtle, J.R. (1990) Knowledge and attitude change as predictors of metabolic improvement in diabetes education. *Social Science and Medicine*, 31 (10), 1135–1141

Etzwiler, D.D. and Robb, J.R. (1972) Evaluation of programmed education among juvenile diabetics and their families. *Diabetes*, **21**, 967–971

Ferguson, G.A. (1976) *Statistical Analysis in Psychology and Education*. 4th ed. Kogakusha: McGraw Hill

Gulliksen, H. (1950) *Theory of mental tests*. New York: Wiley

Hess, G.E. and Davis, W.K. (1983) The validation of a diabetes patient knowledge test. *Diabetes Care*, **6**, 591

Karlander, S.G., Alinder, I., and Hellstrom, K. (1980) Knowledge of diabetes mellitus, diets and nutrition in diabetic patients. *Acta Medica Scandinavica*, **207**, 483–488

Lennon, G.M., Taylor, K.G., Debney, L. and Bailey, C.J. (1990) Knowledge, attitudes, technical competence, and blood glucose control of Type 1 diabetic patients during and after an education programme. *Diabetic Medicine* **7**, 825–832

Lockington, T.J., Farrant, S., Meadows, K.A., Dowlatshahi, D. and Wise, P.H. (1988) Knowledge profile and control in diabetic patients. *Diabetic Medicine*, **5**, 381–386

Maxwell, A.E., Hunt, I.F., and Bush, M.A. (1992) Effects of a social support group as an adjunct to diabetes training on metabolic control and psychosocial outcomes. *Diabetes Educator*, **18** (4), 303–309

Mazzuca, S.A., Moorman, N.H., Wheeler, M.L., Norton, J.A., Fineberg, N.S., Vinicor, F., Cohen, S.J. and Clark, C.M. (1986) The diabetes education study: a controlled trial of the effects of diabetes patient education. *Diabetes Care*, **9**, 1–10

Miller, L.V., Goldstein, J. and Nicolaisen, G. (1978) Evaluation of patients' knowledge of diabetes self–care. *Diabetes Care*, **1**, 275–280

Nunnally, J.C. and Durham, R.L. (1975) Validity, reliability, and special problems of measurement in evaluation research. In E. L. Struening, and M. Guttentag (eds). *Handbook of Evaluation Research*. (Vol. 1). London: Sage Publications

Padgett, D., Mumford, E., Hynes, M. and Carter, R. (1988) Meta-analysis of the effects of educational and psychosocial interventions in the management of diabetes mellitus. *Journal of Clinical Epidemiology*, **41**, 1007–1030

Simon, J.W. and Stewart, M.M. (1976) Assessing patient knowledge about diabetes. *Mount Sinai Journal of Medicine New York*, **43** (2), 189–202

Tu, K-S., McDaniel, G. and Gay, J.T. (1993). Diabetes self-care knowledge, behaviours, and metabolic control of older adults - the effect of a post-educational follow-up program. *The Diabetes Educator*, **19**(1), 25–30

Welborn, T., Garcia-Webb, P., Bonser, A., McCann, V. and Constable, I. (1983). Clinical criteria that reflect C-peptide status in idiopathic diabetes. *Diabetes Care*, **6**, 315

Welch, G., Beeney, L.J., Dunn, S.M. and Smith, R.B.W. (1993) The development of the Diabetes Integration scale: A psychometric study of the ATT39. (in press in *Journal of Multivariate Experimental Clinical Research*)

Williams, T.F., Martin, D.A., Hogan, M.D., Watkins, J.D. and Ellis, E.V. (1967) The clinical picture of diabetes control, studied in four settings. *American Journal of Public Health*, **57**, 441–451

Windsor, R.A., Roseman, J., Gartseff, G. and Kirk, K.A. (1981) Qualitative issues in developing educational diagnostic instruments and assessment procedures for diabetic patients. *Diabetes Care*, **4**, 468–475

Wise, P.H., Dowlatshahi, D.C., Farrant, S., Fromson, S. and Meadows, K.A. (1986) Effect of computer-based learning on diabetes knowledge and control. *Diabetes Care*, **9**, 504

CHAPTER 10

MEASURES OF COGNITIVE FUNCTION

CHRISTOPHER M. RYAN

*Department of Psychiatry, University of Pittsburgh School of Medicine, Western Psychiatric
Institute and Clinic, 3811 O'Hara Street, Pittsburgh, PA 15213, USA*

INTRODUCTION

Both Type 1 and Type 2 diabetic adults have a greatly increased risk of developing mild cognitive impairments. Individuals in poor metabolic control who have a long history of hyperglycaemic-associated biomedical complications (e.g., peripheral neuropathy; retinopathy) may manifest a variety of cognitive deficits. These range from a subtle reduction in mental efficiency (e.g., Ryan *et al.*, 1992) through relatively circumscribed memory impairments (Reaven *et al.*, 1990) to a true "diabetic encephalopathy" characterized by widespread central nervous system (CNS) damage and gross dementia (Reske-Nielsen *et al.*, 1965). Yet the micro- and macrovascular complications of hyperglycaemia are not the only causes or correlates of cognitive impairment in the diabetic adult. Insulin-induced hypoglycaemia can also produce significant neuropsychological dysfunction. Although it has long been known that a single episode of severe hypoglycaemia may be sufficient to cause extensive CNS damage in humans (Chalmers *et al.* 1991; Kalimo & Olsson, 1980) and animals (Auer, 1986), a number of recent reports have suggested that repeated episodes of mild to moderately severe hypoglycaemia may also produce detectable cognitive deficits that are thought to be permanent (Langan *et al.*, 1991; Wredling *et al.*, 1990).

Delineating the nature and extent of cognitive impairment is a primary goal of the neuropsychological, or neurobehavioural, evaluation. By administering a comprehensive battery of tests, the neuropsychologist is not only able to identify cognitive strengths and weaknesses, but can often draw inferences about the integrity of certain brain structures or neural systems. Furthermore, by correlating neuropsychological profiles with biomedical and psychosocial characteristics of the patient, the neuropsychologist may also succeed in identifying those factors that increase the risk of developing significant neuropsychological impairment.

Compared to electroencephalographic (EEG) or neuroimaging techniques like computerised tomography (CT) and magnetic resonance imaging (MRI), the neuropsychological examination has both advantages and disadvantages. Its greatest advantage is that it may be more sensitive to mild brain dysfunction than either EEG or neuroimaging techniques. Its greatest disadvantage is that there is no single neuropsychological test, or battery of neuropsychological tests, that is universally considered as THE measure of cognitive function. Neurologists around the world agree on the basic parameters of an EEG or a CT or an MRI examination; that is not the case with neuropsychologists. As a consequence, any discussion of neuropsychological assessment of diabetic adults (or, in fact, adults with virtually any type of medical or neuropsychiatric disorder) will require a review of myriad tests that vary widely not only in their psychometric properties, but in their "acceptability" within the neuropsychological community.

In this chapter I describe and critically evaluate those neuropsychological tests that have been used most frequently in studies of Type 1 and Type 2 diabetic adults, and provide a brief summary of recent research findings. To help organize this discussion, I shall present measures according to cognitive domain. One should keep in mind that this organisational scheme reflects my own biases and experiences as well as the types of neuropsychological evaluations conducted on diabetic adults. Because any given test may draw on several different cognitive processes, the assignment of test to domain may be a somewhat arbitrary decision.

NEUROPSYCHOLOGICAL MEASURES

Most neuropsychological studies of diabetic adults have been conducted to answer the following series of questions:

1) Is diabetes mellitus associated with neuropsychological impairment?
2) If so, are certain cognitive skills, and specific brain regions, more vulnerable than others?
3) Can biomedical and psychosocial factors be identified that increase the risk of developing such impairment?

To answer those questions, investigators have relied not on a single test, but on a series of tests drawn from different sources, and sensitive to various cognitive domains. With few exceptions, these studies have been cross-sectional; diabetic patients have been evaluated at only one point in time and their performance compared either with published norms or, more frequently, with a demographically similar group of nondiabetic control subjects. Because of time constraints, a limited series of tests has usually been administered – typically during a single session lasting no more than about two hours. Very extensive evaluations requiring four or more hours (e.g. Ryan *et al.*, 1991) tend to be rare.

Measures of Global Neuropsychological Functioning

Ideally, one would like to use a test battery that samples all cognitive processes in a comprehensive fashion. Unfortunately, this ideal has never been fully realised. In the United States, there are only two neuropsychological test batteries that aspire to being comprehensive: the Halstead-Reitan and the Luria-Nebraska. The more recently developed of the two, the Luria-Nebraska Neuropsychological Battery (Golden *et al.* 1981), has two different forms of 269 or 279 items, can be completed in approximately two hours, and yields twelve Clinical Scales, eight Localization Scales, and five Summary Scales (see Golden & Maruish, 1985 for detailed discussion). Although it is now widely used in clinical practice, it has not been used in published studies of diabetic adults. Whether that reflects the preferences (or biases) of certain investigators or whether it reflects inherent limitations of the instrument (e.g. an insensitivity to relatively subtle impairment; a relatively "shallow" sampling of various cognitive domains) is not clear. On the other hand, the Halstead-Reitan Neuropsychological Battery has been used by several investigators studying diabetic adults, and is discussed in more detail below.

Halstead-Reitan Neuropsychological Battery (HRNB)

This battery is still considered by most North American clinicians as the "gold standard" for determining neuropsychological impairment. First developed in the 1930s by Ward Halstead (Halstead, 1947), and subsequently modified somewhat by Ralph Reitan (Reitan & Wolfson, 1993), the HRNB now consists of nine tests. Those tests marked by an asterisk have been used frequently as "stand alone" tests and are described in more detail under specific cognitive domains. The standard HRNB includes 1) Category Test*, 2) Speech-Sounds Perception Test, 3) Seashore Rhythm Test, 4) Tactual Performance Test (TPT)*, 5) Trailmaking Test*, 6) Reitan-Klove Sensory Perceptual Examination, 7) Reitan-Indiana Aphasia Examination, 8) Lateral Dominance Examination (including Grip Strength), and 9) Finger Tapping Test*. In addition, the Wechsler Adult Intelligence Scale (WAIS; WAIS-R), discussed below, is also considered an integral part of the HRNB neuropsychological assessment.

The HRNB was developed before the age of sophisticated neuroimaging techniques, and thus served two diagnostic functions: 1) to determine the presence or absence of clinically significant brain damage, and 2) to estimate its severity. Although a number of different strategies have subsequently been developed for interpreting results from the entire battery (see Golden *et al.* 1981), the most common strategy is to calculate an "Impairment Index". Based on results from several early validation studies, cut-off scores for clinically significant brain damage were established for each test variable. The Impairment Index is the proportion of variables that fall in the "brain damaged" range. Remarkably, there is no consensus as to the number of variables that should comprise this Impairment Index, and anywhere from 7 to 12 different variables have been included. Both Golden and associates (1981) and Reitan and Wolfson (1993) have suggested including the following 7 variables in the Impairment Index. Cut-off values for brain damage are in parentheses: Category Test Errors (51 or more errors); TPT Total Time (15.7 or more minutes); TPT Memory (4 or fewer blocks); TPT Location (5 or fewer blocks); Seashore Rhythm (6 or more errors); Speech Perception (8 or more errors); Nondominant Finger Tapping (< 46 taps/10 sec trial). Thus, an individual with "impaired" or "brain damaged" scores on TPT Total Time, Category Test, Finger Tapping, and Speech Perception would have an Impairment Index of 0.57; any impairment index that exceeds 0.40 is considered to be abnormal. Russell and associates (1970) have published a somewhat different scheme insofar as they include more variables in their Impairment Index, and also rate severity of impairment for each variable on a five point scale, rather than using a normal/abnormal dichotomy.

Although the HRNB is very well validated in the sense that individuals with neurological evidence of brain damage perform poorly on it, there are a number of disadvantages associated with its use. First, it is a very time-intensive procedure; individuals with even mild neurologic involvement may require four or five hours to complete the battery. Second, it does not provide a comprehensive assessment of all cognitive domains. For example, learning and memory processes — which tend to be very sensitive to virtually any type of brain insult (Kapur, 1988) — are examined in a most superficial manner (TPT Memory score), and attentional processes – which are also affected by transient brain dysfunction — are not explicitly tested. For that reason the most reliable information provided by the HRNB is captured by the Impairment Index: the dichotomous diagnostic decision as to whether or not a person has clinically significant neuropsychological impairment. Finally, most earlier work with this battery has neglected to take into account demographic variables like age, education, and gender. Indeed, prior to the publication of norms by Heaton and associates (1991), many normal elderly subjects or normal young subjects with low educational levels were mis-classified as "impaired" because the cut-off scores for brain-damage did not consider the fact that performance on most neuropsychological tests is influenced significantly by both age and education.

To date, three groups of investigators have used the complete HRNB to evaluate neuropsychological status of diabetic adults. In the earliest report, published only as a long abstract, Rennick et al. (1968) attempted to test the hypothesis that the microvascular complications of diabetes, as indexed by clinically significant retinopathy, may adversely affect the central nervous system. Administering the HRNB to a group of 52 diabetic adults (mean age = 40 years) and calculating an Impairment Index comprised of 12 scores, they found that the Impairment Index for subjects with retinopathy was significantly higher (0.515; "impaired") than the Impairment Index for those without retinopathy (0.303; within normal limits). This was interpreted as suggesting that diabetic individuals with retinopathy may have mild chronic cerebral dysfunction.

Using the same test battery, Skenazy and Bigler (1984) compared adults with less and more severe diabetes (as indexed by number of hospitalisations and diabetes-related complications). They did not, however, use an Impairment Index to summarise HRNB scores; rather, they reported results for each of the eighteen HRNB test variables. Compared to subjects who had a less severe course of diabetes, those patients with a more severe form performed worse on some tests, but better on others. The large number of comparisons and the heterogeneous results makes it impossible to draw coherent conclusions about the presence of significant neuropsychological deficit. A better strategy would have been to use a summary measure, like the Impairment Index. An alternate statistical solution would have been to group several related HRNB variables together and use multivariate statistical procedures.

The power of this latter strategy, that is, conducting a multivariate analysis of the HRNB, has been illustrated by Baade (1988). Thirty five diabetic adults were compared with an equal number of controls matched in age (mean = 30 yrs), education (mean = 24.5 yrs) and gender (31% male) on an expanded HRNB. Test variables were assigned to one of four cognitive domains: Cognitive / Motor Speed (Trail Making A & B); Attention / Memory (Seashore Rhythm; Speech Sounds; TPT Memory; TPT Location); Nonverbal Problem Solving (Category Test; TPT Total Time); and Sensory Motor (Grip Strength; Finger Tapping; Finger Recognition; Finger Tip Writing, Tactile Form Recognition). Using Hoteling's Multivariate T^2 statistical procedure, Baade found the diabetic group was more impaired than the control group in all but the Cognitive / Motor Speed domain (and that would have been significant with a somewhat larger sample size). In each domain, when the multivariate t was significant, univariate-ts were computed for each test comprising the domain. Inspection of the eighteen individual HRNB test scores reveals that only six were statistically significant. Had this multivariate procedure not been used, a sceptic could have argued that the pattern of results made no sense conceptually and that the handful of statistically significant differences merely reflected chance. The use of the multivariate procedure leads one to reach a more interpretable conclusion: namely, that because multivariate differences are found on four of five cognitive domains, diabetes mellitus leads to a mild, generalized cognitive dysfunction. However, Baade went on to say that because of the very large standard deviations found in the diabetic group, it is possible that "a subset of the diabetics may have contributed disproportionately to the group differences". The absence of statistically significant between-group differences on the majority of tests suggests that certain tests are far more sensitive than others to neuropsychological impairment. In this particular study, the various subtests from the Tactual Performance Test, and the dominant and nondominant Finger Tapping scores best discriminated between the two groups.

Ascertainment of Intelligence

Wechsler Adult Intelligence Scale (WAIS; WAIS-R)

Performance on virtually any neuropsychological test is likely to be influenced by the individual's general level of intelligence. All other things being equal, a brighter individual will make fewer errors, and perform faster, than someone less bright. It is for that reason that ascertaining the subject's intelligence is critical for interpreting their neuropsychological test results. But how does one do this? The best known individually administered intelligence test is the Wechsler Adult Intelligence Scale (WAIS / WAIS-R; Wechsler, 1955, 1981). With "normal" populations the WAIS is used to estimate intelligence and determine the Intelligence Quotient (IQ). However, because some subtests of the WAIS / WAIS-R are remarkably sensitive to brain dysfunction, the WAIS itself is "contaminated" as a pure measure of IQ in those individuals who have developed brain damage. These characteristics have led to the application of the WAIS / WAIS-R as a global neuropsychological test battery. Amongst clinical researchers studying diabetic adults (and every other kind of patient with a medical or neurologic disorder), the WAIS / WAIS-R, or selected subtests, are the most frequently used measures of neuropsychological functioning (see Lezak, 1983).

Before discussing how the Wechsler Intelligence Scales can be used both to estimate premorbid intelligence (or intellectual potential) and to estimate neuropsychological dysfunction, I will briefly describe relevant characteristics of this measure. An excellent, very detailed description can be found in Kaufman (1990). The WAIS (1955) and WAIS-R (1981) are composed of eleven subtests organised into *Verbal* (Information, Vocabulary, Comprehension, Similarities, Arithmetic, Digit Span) and *Performance* (Picture Completion, Block Design, Object Assembly, Picture Arrangement, and Digit Symbol Substitution) subtest. Scores on both scales are influenced to a very large extent by age and education. A recent report from Kaufman *et al.* (1989) has demonstrated that age alone accounts for 3.1% of the variance in the Verbal IQ score but 28.2% of the Performance IQ, whereas education accounts for 45.1% of the variance in Verbal IQ and 32.9% of the Performance IQ.

Together, three IQ scores can be obtained: a Verbal IQ (VIQ), a Performance IQ (PIQ), and a Full Scale IQ (FSIQ), each normed in such a way that the mean score is 100 and the standard deviation is 15. Because the FSIQ is a composite of the Verbal and the Performance IQ scores, it provides no additional independent information. Thus, in examining between-group differences in IQ, I recommend reporting either the VIQ *and* PIQ scores, or the FSIQ. Each of the eleven subscales yields a raw score which is converted into a "scaled score" (used in the IQ calculation) and an "age scaled score." All scaled scores have a mean of ten and a standard deviation of three. Because the age scaled score compares the individual with others who are similar in age, this is the score that should be used in presenting results from each subtest.

Although the most recent revision of the WAIS (the WAIS-R) was published in 1981, many reports through the 1980s and into the 1990s are based on results from the earlier WAIS. For example, as part of the neuropsychological assessment used by the Diabetes Control and Complications Trial (DCCT), the WAIS, and not the WAIS-R, was administered (see Ryan *et al.*, 1991). Knowing whether the WAIS or the WAIS-R was administered is critical in comparing IQ scores from different studies, and in making neuropsychological interpretations. There is general agreement that the WAIS-R is a more conservative instrument in the sense that it yields IQ scores that are significantly lower (median difference is 5.9 to 6.5 points) than those obtained from the original WAIS (see Ryan *et al.*, 1987).

As stated earlier, the Wechsler Intelligence Scales can be used to estimate premorbid intelligence, and to identify neuropsychological impairment. A useful model that operationalizes those differences has been provided by Horn (1985), who makes a distinction between "crystallized intelligence" (Information, Vocabulary, Comprehension, and Similarities subtests) and "fluid intelligence" (Picture Completion, Picture Arrangement, Block Design, Object Assembly, Similarities and Digit Span). For our purposes, crystallized intelligence reflects education- and experience-based knowledge; this tends to be a well-practiced, highly overlearned knowledge base (which also tends to be largely verbal in nature). Because it draws on highly overlearned information, "crystallized intelligence" tends to be more resistant to the effects of mild diffuse damage, and hence can serve as an estimate of premorbid intelligence in adults. Fluid intelligence, on the other hand, reflects adaptive problem-solving ability. That is, the individual must approach an unfamiliar problem (which more often than not is nonverbal in nature) in a novel way, and reach a solution quickly. Mild diffuse brain damage is far more likely to affect "fluid intelligence" and hence the subtest scores that reflect fluid intelligence tend to be the best indicators of neuropsychological impairment. Stated another way, Performance scales can be thought of as providing an indicator of *current* intellectual functioning. Often, investigators will use the entire Performance scale as an indicator of "fluid intelligence". I think the distinction between crystallized (or premorbid) and fluid intelligence is quite useful from a neuropsychological perspective. Small differences between the two are likely to have little clinical import. On the other hand, when estimates of fluid intelligence are lower than estimates of crystallized (or premorbid) intelligence, *and* when impairments are found on other types of neuropsychological tests, significant neuropsychological dysfunction is likely to be present.

A number of investigators studying diabetic adults have usually found large Verbal / Performance (or crystallized / fluid) differences, with Performance IQ scores being significantly lower. In a recent study comparing 188 diabetic adults with 148 age, education, and socioeconomic status (SES)-matched control subjects (Ryan *et al.*, 1993), we found that the diabetic group earned WAIS-R PIQs that were significantly lower than those earned by controls, whereas there were no statistically reliable differences in VIQ. We have interpreted this pattern as indicating that the two groups were similar in their premorbid (pre-diabetes) level of cognitive functioning or intellectual potential, but that a long history of diabetes has affected the central nervous system subtly, resulting in a reduction in overall neuropsychological efficiency, as indexed by a reduction in fluid intelligence (here defined by PIQ). Using the WAIS, rather than the WAIS-R, Skenazy and Bigler (1984), observed the same VIQ/PIQ pattern when comparing diabetic and nondiabetic subjects.

Other strategies for estimating premorbid intelligence

Because the entire WAIS / WAIS-R may require 60 to 90 minutes to administer, and as much as an additional 30 to 45 minutes to score, there is increasing reluctance to use it in clinical research studies where only a limited amount of time is available for subject assessment. This is especially the case when a battery of other neuropsychological measures is to be administered. As a consequence, more investigators are beginning to use briefer versions of the WAIS-R that include between two and four subtests, are using prediction equations based on demographic data, or are using alternate tests.

Many brief versions of the WAIS-R are now available. In his excellent review of this topic, Kaufman (1990; chapter 5) indicated that a two-subtest battery – Information and Picture Completion – can be completed in twelve minutes or less and correlates 0.88 with Full Scale IQ. Although the Vocabulary and Block Design dyad has a marginally higher average correlation with Full Scale IQ ($r = 0.91$), those two subtests take significantly longer to administer, and are more difficult to score. Correlations between single subtests and WAIS-R summary scores can be found in the WAIS-R Manual (Wechsler, 1981). According to data from the WAIS-R standardization sample averaged across all ages, Information alone correlates 0.79 with VIQ whereas Vocabulary correlates 0.85 with VIQ; Picture Completion alone correlates 0.65 with PIQ whereas Block Design correlates 0.70 with PIQ. This suggests to me that while brief batteries (even single subtests) may provide reasonable estimates of VIQ, no single subtest provides a good estimate of PIQ.

A very different approach to estimating intelligence has been applied by several investigators who have used multiple regression techniques to predict IQ from demographic variables (Crawford, 1989). In an early study, Wilson and associates (1978; 1979) used the following equation to predict WAIS Full Scale IQ: 0.17(age) - 1.53(sex) - 11.33(race) + 2.97(education) + 1.01(occupation) + 74.05. This has been simplified by Karzmark *et al.* (1985), who used only the following: FSIQ = 2.10(education) + 85.34. In a cross-validation study with 246 subjects, Karzmark and associates found that the predicted IQ was within 10 points of the actual WAIS Full Scale IQ in 66% of the cases. More recently, Barona and associates (1984) used the WAIS-R standardisation sample of 1,880 subjects (Wechsler, 1981) to estimate VIQ, PIQ, and FSIQ. For example, VIQ = 54.23 + 0.49(WAIS-R age group) + 1.92(sex) + 4.24(race) + 5.25(education group) + 1.89(occupation group) + 1.24(urban/rural residence). The standard error of estimate of VIQ was found to be 11.79. Similar formulae for PIQ and FSIQ, as well as operational definitions of specific demographic variables, can be found in Barona *et al.* (1984). In the absence of actual IQ test data, these demographic predictor equations provide a reasonable "ball park" estimate not of a numerical IQ score, but of the range (e.g., "average", "bright average," "superior") within which that particular individual is most likely to fall.

An alternate strategy that has recently received much attention is the administration of tests which differ from the traditional Wechsler tests but are thought to provide relatively uncontaminated estimates of premorbid functioning. One measure which is becoming increasingly popular is the NART — the National Adult Reading Test (Nelson, 1982). This oral reading test (sometimes referred to as the *New* Adult Reading Test) consists of between 50 (Nelson, 1982) and 61 (Blair &

Spreen, 1989) short words that do not follow the standard rules of pronunciation (e.g. corps; reify; synecdoche). There is much converging evidence (see Crawford, 1992 for review) to suggest that the NART provides a better estimate of Verbal IQ than does the Vocabulary subtest from the WAIS, especially in patients with dementia who have been followed over time (cf. O'Carroll *et al.*, 1987). The NART also appears to predict WAIS VIQ better than the demographic formulae described above, leading Crawford (1992) to suggest that it is the best available estimate of premorbid functioning.

A very recent study of diabetic adults elegantly illustrates the utility of comparing premorbid intelligence estimates with measures of fluid intelligence to determine whether specific biomedical complications of diabetes adversely affect cognitive functioning. Studying a group of adults who developed Type 1 diabetes after nineteen years of age, Langan *et al.* (1991) categorised subjects either as having no previous history of severe hypoglycaemia (N = 24) or having five or more previous episodes (N = 23). To estimate "decrement" in functioning, they calculated the difference between premorbid IQ (NART estimated IQ) and WAIS-R Performance IQ, which was considered to reflect current level of intellectual efficiency. They found that subjects in the repeated hypoglycaemia group manifested a significantly larger difference (7.9 points) between premorbid and current IQ estimates than did subjects in the no hypoglycaemic group (2.1 point difference) and concluded that repeated episodes of severe hypoglycaemia produce decrements in intelligence. It is important to keep in mind, however, that despite the fact that the two groups were similar on estimates of premorbid intelligence but differed on measures of current or fluid intelligence, we have no *direct* evidence that subjects in the repeated hypoglycaemia group have actually deteriorated intellectually over time. Because these data are cross-sectional rather than longitudinal, the use of the term "decrement" is inappropriate. Nevertheless, the resulting comparisons are consistent with the view that repeated severe hypoglycaemia is likely to affect certain cognitive processes adversely.

Specialized Measures of Attention

Attention is a fundamental cognitive process that is an integral part of every neuropsychological test. Because all tests are "contaminated" to some extent by attentional processes, the identification of attentional dysfunction is a most difficult undertaking. Adding to this difficulty is the fact that attention has never been conceptualized as a unitary process, but is thought of as having a number of components. In their very recent neuropsychological model of attention, Mirsky *et al.* (1991) have identified three major components that can be examined with neuropsychological measures. The first component emphasises the ability to focus, or selectively attend to a single target and screen out irrelevant distractors. "Simple", "choice", and "go/no go" reaction time paradigms provide measures of this very basic attentional process. Tests that provide measures of "mental flexibility" (e.g. Trail Making; Stroop Colour/Word Test) are also often described as being sensitive to selective or focussed attention. The second component emphasises the ability to sustain attention or be alert over an extended period of time. So-called vigilance tests can be used to measure this characteristic. The third component emphasizes the ability to shift attention either from one part of space to another, or from one type of response to another. This attentional component is typically investigated with complex information-processing tasks borrowed from the experimental psychology laboratory. The Posner task (Posner *et al.*, 1984) is one such measure that has been used by a number of investigators, but to my knowledge, not with diabetic patient populations.

Because the structural and neurochemical systems underlying attention are widely distributed throughout the brain, measures of attention are generally considered to be extremely sensitive to brain damage, and for that reason are thought to be an important component of any neuropsychological evaluation. However, because attentional processes are also sensitive to almost any kind of transient organismic (e.g. metabolic; drug-induced) or environmental (e.g., noise) perturbation, tests of attention have been used extensively in recent studies assessing the effects of experimentally-induced changes in plasma blood glucose levels in diabetic children (Ryan *et al.*, 1990) and adults (Hoffman *et al.* 1989; Holmes *et al.*, 1983, 1986, 1988; Herold *et al.*, 1985; Pramming *et al.*, 1986), as well as in adults without diabetes (Mitrakou *et al.*, 1991).

Reaction time

Several different reaction time paradigms have been used. Earlier studies (e.g. Holmes *et al.*, 1983) used equipment manufactured by Lafayette Instruments, but at the present time there are a number of excellent reaction time programmes for personal computers. In all instances, the subject is presented with a warning cue, followed immediately, or after a time period, with the onset of one or more stimuli. The task is to make a particular type of response (usually a key-press; sometimes a verbal response) as quickly as possible. In the "simple reaction time" paradigm, subjects know that each trial will have only a single target; when it appears, they make the designated response. This task can be thought of as providing an estimate of the time needed to register the stimulus (perception; simple attention) and make the appropriate motor response. In the "choice reaction time" paradigm, subjects are presented with two or more stimuli, only one of which is designated as the target. When the target comes on, they make a particular response (e.g. press left key); when a non-target comes on, they make either no response ("go/no go" paradigm) or a different response (e.g. press right key - - "choice" paradigm). Errors made during the "go/no go" paradigm provide an estimate of impulsivity; time taken to make the correct response on the choice paradigm provides an estimate of decision-making efficiency. At a minimum, twenty test trials should be administered and the median response time (in milliseconds), rather than the mean response time across trials, should be used as the outcome measure.

These tasks have been used with a great deal of success in evaluating the effects of transient hypoglycaemia on cognitive functioning in diabetic individuals. Both simple and choice reaction time increase with relatively mild hypoglycaemia in children (e.g. Ryan *et al.*, 1990) and adults (Holmes *et al.*, 1983, 1986). Remarkably, performance on choice reaction time tasks does not recover immediately following return to euglycaemia, but may require as much as forty five minutes or an hour (Herold *et al.*, 1985) for full recovery. Choice reaction time is also significantly slower in euglycaemic diabetic adults who have a history of repeated episodes of severe hypoglycaemia (Langan *et al.*, 1991).

Digit vigilance

This subtest from the Repeatable Cognitive Perceptual Motor Battery (Lewis & Rennick, 1979) consists of two pages of numbers. The subject's task is to cross out all the sixes (or, as an alternate version, all the nines) as quickly as possible. The time taken to complete each page, and the number of omission errors made, are the two variables of interest. This test provides an excellent measure of sustained attention, and has been used in a number of studies with diabetic adults. For example, a recent report from the Pittsburgh group (Ryan *et al.*, 1992) demonstrated that adults with onset of diabetes in childhood performed more slowly (but made no more errors) than a group of demographically similar nondiabetic control subjects. Subsequent regression analyses indicated that the best predictor of slowed responding was a diagnosis of clinically significant peripheral neuropathy. The Diabetes Control and Complications Trial has also had extensive experience with this measure, and have found it to be extremely effective in identifying those diabetic subjects who manifest clinically significant neuropsychological deterioration over time (Lan *et al.* in press).

The Digit Vigilance Test can be thought of as a "low-tech" measure of sustained attention. Mirsky and associates (1991) have developed a number of continuous performance tests that have a similar goal. The subject sits in front of a computer terminal and responds every time a designated target occurs. The sensitivity of the task can be increased by increasing the complexity of the target (e.g. only respond when a X appears immediately after the letter A). A number of manufacturers now produce such software for use with various types of personal computers.

WAIS Digit Span

This provides a clinical measure of "span of apprehension". The classic view (Norman, 1969) is that one can attend to seven (plus or minus two) items at one time. Individuals with psychiatric illness or moderately severe brain dysfunction tend to have a significantly lower attention span. The Wechsler Digit Span subtest, which is the most commonly used span measure, actually has two components: Forward Digit Span (repeating up to nine digits immediately after having heard them), and Backward Digit Span (immediately after hearing up to eight digits, repeating them backward). Typically, the total of the two component scores is used for the calculation of the Digit Span Scaled Score. However, it is only the Forward Span (i.e. the longest digit span repeated by the subject) which provides an estimate of attention. On the other hand, Backward Span is a far more complex test because it requires both attention and mental reorganization. One may be better off considering this as a measure of "mental flexibility" or "working memory". Again, the best way to record backward span is either longest span, or total number of trials prior to a failure (missing two trials in a row). Although span measures have been used by a number of investigators, studies using either a composite WAIS-R scaled score or only Digits Forwards have usually failed to differentiate diabetic adults from nondiabetic control subjects (e.g. Dejgaard *et al.*, 1991; Reaven *et al.*, 1990; Mattlar *et al.*, 1985; Mooradian *et al.* 1988). It is noteworthy, however, that Wredling and associates (1990) found that Forward Digit Span was apparently reduced by repeated episodes of severe hypoglycaemia.

Psychomotor Efficiency and "Mental Flexibility"

Mental flexibility and psychomotor efficiency are terms that refer to a construct or cognitive process that is not well defined or conceptualised. We have used the term to include measures that require the individual not only to pay attention but also to engage in additional mental reorganization, and then respond as rapidly as possible (e.g. Ryan *et al.*, 1992). Excellent examples of this would be tasks like an Embedded Figures Test (find the design hidden in the complex pattern as quickly as possible) or Digit Span Backwards. Tasks which require the subject to engage in complex eye/hand coordination (pick the key shaped peg, use visual and tactile information to rotate it so that it fits into the keyhole, and do this as quickly as possible) would also fall under that category. Many writers do not regard "mental flexibility" to be a viable cognitive domain. For example, Mirsky and associates (1991) would consider some of these tasks to be attentional, and to fall specifically under the "selective attention" rubric.

Our work with adults has demonstrated that many measures of "mental flexibility" differentiate Type 1 diabetic from nondiabetic adults (e.g. Ryan *et al.*, 1992; 1993). It is noteworthy that many diabetic adolescents also tend to perform slower on these types of tasks (e.g. Grooved Pegboard; Digit Symbol Substitution) as compared with their nondiabetic siblings and peers (Ryan *et al.*, 1984). Further, these tasks tend to be very sensitive to transient changes in ambient blood glucose level. Diabetic adolescents show significant psychomotor slowing at relatively mild (ca. 65 mg/dl; 3.6 mM) levels of hypoglycaemia (Ryan *et al.*, 1990), whereas diabetic and nondiabetic adults do not show changes until blood glucose levels have fallen into the moderate (ca. 45 mg/dl; 2.5 mM) hypoglycaemia range (e.g. Mitrakou 202*et al.* 1991).

WAIS Digit Symbol Substitution Test

On this Wechsler Performance subtest, the individual is presented with a series of nine digits, each paired with a symbol. Below the code are a series of numbers alone; the subject is told to draw the correct symbol underneath each number as quickly as possible. This task places a premium on attention, rapid responding, visual scanning (keeping track of where one is on the page) and associative learning (learning the digit-symbol code), and has proven to be extremely sensitive to even mild brain dysfunction (Lezak, 1983). One can either convert the raw score (total number of items completed in 90 seconds) into a Wechsler Age-scaled score, or one can use the ninety second raw score, or a time score (time taken to complete the entire array). Because the measure is extremely sensitive to the effects of normal aging, raw scores must be age-corrected in some fashion.

The Digit Symbol Substitution Test has been used in studies of both Type 1 and Type 2 diabetic adults. It appears that older Type 2 subjects are more likely to manifest significant performance decrements, relative to nondiabetic comparison subjects (e.g. Perlmuter et al., 1984; Reaven et al., 1990), than are younger Type 1 diabetic subjects (e.g. Ryan et al., 1992; Franceschi et al. 1984). Studies examining the effects of experimentally induced hypoglycaemia have also used this task. For example, Stevens et al. (1989) noted large decrements in performance on this task when blood glucose levels fell from 4.9 mM (88 mg/dl) to 3.4 mM (61 mg/dl).

The Symbol Digit Modalities Test (SDMT)

This test, developed by Smith (1973), can be thought of as an alternate version of Digit Symbol Substitution Test. On this task, the individual is presented with symbols and has to substitute numbers as quickly as possible. The advantage to this particular version is that the response measure (writing or saying numbers) is more familiar to individuals, and hence may be less threatening, particularly to individuals who are quite impaired. Unlike the DSST, an oral response can be made on the SDMT; for that reason, the test can also be administered to individuals with finger or hand mobility problems. Like the DSST, the SDMT has excellent psychometric properties, with normative data available on subjects 18 to 74 years of age. This test has been used in studies of both Type 1 (Dejgaard et al. 1991) and Type 2 (U'ren et al., 1990) diabetic adults. As was the case with the DSST, elderly Type 2 diabetic adults are more likely to show impairment on this measure than are younger Type 1 subjects.

Trail Making Test

Trail making is a widely used paper and pencil test that is appropriate for subjects of all ages (Boll, 1981). The task has two components. Part A presents the subject with a page on which the numbers 1 to 25 are arranged randomly. The task is to draw a line connecting the numbers as quickly as possible. Part B presents the subject with both numbers and letters. Here the task is to alternate between numbers and letters sequentially (1-A-2-B etc), again, as quickly as possible. The primary outcome measure is time taken to complete the task. When subjects make an error they are corrected by the examiner (who does not stop the clock), and they go on. This task places an emphasis on a number of cognitive processes (e.g. attention, visual tracking, sequencing, mental and motor speed) and for that reason is quite sensitive to any type of mild, diffusely distributed CNS dysfunction. Indeed, because this test has been used widely in many clinical settings, cut-off scores for clinically significant impairment have been established. Heaton and associates (1991) provide excellent age-, education-, and gender-corrected norms in that regard. Unfortunately, one needs to keep in mind that performance decrements are not unequivocally diagnostic of brain dysfunction. For example, individuals with psychomotor retardation secondary to depression are likely to perform quite poorly on this task. This test has been used very successfully in a number of small scale studies examining the acute effects of hypo- and hyperglycaemia both in children (Ryan et al., 1991) and adults (Hoffman et al., 1989; Ipp & Forster, 1987; Mitrakou et al. 1991; Pramming et al. 1986). Our work with diabetic children (Ryan et al., 1991) indicated that Trails B performance was perfectly correlated with glycaemic level. As blood glucose levels dropped into the mild hypoglycaemic range (65 mg/dl; 3.6 mM), Trails B times increased, falling in the clinically impaired range. Immediately upon restoration of euglycaemia, Trails B scores returned to the pre-study baseline level. Trail Making has been less successful in large-scale studies comparing euglycaemic diabetic children (Ryan et al., 1984) or adults (Dejgaard et al., 1991) with age-appropriate nondiabetic comparison subjects (but see Skenazy & Bigler, 1984). For example, we have rarely found statistically reliable between-group differences in those types of comparisons (Ryan et al., 1992). This failure may reflect the fact that Trails B is so sensitive to so many kinds of "aberrations" that the within-group variance is excessive – for patient groups as well as for comparison groups drawn from the general population. On the other hand, at least one research group has noted significant differences between Type 2 diabetic adults and age-matched nondiabetic comparison subjects on this measure (Reaven et al., 1990). Several investigators have recently modified the test so that it can be administered on a computer (e.g. Reichard et al. 1991; Stevens et al. 1989). While the computerized Trails tests may provide excellent "stand alone" measures of mental efficiency, their clinical comparability to the standard paper and pencil version of Trail Making has not yet been thoroughly investigated.

Stroop Colour-Word Interference Test

Several different versions of this test exist. The version developed by Golden (1978) may be used most frequently, perhaps because it is readily available. The task is usually composed of three subtests: reading a page of names of colours ("red," "green," "blue"), naming a page of the same colours (as Xs or colour squares), and naming the colour of the ink in which a different colour word is written. That is, when the word "green" is printed in red ink, the correct response is "red". This third, or interference, subtest serves as the most informative outcome measure. Because this task examines how well the individual can inhibit a highly overlearned or salient response (reading a word) and substitute a less salient response (naming the ink colour), it is often considered to be sensitive to damage to the so-called "frontal system". The number of correct responses made in forty five seconds on each subtest are converted into T scores according to a formula provided by Golden (1978).

This measure has been used only occasionally by investigators studying diabetic and nondiabetic adults. Both Holmes and associates (1984) and Mitrakou *et al.* (1991) found that performance on the colour naming and ink reading (or "interference") subtests were impaired during relatively mild experimentally-induced hypoglycaemia. Unfortunately, because hypoglycaemia may adversely affect normal colour vision (Harrad *et al.*, 1985), it is possible that the response slowing seen on several Stroop subtests during hypoglycaemia is not due to changes within the so-called frontal system, but is secondary to difficulties with hue discrimination.

Grooved Pegboard

At first glance, this motor task appears out of place in a discussion of "mental flexibility". Yet it requires the subject to integrate visuospatial information with fine motor control to make a response as quickly as possible (Rourke *et al.*, 1973). The individual is presented with a series of key-like metal pegs and told to insert them, as quickly as possible, into a board covered with twenty five keyhole-like shapes. The subject first does this with the dominant hand, and then with the nondominant hand. The time taken to complete each trial is the primary outcome measure of interest. Seeing the board and feeling the peg, it is necessary for the subject to rotate the peg between thumb and finger so that it is inserted correctly as rapidly as possible. Our work has indicated that diabetic adults perform this task far more slowly than nondiabetic control subjects (Ryan *et al.*, 1992).

Learning and Memory

Learning and memory measures examine the ability of the individual to acquire or encode new information, store it for a period of time, and retrieve or recall it on demand. Numerous theories have been developed to describe these processes, yet none are entirely satisfactory (for review, see Squire & Butters, 1992). From a neuropsychological perspective, the assessment of learning and memory skills is a critical part of any evaluation, since memory changes often provide the earliest evidence of brain dysfunction (Kapur, 1988).

Most tests of learning require the individual to form associations between unfamiliar items, which are presented repeatedly. The expectation is that with repetition, performance will improve gradually. For example, subjects may be asked to learn a list composed of pairs of unrelated words (e.g. neck/salt; gate/native). In the typical paired-associate learning paradigm, the subject studies (i.e., is presented with) the list of to-be-learned word pairs, and is then tested by presenting the first item of each pair as a clue or cue (Ryan *et al.*, 1987). This study/test procedure is repeated either until the subject masters the list, or until some pre-determined number of study trials occur (usually three to five repetitions of the list). On each subsequent trial, the order of word-pair presentation changes. Paired-associate procedures are very powerful because they provide a great deal of examiner control: a stimulus is presented each time, and one can observe how well the subject is actually able to form stimulus-response associations. An alternate version of this technique is provided by the serial learning paradigm. Here, a single list of words is presented in the same order each time. The task is to learn the word list in order; in a sense, the preceding word becomes the stimulus cue for the next word in the list. In the free recall paradigm, subjects are not provided by the examiner with cuing; rather they must impose their own "subjective" organization onto the list. Memory is assessed by asking the subject to recall recently learned information after a delay. Typically, a delay of thirty minutes is used, but very brief delays may also be used, as a way of examining the integrity of short-term memory.

Wechsler Memory Scale (WMS; WMS-R)

The most widely used "battery" of memory tests is the Wechsler Memory Scale. The earlier scale (Wechsler, 1945) is composed of subtests that examine Orientation to time and place, Mental Control (e.g. count by three beginning with one), Logical Memory (or story recall), Paired-Associate Learning, Digit Span, and Visual Reproductions (immediate recall of four geometric designs). There are numerous problems with this version of the WMS (for critical reviews see Russell, 1981; Prigatano, 1977, 1978). Nevertheless, investigators studying diabetic adults have administered either the entire battery (e.g. Franceschi *et al.*, 1984; Lawson *et al.*, 1984; Skenazy & Bigler, 1984) or selected subtests (e.g. Ryan *et al.* 1992). With the exception of the report of Franceschi *et al.*, there is no evidence that Type 1 diabetic adults show significant impairments on these measures. At the present time, the revised version of the Wechsler Memory Scale (Wechsler, 1987) is in wide clinical use. To my knowledge, it has not yet been used in studies of diabetic adults.

Rey Auditory Verbal Learning Test (AVLT)

This is a free-recall learning test in which the subject hears a list of fifteen words, read at the rate of one word per second (Lezak, 1983). Immediately after hearing the last word, the subject recalls the list in any order. Five such free-recall trials are provided. After the fifth trial, a second list is read as a "distracter" trial, and the subject asked to recall those words. The subject is then asked to recall as many words from the first list as possible. A thirty minute delayed recall, and/or a recognition test ("circle all the words in this paragraph that were in the first list") may also be administered. Norms for healthy adults have recently been published by Wiens *et al.*, (1988) and versions of the word list are now available for English and French children (Bishop *et al.* 1990). Lezak (1983) characterized the AVLT as an excellent test of memory because it not only measures immediate memory span and yields a learning curve, but it has the potential to examine the kinds of organizational or mnemonic strategies the subject uses, and their sensitivity to both proactive and retroactive interference.

This measure has been used by a number of investigators studying verbal learning in both Type 1 and Type 2 diabetic adults. Langan and associates (1991) compared Type 1 adults with and without a history of repeated episodes of severe hypoglycaemia and found no evidence of a hypoglycaemic-induced verbal learning deficit: the two groups performed similarly on the AVLT. In contrast, Mooradian and associates (1988) compared forty three elderly Type 2 diabetic adults with forty one age-matched nondiabetic control subjects and found the diabetic subjects recalled significantly fewer words by the end of the fifth trial.

California Verbal Learning Test (CVLT)

This task is very similar to the AVLT. Using a free-recall paradigm, a sixteen item list is read to the subject five times, followed by a second list of 16 items. Like the AVLT, a sixth recall of the first list is requested immediately after recalling the second list; both long-term free recall of the first list, and long-delay recognition memory are also evaluated. A major difference between the CVLT and the AVLT is that the CVLT words are drawn from four categories: clothing, fruits, tools, and spices and herbs. This allows the examiner to determine whether category cuing will facilitate performance in any way. The test has several advantages over most other learning and memory tests. In addition to the completion of a number of studies demonstrating its excellent psychometric properties, the test can be administered and scored by computer, and a large number of memory and performance measures can be obtained (Delis *et al.*, 1987).

This test has been used by Reaven and associates (1990), in their study of elderly Type 2 diabetic adults. Compared to demographically similar nondiabetic control subjects, their diabetic subjects made fewer correct responses. Of particular interest is the fact that the number of correct responses was correlated with glycosylated haemoglobin level for both the diabetic ($r = -0.57$) and nondiabetic ($r = -0.43$) control subjects: the better the degree of metabolic control, the more words that were recalled.

Benton Visual Retention Test (BVRT)

On this visual memory test, the individual is presented with a series of ten cards, each of which contains two or three geometric designs that differ in size, and in placement on the card. The card is exposed for a period of time, and the subject is asked to draw it from memory either immediately after the end of the exposure period, or after a five to fifteen second delay. Three alternate versions of the test materials are available. Norms that take into account age and level of intelligence are available for administration A (ten sec exposure for each card; immediate recall by drawing), administration B (five sec exposure; immediate recall by drawing) and administration C (copy the design). Detailed scoring criteria permit the identification of six different types of errors (Benton, 1974). An excellent discussion of this measure can be found in Lezak (1983). This test is in wide clinical use, and may be one of the better measures of purely nonverbal memory.

The BVRT has been used in studies of both Type 1 and Type 2 diabetic adults. Mooradian and associates (1988) found that elderly Type 2 diabetic subjects reproduced fewer drawings correctly, and made more errors, than age-matched nondiabetic control subjects. Although Meuter and associates (1980) administered this to younger Type 1 and Type 2 subjects as part of a larger assessment of memory and concentration, they did not report results from this particular test.

Problem-solving and Abstract Reasoning

One of the unfortunate problems besetting neuropsychologists is the absence of good measures of abstract reasoning ability. Although many tests have a significant problem-solving component (e.g., Block Design subtest from the WAIS-R; Raven's Progressive Matrices) there are only three "stand alone" measures of reasoning that are widely accepted clinically and are appropriate for people of "average" intelligence: the Wisconsin Card Sorting Test; the Category Test; and the Tactual Performance Test. One advantage in using any of these three measures is the recent publication by Heaton *et al* (1991) of age- and education-corrected norms.

Wisconsin Card Sorting Test

This deductive reasoning task is generally considered to be an excellent measure of "frontal lobe" function (Robinson *et al.*, 1980). The individual is presented with a series of four "key" cards (one red triangle; two green stars; three yellow crosses; four blue circles), and given a deck of cards. Subjects are told to take a card off the deck and place it under one of the four key cards. If the placement is correct, they will be told; if it is incorrect, they will be informed that it is wrong (but will not be given the correct response). After ten correct responses are made in succession, the examiner shifts to a different organising principle, without informing the subject. Three sorting rules (colour, shape, number) are used twice, and the subject continues until all six are discovered, or until 128 cards (trials) are placed. This task requires the subject to use feedback to modify behaviour, and to use various planning and problem-solving strategies. Although the task is difficult to administer manually, computerised versions of the test are now available, making administration error-free, and providing detailed counts of different types of errors.

This test has been used in studies of both Type 1 and Type 2 diabetic adults, and in each case, has successfully differentiated diabetic from nondiabetic control subjects. Reaven and associates (1990) found that elderly Type 2 diabetic subjects discovered significantly fewer categories than control subjects (3.3 vs 4.9). Similarly, Dejgaard and associates (1991) found that middle-aged adults with diabetes of long duration performed significantly more poorly than the norm.

Category Test

This subtest from the Halstead-Reitan Neuropsychological Battery is a challenging, often frustrating problem-solving task that consists of seven subtests. Like the Wisconsin Card Sorting Test, the subject has to discover the underlying organising principle by making a response (pressing one of four buttons) and using feedback to guide subsequent responses. Unlike the Wisconsin, the Category Test uses stimuli that may be quite complex visually, and may change within a subtest. As a consequence, subjects who are not paying attention to details (or have a visual acuity problem) may perform poorly not because they cannot reason clearly, but because they have missed certain stimulus details. On the other hand, this complexity makes the test extremely sensitive to the effects of virtually any kind of mild, diffusely distributed brain damage. Because it is part of the Halstead-Reitan Battery, cutoff scores for clinically significant impairment are available: more than fifty errors (out of 220 total responses) is generally indicative of clinically significant impairment.

The Category Test has been used by a number of investigators studying diabetic adults. Although Skenazy and Bigler (1984) and Rennick *et al.* (1968) found that Type 1 diabetic adults made more errors than nondiabetic comparison subjects, neither Baade (1988) nor Ryan and associates (1992) were able to replicate those findings. These differences may reflect the fact that the subjects studied by Rennick *et al.* and Skenazy and Bigler tended to be older and have more severe biomedical complications than those studied by Baade and Ryan *et al.*

Tactual Performance Test (TPT)

The Tactual Performance Test is a complex cognitive task that requires the integration of spatial and kinesthetic / proprioceptive skills, as well as good memory and problem-solving skills. Because it draws on so many processes, it has proven to be extremely sensitive to diffusely distributed brain damage. This test is an important component of the Halstead-Reitan Neuropsychological Battery; indeed, three of the seven HRNB scores comprising the Impairment Index are drawn from the TPT (Total Time; Memory; Location scores). The task itself requires the blindfolded subject to place a series of geometric shapes into a formboard, first with the dominant hand, then with the nondominant hand, and then with both hands. As a measure of problem-solving, the primary response measure of interest is the total time taken by the subject (in minutes) to complete all three trials ("Total Time"). Following the third trial, the subject removes the blindfold and is asked to draw the board from memory, and draw the shapes in the correct location. Separate scores for number of correct shapes ("Memory") and accurate placement ("Location") are also obtained.

This test has been used in several studies of Type 1 diabetic adults (e.g. Skenazy & Bigler, 1984; Rennick *et al.*, 1968; Baade, 1988) and a poorer level of performance appears to be associated with the occurrence of hyperglycaemic complications such as peripheral neuropathy. Although the slowed responses seen in many diabetic subjects are consistent with the view that chronic hyperglycaemia induces a "central neuropathy" (i.e. CNS dysfunction largely affecting white matter — see Ryan *et al.*, 1992), researchers have not completely succeeded in ruling out the possibility that the slowed responses are merely a consequence of sensory-motor problems secondary to diabetic peripheral neuropathy.

Motor Speed

Many of the tests described in this chapter have a significant motor component. Whether the test is measuring mental flexibility (e.g. Trail Making), problem-solving (e.g. Tactual Performance) or attention (e.g. Digit Vigilance; Reaction Time), in each case the subject must make some motor response and do so as quickly as possible. Relatively little effort has been devoted to developing tests that measure simple motor responding. Indeed, only one measure is currently in wide use: the Finger Tapping or Finger Oscillation Test.

Finger Tapping

This subtest from the Halstead-Reitan Battery requires the subject to tap a telegraph key for ten seconds. Usually five trials with the dominant hand and five trials with the nondominant hand are administered. Comparisons between dominant and nondominant tapping speed allow one to draw inferences about the possibility of lateralised brain damage. Because females tend to perform significantly slower than males on this task, test scores must be corrected for gender differences (e.g. Heaton *et al.*, 1991). This test provides a measure of simple motor speed, and has been used extensively, but with little success, in studies of euglycaemic diabetic adults (e.g. Reaven *et al.*, 1990; Ryan *et al.*, 1992), and in studies of adults during experimentally-induced hypoglycaemia (e.g. Holmes *et al.*, 1986). To date, only Baade (1988) has reported between-group differences on this measure, with diabetic adults tapping more slowly with both the dominant and nondominant hands.

Language Processes

One domain that is routinely assessed during a standard neuropsychological evaluation, but has not been evaluated extensively in studies of diabetic adults, is language. Indeed, formal language assessments (e.g. emphasising confrontation naming; phrase or sentence repetition; writing) have never been conducted systematically in groups of diabetic subjects. To some extent this may reflect the fact that these highly overlearned skills are rarely disrupted unless an individual suffers a stroke that affects the language areas of the brain (e.g. Broca's area; Wernicke's area) *or* unless the individual has developed a degenerative disorder like Alzheimer's disease. However, given the heightened incidence of cardiovascular and cerebrovascular disorders in older diabetic adults, one might *expect* to find an increased occurrence of subclinical language disorders in that patient population. The only language skill that has been evaluated to date in diabetic adults is verbal fluency ('name all the words you can think of that begin with a particular letter of the alphabet'). However, many writers (including this one) would not consider that test to measure the integrity of language skills. Rather, it may be better conceptualized as providing an estimate of general mental efficiency or a measure of the ability to retrieve information from semantic memory.

Verbal fluency

This task requires the individual to name as many words as possible that begin with a particular letter of the alphabet. Typically three trials are administered, with one minute for each of the three letters. Different investigators use different letter triads with F, A, and S, or C, F, and L, or P, R, and W being the three most popular. Norms for each letter of the alphabet have been published by Borkowski *et al.* (1967), and tables have been provided by Lezak (1983, p 33) to convert raw scores into percentiles. Verbal Fluency is generally considered to be very sensitive to brain damage, particularly to damage in the frontal regions of the brain (Perret, 1974).

Although this test has not been widely used with diabetic adults, at least one study has suggested that Type 1 patients perform more poorly than age-matched nondiabetic control subjects (Baade, 1988). Tun and associates (1987) examined verbal fluency in elderly Type 2 diabetic adults, and while they found no differences in number of words produced, the diabetic subjects produced more repetition errors than nondiabetic comparison subjects. Verbal fluency is also disrupted during a period of experimentally-induced hypoglycaemia (Holmes *et al.*, 1984).

Table 1 provides a general summary of specific neuropsychological tests that have discriminated between diabetic and nondiabetic subjects, or those with and without complications.

Table 1. A summary of neuropsychological tests that have successfully discriminated be-tween diabetic and nondiabetic subjects, or those with and without complications

Test	Study	Findings
Diabetic vs non-diabetic control groups		
Type 1 adults:		
Tactual Performance Time	Baade, 1988	Diabetic subjects are slower
Tactual Performance Location	Baade, 1988	Diabetic adults are less accurate
WAIS Performance IQ	Skenazy & Bigler, 1984	Lower PIQ in diabetic group
WAIS Block Design	Franceschi *et al.*, 1984	Diabetic subjects earn lower scores
WAIS Similarities	Franceschi *et al.*, 1984	Diabetic subjects earn lower scores
WAIS-R Object Assembly	Ryan *et al.*, 1992	Diabetic subjects earn lower scores
WAIS-R Picture Completion	Ryan *et al.*, 1992	Diabetic subjects earn lower scores
Wechsler Memory Scale	Franceschi *et al.*, 1984	Lower MQs in diabetic group
Digit Vigilance Test	Ryan *et al.*, 1992	Diabetic subjects are slower
Grooved Pegboard	Ryan *et al.*, 1992	Diabetic subjects are slower
Finger Tapping	Baade, 1988	Slower tapping by diabetic subjects
Wisconsin Card Sorting	Dejgaard *et al.*, 1991	Diabetic adults with retinopathy or neuropathy performed worse than nondiabetic normative sample
Type 2 adults:		
California Verbal Learning	Reaven *et al.*, 1990	Poorer recall in diabetic group
Serial Learning Test	Perlmuter *et al.*, 1984	Slower learning by diabetic subjects
Rey Auditory Learning Test	Mooradian *et al.*, 1988	Fewer words recalled on trials 5 or 6 by diabetic subjects
Benton Visual Retention Test	Mooradian *et al.*, 1988	Fewer correct drawings and more errors made by diabetic group
Wisconsin Card Sorting	Reaven *et al.*, 1990	Fewer categories discovered by diabetic subjects
Trail Making Test	Reaven *et al.*, 1990	Slower responding on Trails A and B in diabetic group
Digit Symbol Substitution Test	Reaven *et al.*, 1990	Slower responding by diabetic group
Verbal Fluency	Tun *et al.*, 1987	Older diabetic subjects make more repetition errors
Hyperglycaemic complications vs no complications		
Halstead-Reitan Battery	Rennick et al. 1968	Diabetic adults with retinopathy earned higher Impairment Index scores than those without retinopathy
Grooved Pegboard Test	Ryan et al. 1993	Diabetic adults with one or more complications performed more slowly than those with no complications

Table 1 (Continued) A summary of neuropsychological tests that have successfully discriminated between diabetic and nondiabetic subjects, or those with and without complications

Test	Study	Findings
Degree of metabolic control (glycosylated haemoglobin)		
Simple Reaction Time	Holmes *et al.*, 1988	Adults in good metabolic control (HbA1c ≤ 7) showed slower reaction time than those in average control
California Verbal Learning	Reaven *et al.*, 1990	Better recall associated with lower GHb in elderly adults with or without Type 2 diabetes
Recurring and/or severe hypoglycaemic episodes vs no such history		
Four Choice Reaction Time	Langan *et al.*, 1991	Diabetic adults with 5 or more episodes of severe hypoglycaemia are slower than those with no episodes
WAIS Performance IQ	Langan *et al.*, 1991	Repeated hypoglycaemia associated with larger differences between NART and PIQ scores, compared to those without hypoglycaemia
Forward Digit Span	Wredling *et al.*, 1990	Repeated hypoglycaemia associated with shorter spans

THE UTILITY OF ASSESSING THE NEUROPSYCHOLOGICAL STATUS OF DIABETIC ADULTS

There is no doubt in my mind that diabetes is associated with an increased risk of cognitive dysfunction. It is important to keep in mind, however, that the magnitude of this dysfunction is relatively small. Rarely are these impairments so severe as to prevent the individual from living independently, although they can certainly reduce mental efficiency and potentially affect job performance adversely. In young and middle-aged Type 1 diabetic adults, the most commonly found cognitive impairments appear on measures of "mental flexibility"; in elderly Type 2 diabetic adults, learning and memory skills seem to be most disrupted. Both recurrent hypoglycaemia and chronic hyperglycaemia (indexed either by the presence of biomedical complications like distal symmetrical polyneuropathy or elevated glycosylated haemoglobin levels) appear to be associated with an increased risk of developing such impairments.

If Type 1 and Type 2 diabetic adults are at risk for developing detectable cognitive impairments, then any comprehensive psychological evaluation should incorporate some kind of neuropsychological assessment. Given our current state of knowledge, such an assessment battery should include, at a minimum, measures that estimate premorbid intelligence (e.g. the NART), learning and memory (e.g. AVLT or CVLT), "fluid intelligence" or "mental flexibility" (e.g. WAIS/WAIS-R Performance subtests; Trail-Making Test; Grooved Pegboard), attention (e.g. Digit Vigilance; Choice Reaction Time), and problem-solving (e.g. Wisconsin Card Sorting Test). This type of battery could be completed in ninety minutes or less, on average, and could be used to identify those Type 1 and Type 2 diabetic adults who are beginning to manifest decrements in mental efficiency that may be secondary to diabetes or its biomedical complications. It is reasonable to believe that interventions designed to improve metabolic control may reverse cognitive decrements, or at least prevent further worsening, although that belief has not yet been subjected to a formal empirical test.

To determine the nature and duration of cognitive dysfunction induced by a *transient* episode of hypoglycaemia, one could profitably use a more limited battery of tests. Measures of attention and mental flexibility (e.g., Choice Reaction Time; Trail Making; Stroop Colour Word Test) would be particularly appropriate because they are brief enough to be administered during a hyperinsulinaemic clamp study of the sort described by Mitrakou *et al.*, (1991). Having conducted such assessments with both diabetic children (Ryan *et al.*, 1990) and adults (Ryan *et al.*, 1992) during experimentally-induced hypoglycaemia, I find that these measures can be used to identify those individuals who have the greatest risk of experiencing cognitive impairment so severe that it could interfere with their ability to treat a hypoglycaemic episode. Type 1 and 2 diabetic adults who are found to have a heightened susceptibility to significant cognitive impairment during experimentally-induced hypoglycaemia may not be good candidates for intensive insulin therapy, given the increased risk of severe hypoglycaemia that is associated with such a regimen (DCCT, 1991). The fact that mental efficiency usually declines somewhat during acute hypoglycaemia also suggests that during any extended assessment of cognitive functioning, one should periodically take a finger-stick blood glucose reading. This may be particularly crucial if the subject is in very good metabolic control and hence prone to hypoglycaemia without symptom awareness.

Although much has been published recently on neuropsychological functioning in diabetic adults, one must keep in mind that virtually all of this work has appeared since 1980. The relative youth of this subspeciality area is apparent in the measures used by investigators to document cognitive decrements. For example, neuropsychological tests that are specific to diabetes-related cognitive impairment have not been developed. Rather, investigators have borrowed neuropsychological measures, generally from the clinic, and have applied them to a new patient population under the assumption that the assessment and delineation of cognitive dysfunction requires no knowledge of the disease process causing that dysfunction. In that sense, this chapter is quite different from most of the others in this volume which emphasise the development and use of measures that are specific to adults having diabetes mellitus.

The development of new measures requires the demonstration that they be psychometrically sound. Another difference between this chapter and many of the others is the absence of carefully conducted studies that examine the reliability and validity of most of the neuropsychological measures described herein. Franzen (1989) has prepared the first comprehensive review of the psychometric properties of the most frequently used neuropsychological tasks and points out that the vast majority of these measures have never been adequately evaluated using the methods of modern psychometric theory. To some extent, this may reflect the fact that many measures (e.g. Halstead-Reitan Neuropsychological Battery) were developed long before sophisticated psychometric techniques had been developed. Moreover, because those tests were for use by highly trained clinicians, there may have been less concern about issues of reliability and validity. These comments are meant to serve as a warning to those readers who wish to include a neuropsychological component in their assessment of diabetic adults. Although the administration and interpretation of neuropsychological tests is not an extraordinarily complex undertaking, their often less-than-optimal (or unknown) psychometric properties suggests that their use be restricted to those individuals who have received adequate training and continuing supervision from an experienced clinical neuropsychologist.

SUMMARY

Increasing evidence indicates that both Type 1 and Type 2 diabetic adults have an elevated risk of developing cognitive impairments. Deficits on neuropsychological tests are associated with chronic hyperglycaemia as well as with repeated episodes of severe hypoglycaemia. In addition, acute episodes of mild or moderate hypoglycaemia may trigger transient decrements in mental efficiency. This chapter describes those neuropsychological tests that have been used most frequently in previous clinical studies of diabetic adults and attempts to identify, wherever possible, specific biomedical factors (e.g, degree of metabolic control; presence of certain complications) that appear to increase the risk of impairment. Specific tests are organised by cognitive domain: intelligence, attention, psychomotor efficiency and mental flexibility, learning and memory, problem-solving and abstract reasoning, motor speed, and language processes. In general, tests of attention and psychomotor efficiency are most sensitive to diabetes-related variables. During an acute episode of experimentally-induced hypoglycaemia, performance on certain tests (e.g. Reaction Time; Digit Vigilance; Trail Making B) is most likely to deteriorate in both diabetic and nondiabetic research subjects. These same types of measures are also likely to differentiate young and middle-aged Type 1 diabetic adults from demographically similar nondiabetic control subjects. In contrast, tests of learning and memory are most likely to distinguish elderly Type 2 diabetic adults from nondiabetic comparison subjects. Studies of both Type 1 and Type 2 diabetic adults indicate that the best biomedical predictor of cognitive dysfunction appears to be chronic hyperglycaemia (as indexed by elevated glyco-sylated haemoglobin levels or the presence of certain complications like periph-eral neuropathy). For younger Type 1 diabetic adults, repeated episodes of severe hypoglycaemia are also associated with a reduction in mental efficiency.

REFERENCES

Auer, R.B. (1986) Progress review: Hypoglycemic brain damage. *Stroke*, **17**, 699–708

Baade, L. (1988) Neuropsychological test differences between insulin- dependent diabetic adults and matched controls. Presented at the 16th annual meeting of the International Neuropsy-chological Society, New Orleans, LA, February, 1988

Barona, A., Reynolds, C.R. and Chastain, R. (1984) A demographically based index of premorbid intelligence for the WAIS-R. *Journal of Consulting and Clinical Psychology*, **52**, 885-887

Benton, A.L. (1974) *Revised Visual Retention Test (4th ed.).* New York: Psychological Corporation

Bishop, J., Knights, R.M., and Stoddart, C. (1990) Rey Auditory-Verbal Learning Test: Perfor-mance of English and French children aged 5 to 16. *The Clinical Neuropsychologist*, **4**, 133–140

Blair, J.R., and Spreen, O. (1989) Predicting premorbid IQ: A revision of the national adult read-ing test. *The Clinical Neuropsychologist*, **3**, 129–136

Boll, T. (1981) The Halstead-Reitan Neuropsychological Battery. In S.l Filskov and T. Boll (Eds.) *Handbook of Clinical Neuropsychology*, New York: Wileypp. 577–607

Borkowski, J.G., Benton, A.L. and Spreen, O. (1967) Word fluency and brain damage. *Neuropsy-chologia*, **5**, 135–140

Chalmers, J., Risk, M.T.A., Kean, D.M., Grant, R., Ashworth, B., and Campbell, I.W. (1991) Severe amnesia after hypoglycemia: Clinical, psychometric and magnetic resonance imaging corre-lations. *Diabetes Care*, **14**, 922–925

Crawford, J.R. (1989) Estimation of premorbid intelligence: A review of recent developments. In J.R. Crawford and D.M. Parker (eds.), *Developments in Clinical and Experimental Neuropsychology* New York: Plenum Press. pp.55–74

Crawford, J.R. (1992) Current and premorbid intelligence measures in neuropsychological as-sessements. In J.R. Crawford, D.M. Parker and W.W. McKinlay (eds.), *Handbook of Neuropsy-chological Assessment* Hillsdale, NJ: Lawrence Erlbaum. pp 21–49

DCCT Research Group. (1991) Epidemiology of severe hypoglycemia in the Diabetes Control and Complications Trial. *American Journal of Medicine*, **90**, 450–459

Dejgaard, A., Gade, A., Larsson, H., Balle, V., Parving, A. and Parving, H. (1991) Evidence for diabetic encephalopathy. *Diabetic Medicine*, **8**, 162– 167

Delis, D.C., Kramer, J.H., Kaplan, E. and Ober, B.A. (1987) *California Verbal Learning Test Research Edition.* San Antonio: Psychological Corporation

Franceschi, M., Cecchetto, R., Minicucci, F., Smizne, S., Baio, G. and Canal, N. (1984) Cognitive processes in insulin-dependent diabetes. *Diabetes Care*, **7**, 228–231

Franzen, M. (1989) Reliability and Validity in Neuropsychological Assessment. New York: Plenum Press

Golden, C.J. (1978) *Stroop Color and Word Test: A Manual for Clinical and Experimental Use.* Chicago: Stoelting

Golden, C.J., Osmon, D.C., Moses, J.A. and Berg, R.A. (1981) *Interpretation of the Halstead-Reitan Neuropsychological Test Battery: A Casebook Approach.* New York: Grune and Stratton

Golden, C.J. and Maruish, M. (1985) The Luria-Nebraska Neuropsychological Battery. In T. In-cagnoli, G. Goldstein and C.J. Golden (eds.), *Clinical Application of Neuropsychological Test Bat-teries. New York: Plenum*

Halstead, W.C. (1947) *Brain and Intelligence.* Chicago: University of Chicago Press

Harrad, R.A., Cockram, C.S., Plumb, A.P., Stone, S., Fenwick, P. and Sonksen, P.H. (1985) The effect of hypoglycaemia on visual function: A clinical and electrophysiological study. *Clinical Science,* **69,** 673–679

Heaton, R.K., Grant, I. and Matthews, C.G. (1991) *Comprehensive Norms for an Expanded Halstead-Reitan Battery: Demographic Corrections, Research Findings, and Clinical Applications.* Odessa FL: Psychological Assessment Resources

Herold, K.C., Polonsky, K.S., Cohen, R.M., Levy, J. and Douglas, F. (1985) Variable deterioration in cortical function during insulin-induced hypoglycemia. *Diabetes,* **34,** 677–685

Hoffman, R.G. Speelman, D.J., Hinnen, D.A., Conley, K.L., Guthrie, R.A. and Knapp, R.K. (1989) Changes in cortical functioning with acute hypoglycemia and hyperglycemia in Type I diabetes. *Diabetes Care,* **12,** 193–197

Holmes, C.S., Hayford, J.T., Gonzales, J.L. and Weydert, J.A. (1983) A survey of cognitive functioning at different glucose levels in diabetic persons. *Diabetes Care,* **6,** 180–185

Holmes, C.S., Koepke, K.M., Thompson, R.G., Gyves, P. and Weydert, J.A. (1984). Verbal fluency and naming skills in type I diabetes at different glucose levels. *Diabetes Care,* **7,** 454–459

Holmes, C.S., Koepke, K.M. and Thompson, R.G. (1986). Simple versus complex neuropsychological impairments during three blood glucose levels. *Psychoneuroendocrinology,* **11,** 353–357

Holmes, C.S., Tsalikian, E., and Yamada, T. (1988) Blood glucose control and visual and auditory attention in men with insulin-dependent diabetes. *Diabetic Medicine,* **5,** 634–639

Horn, J.L. (1985) Remodeling old models of intelligence. In B.B. Wolman (ed.), *Handbook of Intelligence.* New York: Wiley. pp 267–300

Ipp, E. and Forster, B. (1987) Sparing of cognitive function in mild hypoglycemia: Dissociation from the neuroendocrine response, *Journal of Clinical Endocrinology and Metabolism,* **65,** 806–810

Kalimo, H., and Olsson, Y. (1980). Effects of severe hypoglycemia on the human brain. *Acta Neurologica Scandinavica,* **62,** 345–356

Kapur, N. (1988) *Memory Disorders in Clinical Practice.* London: Butterworths

Karzmark, P., Heaton, R.K., Grant, I. and Matthews, C.G. (1985) Use of demographic variables to predict full scale IQ: A replication and extension. *Journal of Clinical and Experimental Neuropsychology,* **7,** 412–420

Kaufman, A.S. (1990) *Assessing Adolescent and Adult Intelligence.* Boston: Allyn and Bacon

Kaufman, A.S., Reynolds, C.R. and McLean, J.E. (1989) Age and WAIS-R intelligence in a national sample of adults in the 20- to 74-year age ranges: A cross-sectional analysis with education level controlled. *Intelligence,* **13,** 235–253

Lan, S-P., Ryan, C.M., Adams, K., Grant, I., Heaton, R., Rand, L.I., Jacobson, A.M., Nathan, D.M. and Cleary, P.A. (In press) A screening algorithm to identify clinically significant changes in neuropsychological functions in the diabetes control and complications trial. *Journal of Clinical and Experimental Neuropsychology*

Langan, S., Deary, I., Hepburn, D. and Frier, B. (1991) Cumulative cognitive impairment following recurrent severe hypoglycaemia adult patients with insulin-treated diabetes mellitus. *Diabetologia,* **34,** 337–344

Lawson, J., Williams Erdahl, D., Monga, T., Bird, C., Donald, M., Surridge, D. and Letemendia, F. (1984) Neuropsychological function in diabetic patients with neuropathy. *British Journal of Psychiatry,* **145,** 263–268

Lewis, R. and Rennick, P. (1979) *Manual for the Repeatable Cognitive-Perceptual-Motor Battery.* Gross Point Park MI: Axon

Lezak, M. D. (1983) *Neuropsychological Assessment.* (2nd ed.) New York: Oxford University Press

Mattlar, C-E., Falck, B., Ronnemaa, T., and Hyyppa, M.T. (1985) Neuropsychological cognitive performance of patients with Type 2 diabetes. Scandinavian Journal of Rehabilitation Medicine, **17,** 101–105

Meuter, F., Thomas, W., Gruneklee, D., Gries, F. and Lohmann, R. (1980) Psychometric evaluation of performance in diabetes mellitus. *Hormone and Metabolic Research* **9 (Suppl)**, 9–17

Mirsky, A.F., Anthony, B.J., Duncan, C.C., Ahern, M.B, and Kellam, S.G. (1991) Analysis of the elements of attention: A neuropsychological approach. *Neuropsychology Review*, **2**, 109–145

Mitrakou, A., Ryan, C., Veneman, T., Mokan, M., Jenssen, T., Kiss, I., Durrant, J., Cryer, P. and Gerich, J. (1991). Hierarchy of glycemic thresholds for counterregulatory hormone secretion, symptoms, and cerebral dysfunction. American Journal of Physiology, **260**, E67–E74

Mooradian, A., Perryman, K., Fitten, J., Kavonian, G. and Morley, J. (1988) Cortical function in elderly non-insulin dependent diabetic patients. Archives of Internal Medicine, **148**, 2369–2372

Nelson, H.E. (1982) *National adult reading test (NART): Test manual.* Windsor: NFER-Nelson

Norman, D.A. (1969) *Memory and Attention.* New York: Wiley

O'Carroll R.E., Baikie E.M. and Hittick J.E. (1987) Does the National Adult Reading Test hold in dementia? *British Journal of Clinical Psychology*, **26**, 315–316

Perlmuter, L.C., Hakami, M., Hodgson-Harrington, C., Ginsberg, J., Katz, J., Singer, D.E. and Nathan, D.M. (1984) Decreased cognitive function in aging non-insulin-dependent diabetic patients. *American Journal of Medicine*, **77**, 1043–1048

Perret, E. (1974) The left frontal lobe of man and the suppression of habitual responses in verbal categorical behavior. *Neuropsychologia*, **12**, 323–390

Posner, M.I., Walker, J.A., Friedrich, F.J and Rafal, R.D. (1984) Effects of parietal lobe injury on covert orienting of attention. *Journal of Neuroscience*, **4**, 1863–1874

Pramming, S., Thorsteinsson, B., Theilgaard, A., Pinner, E.M., and Binder, C. (1986) Cognitive function during hypoglycaemia in type I diabetes mellitus. *British Medical Journal*, **292**, 647–650

Prigatano, G.P. (1977) Wechsler Memory Scale is a poor screening test for brain dysfunction. *Journal of Clinical Psychology*, **33**, 772–777

Prigatano, G.P. (1978) Wechsler Memory Scale: A selective review of the literature. *Journal of Clinical Psychology*, **34**, 816–832

Reaven, G., Thompson, L., Nahum, D. and Haskins, E. (1990) Relationship between hyperglycemia and cognitive function in older NIDDM patients. *Diabetes Care*, **13**, 16–21

Reichard, P., Berglund, A., Britz, A., Levander, S. and Rosenqvist, U. (1991) Hypoglycaemic episodes during intensified insulin treatment: increased frequency but no effect on cognitive function. *Journal of Internal Medicine*, **229**, 9–16

Reitan, R.M. and Wolfson, D. (1993) *The Halstead-Reitan Neuropsychological Test Battery: Theory and Clinical Interpretation.* Tuscon AZ: Neuropsychology Press

Rennick, P., Wilder, R., Sargent, J. and Ashley, B. (1968) Retinopathy as an indicator of cognitive-perceptual-motor impairment in diabetic adults [Summary]. Proceedings of the 76th Annual Convention of the American Psychological Association, pp. 473–474

Reske-Nielson, E., Lundbaek, K., and Rafaelsen, O. (1965) Pathological changes in the central and peripheral nervous systems of young long-term diabetics. *Diabetologia*, **1**, 232–241

Robinson, A.L., Heaton, R.K., Lehman, R.A.W., and Stilson, D.W. (1980) The utility of the Wisconsin Card Sorting Test in detecting and localizing frontal lobe lesions. *Journal of Consulting and Clinical Psychology*, **48**, 605–614

Rourke, B., Yanni, D, MacDonald, G., and Young, G. (1973) Neuropsychological significance of lateralized deficits on the Grooved Pegboard Test for older children with learning disabilities. *Journal of Consulting and Clinical Psychology*, **41**, 128–134

Russell, E.W. (1981) The pathology and clinical examination of memory. In S.B. Filskov and T.J. Boll (eds.), Handbook of Clinical Psychology. New York: Wiley. pp287–318

Russell, E.W., Neuringer, C. and Goldstein, G. (1970) *Assessment of Brain Damage: A Neuropsychological Key Approach.* New York: Wiley

Ryan, C. Vega, A., Longstreet, C. and Drash, A. (1984) Neuropsychological changes in adolescents with insulin-dependent diabetes. *Journal of Consulting and Clinical Psychology,* **52**, 335–342

Ryan, C. Morrow, L., Bromet, E. and Parkinson, D. (1987) Assessment of neuropsychological dysfunction in the workplace: Normative data from the Pittsburgh Occupational Exposures Test Battery. *Journal of Clinical and Experimental Neuropsychology,* **9**, 665–679

Ryan, C., Atchinson, J., Puczynski, S., Puczynski, M., Arslanian, S., and Becker, D. (1990) Mild hypoglycemia associated with deterioration of mental efficiency in children with insulin-dependent diabetes mellitus. *Journal of Pediatrics,* **117**, 32–38

Ryan, C., Adams, K.M., Heaton, R.K., Grant, I., Jacobson, A. and the DCCT Study Group. (1991) Neurobehavioral assessment of medically ill patients: The DCCT experience. In E. Mohr and P. Brouwers (eds.), *Handbook of Clinical Trials: The Neurobehavioral Approach.* Lisse: Swets and Zeitlinger. pp 215–241

Ryan, C., Williams, T., Orchard, T. and Finegold, D. (1992) Psychomotor slowing is associated with distal symmetrical polyneuropathy in adults with diabetes mellitus. *Diabetes,* **41**, 107–113

Ryan, C., Williams, T.M., Finegold, D.N. and Orchard, T.J. (1993) Cognitive dysfunction in adults with Type I (insulin-dependent) diabetes mellitus of long duration: effects of recurrent hypoglycaemia and other chronic complications. *Diabetologia,* **36**, 329–334

Ryan, J.J., Nowak, T.J. and Geisser, M.E. (1987) On the comparability of the WAIS and the WAIS-R: Review of the research and implications for clinical practice. *Journal of Psychoeducational Assessment,* **5**, 15–30

Skenazy, J. and Bigler, E. (1984) Neuropsychological findings in diabetes mellitus. *Journal of Clinical Psychology,* **40**, 246–258

Smith, A. (1973) *Symbol Digit Modalities Test: Manual.* Los Angeles: Western Psychological Services

Squire, L.R. and Butters, N. (1992) *Neuropsychology of Memory* (2nd ed.). New York: Guilford Press

Stevens, A.B., McKane, W.R., Bell, P., King, D. and Haynes, J. (1989) Psychomotor performance and counterregulatory responses during mild hypoglycemia in healthy volunteers. *Diabetes Care,* **12**, 12–17

Tun, P.A., Perlmuter, L.C., Russo, P. and Nathan, D.M. (1987) Memory self-assessment and performance in aged diabetics and non-diabetics. Experimental Aging Research, **13**, 151–157

U'Ren, R., Riddle, M. Lezak, M. and Bennington-Davis, M. (1990) The mental efficiency of the elderly person with type II diabetes mellitus. *Journal of the American Geriatric Society,* **38**, 505–510

Wechsler, D. (1945) A standardized memory scale for clinical use. *Journal of Psychology,* **19**, 87–95

Wechsler, D. (1955) *Manual for the Wechsler Adult Intelligence Scale.* New York: Psychological Corporation

Wechsler, D. (1981) *Manual for the Wechsler Adult Intelligence Scale, Revised.* Cleveland, OH: Psychological Corporation

Wechsler, D. (1987) *Manual for the Wechsler Memory Scale - Revised.* San Antonio, TX: Psychological Corporation

Wiens, A.N., McMinn, M.R. and Crossen, J.R. (1988) Rey Auditory-Verbal Learning Test: Development of norms for healthy young adults. *The Clinical Neuropsychologist,* **2**, 67–77

Wilson, R.S., Rosenbaum, G., and Brown, G. (1979) The problem of premorbid intelligence in neuropsychological assessment. *Journal of Clinical Neuropsychology,* **1**, 49–53

Wilson, R.S., Rosenbaum, G., Brown, G., Rourke, D., Whittman, D., and Grisell, J. (1978) An index of premorbid intelligence. *Journal of Consulting and Clinical Psychology,* **46**, 1554–1555

Wredling, R., Levander, S., Adamson, U. and Lins, P. (1990) Permanent neuropsychological impairment after recurrent episodes of severe hypoglycaemia in man. *Diabetologia,* **33**, 152–157

SECTION 4

MEASURES OF ATTITUDES
AND BELIEFS

## CHAPTER 11

THE ATT39: A MEASURE OF PSYCHOLOGICAL ADJUSTMENT TO DIABETES

GARRY WELCH[1], STEWART M. DUNN[2] and LINDA J. BEENEY[3]

[1]Mental Health Unit, Joslin Diabetes Centre, One Joslin Place, Boston, Massachusetts, MA 02215, USA; [2]Medical Psychology Unit, Royal Prince Alfred Hospital and Department of Medicine, University of Sydney, NSW 2006, Australia; [3]Medical Psychology Unit, Department of Medicine, University of Sydney, NSW 2006, Australia.

INTRODUCTION

The ATT39 (Dunn et al., 1986) is a measure of psychological adjustment to diabetes that was developed in response to the need for more specific measurement tools for the assessment of psychosocial issues in diabetes. Specific instruments were expected to provide more sensitive measurement of the dynamic psychological processes unique to diabetes and greater predictive validity than was available from the broad personality measures then in use. Early studies of psychological adjustment to diabetes at that time had focused on efforts to identify both a "diabetes personality" and a "compliant personality". These studies proved unproductive (Simonds, 1981; Dunn & Turtle, 1981, Wilkinson, 1987; Dunn, 1986). More recently, there has been interest in the cognitive and behavioural strategies patients use to manage diabetes and emotional response.

The rationale for measuring this more broadly defined adjustment to diabetes is that such characteristics may impact on blood sugar control both directly, i.e. through stress-related hormonal and sympathetic nervous system activity that mediates gluconeogenesis and insulin utilisation, or indirectly, through the effect of day to day patient behaviours.

Clinical opinion on what constitutes appropriate psychological adjustment to diabetes is conflicting and attempted validation against criteria such as "good adjustment equals good control" is certainly an over-simplification. Emotional adjustment is, by definition, dynamic and fluctuating and presents a challenge to researchers in diabetes aiming to develop reliable and valid measures of this complex adjustment process.

With these issues in mind, the ATT39 has been developed specifically to provide clinicians and researchers with an assessment tool to assess psychological adjustment to diabetes (see Figure 1). It may be used to augment the clinical and educational assessment of diabetes patients, to detect change in psychological functioning following short term interventions (e.g. diabetes education programmes) and to investigate the correlates of psychological adjustment to diabetes. Measures such as the ATT39 may provide a basis for psychological

intervention among patients with poor psychological adjustment and poor metabolic control (and those patients with good metabolic control who are adjusted
poorly). Ultimately, of course, we would hope that the early application of measures such as the ATT39 would help in the *prevention* of poor psychological adjustment to diabetes.

NAME: ....AGE: ....   SEX: M/F(circle one) DATE:......................
How long have you had diabetes? ....
How is it treated? (tick one)   Diet .... Diet & tablets...............Diet & insulin............

INSTRUCTIONS: This form contains 39 questions to see how you feel about diabetes and its effect on
your life. There are no "right " or "wrong" answers because everyone has the right to his or her own
views. You are asked not to spend too long on each question. There are five possible answers to choose
from:

I DISAGREE or,	I DISAGREE or,	I DON'T KNOW or,	I AGREE or,	I AGREE
COMPLETELY				COMPLETELY
(DC)	(D)	(?)	(A)	(AC)

For each question, circle the **ONE** answer that is right for you. Give your first, natural answer as it
occurs to you.

	I disagree completely	I disagree	I don't know	I agree	I agree completely	OFFICE USE
EXAMPLE: There are no "right "or "wrong" answers to these questions.....................	DC	D	?	A	(AC)	....
1. If I did not have diabetes I think I would be quite a different person........................	DC	D	?	A	AC	....
2. Diabetes has made no difference to my life at all........	DC	D	?	A	AC	....
3. I dislike being referred to as "A DIABETIC"............................	DC	D	?	A	AC	....
4. Diabetes is the worst thing that has ever happened to me..	DC	D	?	A	AC	....
5. I feel quite capable of looking after my diabetes with minimum outside help.............	DC	D	?	A	AC	....
6. I know as much as I need to know about diabetes.................	DC	D	?	A	AC	....
7. I believe that research will discover a cure for diabetes before too long.........................	DC	D	?	A	AC	....
8 Most people would find it difficult to adjust to having diabetes.....................................	DC	D	?	A	AC	....
9. I often feel embarrassed about having diabetes..........................	DC	D	?	A	AC	....
10. Most people would be a lot healthier if they followed a diabetic diet............................	DC	D	?	A	AC	....

PLEASE TURN OVER TO COMPLETE REMAINING QUESTIONS

	I disagree completely	I disagree	I don't know	I agree	I agree completely	OFFICE USE
11. Talking to my doctor about my diabetes usually makes me feel better..................................	DC	D	?	A	AC	....
12. There is not much I seem to be able to do to control my diabetes..................................	DC	D	?	A	AC	....
13. I like to be told when my diabetes has been well controlled..................................	DC	D	?	A	AC	....
14. There is little hope of leading a normal life with diabetes..................................	DC	D	?	A	AC	....
15. The proper control of diabetes involves a lot of sacrifice and inconvenience............................	DC	D	?	A	AC	....
16. Having diabetes means accepting responsibility for your own treatment...................	DC	D	?	A	AC	....
17. The thought of giving myself an injection does not bother me	DC	D	?	A	AC	....
18. Food is very important in my life	DC	D	?	A	AC	....
19. I try not to let people know about my diabetes......................	DC	D	?	A	AC	....
20. Being told you have diabetes is like being sentenced to a life time of illness............................	DC	D	?	A	AC	....
21. Hypo's are not really as frightening as people seem to think...	DC	D	?	A	AC	....
22. Most people do not understand the problems associated with having diabetes..........................	DC	D	?	A	AC	....
23. My diabetic diet does not really spoil my social life............	DC	D	?	A	AC	....
24. Weight-control is not a problem for me...........................	DC	D	?	A	AC	....
25. In general, doctors need to be a lot more sympathetic in their treatment of people with diabetes...............................	DC	D	?	A	AC	....
26. Having diabetes over a long period changes the personality..	DC	D	?	A	AC	....
27. A person should learn to live with diabetes, without involving other members of the family.....	DC	D	?	A	AC	....
28. I often find it difficult to decide whether I feel sick or well..........	DC	D	?	A	AC	....
29. Most doctors really don't understand what it's like to have diabetes..........................	DC	D	?	A	AC	....
30. I often forget that I even have diabetes..................................	DC	D	?	A	AC	....

PLEASE TURN OVER TO COMPLETE REMAINING QUESTIONS

	I disagree completely	I disagree	I don't know	I agree	I agree completely	OFFICE USE
31. Diabetes is not really a problem because it can be controlled........	DC	D	?	A	AC	....
32. Sometimes I have used my diabetes as an excuse to get my own way..................................	DC	D	?	A	AC	....
33. I do not like being told what to eat, when to eat, and how much to eat..........................	DC	D	?	A	AC	....
34. I think that I have a good relationship with my doctor........	DC	D	?	A	AC	....
35. There is really nothing you can do if you have diabetes.........	DC	D	?	A	AC	....
36. I would like to be told if my diabetic control had been poor..	DC	D	?	A	AC	....
37. There is really no-one I feel I can talk to openly about my diabetes..............................	DC	D	?	A	AC .	....
38. I believe I have adjusted well to having diabetes.......................	DC	D	?	A	AC	....
39. I often think it is unfair that I should have diabetes when other people are so healthy........	DC	D	?	A	AC	....

ATT39 ©Diabetes Centre, Royal Prince Alfred Hospital, Camperdown, NSW 2050, Australia

Since its development, the ATT39 has been used to evaluate the impact of diabetes education programmes in Australia (Dunn *et al.*, 1985; Dunn, 1986; Seal, 1992, personal communication), Germany (Bott *et al.*, 1988) and Canada (Gosselin & Bergeron, submitted for publication). It has also been used to investigate patient psychological typologies by cluster analysis (Dunn *et al.*, 1986a), to measure changes in stability of psychological adjustment over the course of diabetes (Dunn *et al.*, 1985a) and to explore ethnic differences in diabetes adjustment between Australian and Greek patients (Papadam *et al.*, 1985).

Given that the ATT39 was empirically-derived, it is not surprising that there have also been a number of studies that have further examined the measure's psychometric characteristics and subscale structure. This series of studies has thrown some interesting light on the nature of the internal structure of the ATT39, with the more recent studies applying rigorous psychometric criteria that have highlighted the unidimensional nature of the ATT39 as an index of psychological adjustment to diabetes. However, as will be described later, the emphasis to date in terms of the clinical application of the ATT39 has been on the earlier multidimensional forms of the scale and the relationship of these subscales to important demographic and clinical variables.

In addition to the original English form, the ATT39 has been translated into German (Bott *et al.*, 1988), French-Canadian (Gosselin & Bergeron, submitted for publication), Greek (Papadam *et al.*, 1985) and Italian (developed by the Diabetes Centre, Royal Prince Alfred Hospital, Sydney).

THE ATT39 SCALE

Design

The ATT39 is a thirty-nine item self-report measure comprising a range of attitudinal statements related to a patient's perception of diabetes and its treatment (see Figure 1). The ATT39 item pool generated by Dunn *et al.* (1986) came from three sources: 1) the results of two factor analyses on demographic, personality and treatment data; 2) a review of the diabetes psychological literature; and 3) patient interviews and clinical experience on patient adjustment in diabetes (Dunn *et al.*, 1986). In addition to the full thirty-nine item scale and six subscales, three short parallel forms have been described (i.e. ATTA, ATTB and ATTC) the latter each comprising fourteen items extracted from the full scale. The items for each were obtained by matching individual items from the total test and forming these into three pools on the basis of similar content, difficulty and item-total test correlation. More recent analyses have identified a new nineteen item subscale (labelled the ATT19 or "Diabetes Integration") as the central and replicable core of the ATT39 for both IDDM and NIDDM patient groups (see Scoring, Structure and Interpretation).

Scoring, Structure and Interpretation

The ATT39 is a self-report measure whose items are scored on a five-point Likert scale that ranges from "I disagree completely" (scored 1) through to "I agree completely" (scored 5). A patient completing the measure is instructed to indicate "how you feel about diabetes and its effect on your life". It is stressed that there are no right or wrong answers to the questions and patients are asked not to dwell too long on their answers to each question. Twenty three items are reverse scored (i.e. items 1, 3, 4, 6, 7, 8, 9, 12, 14, 15, 19, 20, 22, 25, 26, 27, 28, 29, 32, 33, 35, 37 and 39) so that a high score consistently reflects a positive attitude to diabetes.

The original ATT39 yielded an unweighted total score and six weighted subscales, the latter calculated from factor scores based on responses from a sample of 170 patients attending the Outpatient Diabetic Clinic, Royal Prince Alfred Hospital, Sydney. The original six ATT39 subscales (with items loading greater than 0.35 on each factor) were described as follows:

1. **Factor 1: "Diabetes stress"** (Items 1, 2, 4, 8, 9, 14, 15, 20, 26, 28, 39) includes items which show the degree to which respondents feel that diabetes creates stress and feelings of disintegration.

2. **Factor 2: "Coping"** (Items 10, 11, 13, 14, 31, 32, 34, 36, 38) items assess the individual's perception of his or her ability to cope with these stresses, and to feel competent to deal with diabetes.

3. **Factor 3: "Guilt"** (Items 3, 9, 12, 19, 25, 37) measures guilt and embarrassment associated with diabetes and includes items like "I try not to let people know that I have diabetes".

4. **Factor 4: "Alienation - Cooperation"** (Items 10, 16, 25, 26, 29) is more complex: some items indicate dissatisfaction with the empathy and understanding shown by medical personnel, and other items show a conviction that one can cope independently. Our interpretation of this factor is that it assesses the adoption of an independent approach to diabetes management versus a more medically-dependent, cooperative attitude.

5. **Factor 5: Illness conviction** (Items 7, 10, 13, 16, 17, 24) is a bipolar factor very similar to a factor identified in patients with chronic pain, called "disease conviction". People who score negatively on this factor reject the notion that they have a chronic disease and find the whole routine of daily management abnormal and distasteful. They also anticipate that diabetes will be cured in the near future. Positive scores indicate acceptance of the daily regimen as a normal part of life and reconciliation to the belief that diabetes will never go away.

6. **Factor 6: "Tolerance for ambiguity"** (Items 5, 6, 21, 35) includes items like "I know as much as I need to know about diabetes" and "I can look after my diabetes with minimum outside help". The person who agrees strongly with these items shows a marked lack of flexibility and a resistance to new input. Diabetes is fraught with possibilities, ambiguities and unanswered questions and such a person has a poor tolerance for the ambiguities. Conversely, the positive-scoring person tolerates the ambiguities and associated anxiety.

A German study (Bott *et al.*, 1988) also described six subscales for the ATT39, using the same factor extraction and rotation techniques employed by Dunn *et al.* (1986). Bott *et al.* labelled their six factors: "Diabetes-related stress", "Deficient coping and isolation", "Relationship to medical practitioner", "Personal responsibility", "Self-competence conviction" and "Unrealistic optimism". As will be noted below in the summary of ATT39 factor analytic studies, there is overlap between some of the factors identified here by Bott *et al.* and those in the original ATT39 but there is also significant blurring and lack of replication of some other factors.

The parallel forms ATTA, ATTB and ATTC consist of fourteen items each extracted from the full ATT39 scale. These short scales have been scored both as unweighted sums of the items and as sten scores with a mean of 5.5 and an s.d. of 1.0 (Dunn *et al.*, 1990). Also, Maxwell *et al.* (1992) have reported a shortened fifteen item form of the measure that excluded items with a high number of undecided responses and those that did not load significantly on the first four factors of a six-factor solution.

A recent Australian-New Zealand study (Welch *et al.*, 1994) described a single subscale for the ATT39 which was based on twenty one items. Other more recent analyses carried out for the first time on IDDM and NIDDM patient groups separately (Welch *et al.*, in preparation), showed that the ATT39 can be scored as a single nineteen item scale for both IDDM and NIDDM patient groups. This new scale has been named the "ATT19" or "Diabetes Integration" (see Figure 2) and is scored as a sum of unit weights (rather than using factor scores) to simplify its scoring. Apart from its practical advantage, the move to this method of scoring was based on recent evidence that factor weights and unit weights provide similar scores (Cohen, 1990).

Based on these recent and comprehensive factor analyses, the revised nineteen-item version (the ATT19) is potentially more reliable and practical for clinical use. The ATT19 items are scored on a five-point Likert scale ranging from "I disagree completely" scored "1" through to "I agree completely" (scored 5) as for the thirty-nine item scale with all items except 11, 15 and 18 being reverse scored. Raw scores (reversed as required) on the nineteen items are summed to produce a total score that ranges from 19 to 95.

NAME: ....AGE: ....   SEX: M/F(circle one) DATE:........................

How long have you had diabetes? ....

How is it treated? (tick one)   Diet ....   Diet & tablets...............Diet & insulin............

INSTRUCTIONS: This form contains 19 questions to see how you feel about diabetes and its effect on your life. There are no "right " or "wrong" answers because everyone has the right to his or her own views. Please do not spend too long on each question. There are five possible answers to choose from:

I DISAGREE or,	I DISAGREE or,	I DON'T KNOW or,	I AGREE or,	I AGREE
COMPLETELY				COMPLETELY
(DC)	(D)	(?)	(A)	(AC)

For each question, circle the **ONE** answer that is right for you . Give your first, natural answer as it occurs to you.

	I disagree completely	I disagree	I don't know	I agree	I agree completely	OFFICE USE
1. If I did not have diabetes I think I would be quite a different person...........................	DC	D	?	A	AC	....
2. I dislike being referred to as "A DIABETIC".............................	DC	D	?	A	AC	....
3. Diabetes is the worst thing that has ever happened to me....	DC	D	?	A	AC	....
4. Most people would find it difficult to adjust to having diabetes..	DC	D	?	A	AC	....
5. I often feel embarrassed about having diabetes.................	DC	D	?	A	AC	....
6. There is not much I seem to be able to do to control my diabetes	DC	D	?	A	AC	....
7. There is little hope of leading a normal life with diabetes.........	DC	D	?	A	AC	....
8. The proper control of diabetes involves a lot of sacrifice and inconvenience.............................	DC	D	?	A	AC	....
9. I try not to let people know about my diabetes......................	DC	D	?	A	AC	....
10. Being told you have diabetes is like being sentenced to a lifetime of illness........................	DC	D	?	A	AC	....
11. My diabetic diet does not really spoilt my social life............	DC	D	?	A	AC	....
12. In general, doctors need to be a lot more sympathetic in their treatment of people with diabetes	DC	D	?	A	AC	....
13. Having diabetes over a long period changes the personality..	DC	D	?	A	AC	....

	I disagree completely	I disagree	I don't know	I agree	I agree completely	OFFICE USE
14. I often find it difficult to decide whether I feel sick or well............ DC		D	?	A	AC	....
15. Diabetes is not reallya problem because it can be controlled .... DC		D	?	A	AC	....
16. There is really nothing you can do if you have diabetes.......... DC		D	?	A	AC	....
17. There is really no-one I feel I can talk to openly about my diabetes.................................. DC		D	?	A	AC	....
18. I believe I have adjusted well to having diabetes......................... DC		D	?	A	AC	....
19. I often think it is unfair that I should have diabetes when other people are so healthy.......... DC		D	?	A	AC	....

SCALE DEVELOPMENT

Subject Samples

Dunn et al. (1986)

The original item development sample comprised two heterogeneous samples of diabetes patients (n = 205, n = 107) and the subscale development sample a further group of 170 patients. The three samples were similar in demographic and clinical characteristics and were drawn from the Royal Prince Alfred Hospital Outpatient Diabetes Clinic, Sydney, Australia. For example, the mean age of the third sample (n = 170) was 48 years, the gender ratio for male to female 3:2, average duration of diabetes was 11 years and the ratio of IDDM to NIDDM was 2:1.

German DTTP study (Bott et al., 1988)

The authors used 546 Type 1 diabetes patients attending consecutive structured five-day inpatient Diabetes Teaching and Treatment Programmes (DTTP) conducted in nine German cities. Exclusion criteria included blindness and renal insufficiency. Mean patient age was 26 years (±7) and mean duration of diabetes was 9 years (±7).

Canadian study (Gosselin & Bergeron, submitted for publication)

These authors used a study sample of 144 Type 1 and Type 2 diabetes patients attending a diabetes education programme at the Diabetes Daycare Center of Cité de La Sante de Laval Hospital in Montreal, Canada. Patients were eighteen years or older, French speaking and free from serious physical complications related to diabetes. In addition, pregnant women and newly diagnosed patients were excluded. The sample had a gender ratio for male to female of 3:2, 29% were Type 1 and 71% Type 2 and the patients had a mean age of 48.9 years and a mean duration of diabetes of 10.4 years.

New Zealand study (Welch et al., 1992)

The authors examined the factor structure of the ATT39 using two samples (both n = 155) of insulin-using patients attending the Wellington Diabetes Service, Wellington Hospital who were randomly allocated to one of two groups to form replication samples for a series of factor analyses. Mean ages were 45.4 (±17.9) years and 47.9 (±16.9) years for the two groups. These patients represented the 79% of patients registered with the service who had returned the study questionnaire. The authors also made use of data from the mixed sample of 170 IDDM and NIDDM patients from the original study of Dunn *et al.* (1986).

1992 Sydney analyses

In this study, four diabetes patient samples from two Metropolitan hospital districts in Australia and New Zealand were used (see Table 1). Patients were classified as having IDDM or NIDDM using the criteria of Welborn *et al.* (1983). Patients with IDDM were forty years or younger at diagnosis and on permanent insulin therapy within two years of diagnosis. Patients with NIDDM had an onset of diabetes after forty years of age. Welborn *et al.* found a sensitivity of 84%, a specificity of 96%, a positive predictive value of 96% and a negative predictive value of 84% for their criteria against a serum C-peptide assay and using adult Caucasian patients. C-peptide was used by Welborn *et al.* as the standard measure of residual endogenous insulin production against which the new criteria were compared. Two of the four samples (IDDM, n = 142; NIDDM, n = 303) comprised patients attending Diabetes Education Programmes at five public hospitals in Sydney, Australia. Patients were consecutive referrals to these programmes and 90% agreed to take part in the study. The NIDDM patient sample had a mean age of 49.5 years (±17.1), a mean age at onset of diabetes of 41.0 years (±17.6) and a mean duration of diabetes of 8.5 years (±9.4). The mean glycosylated haemoglobin for NIDDM patients described in Table 1 would be classified as "good" according to Eross *et al.*'s (1984) classification. The IDDM patients had a mean age of 36 years (±13.8), a mean age of onset of diabetes of 25.3 years (±9.9) and a mean duration of diabetes of 10.7 years (±11.7). Mean GHb for IDDM patients described in Table 1 would be classified as "fair".

Table 1 Demographic and clinical characteristics of IDDM and NIDDM patient groups for Sydney and Wellington treatment centres

N	Diabetes type	Sex ratio (M/F)	Age Mean (s.d.)	Age of onset Mean (s.d.)	Duration of diabetes Mean (s.d.)	Glycosylated haemoglobin Mean (s.d.)
Sydney samples						
142	IDDM	63/79	36.0 (±13.8)	25.3 (±9.9)	10.7 (±11.7)	1637.2 (±420.1)
303	NIDDM	127/176	49.5 (±17.1)	41.0 (±17.6)	8.5 (±9.4)	1522.2 (±341.9)
Wellington samples						
198	IDDM	89/109	35.4 (±11.7)	19.8 (±9.1)	18.5 (±10.7)	9.2% (±1.5)
177	NIDDM	95/82	58.4 (±13.2)	46.4 (±12.1)	15.7 (±8.1)	9.5% (±1.6)

Note: Glycosylated haemoglobin was measured as a modified thiobarbituric acid assay for the Sydney samples (Eross *et al.*, 1984). The GHb normal range for this assay is 700 to 1100 pmol HMF/mg Hb. For the Wellington samples HbA_1 represented a mean % GHb gathered over the previous year (Simon & Elssler, 1980). The mean value for the Wellington IDDM group of 9.2% and the mean value of 9.5% for the NIDDM group are both classified clinically as "good" by Simon and Elssler's classification.

In addition to these Sydney samples, further IDDM (n = 198) and NIDDM (n = 177) samples were obtained to provide replication samples for the factor analyses. These patients were drawn from patient files at the Wellington Diabetes Service, Wellington Hospital, New Zealand. Mean HbA1 (Simon & Elssler, 1980) data available for these groups represented average readings over the previous year. These were 9.2% (±1.5) for IDDM and 9.5% (±1.6) for NIDDM. Seventy six percent of the patients returned the ATT39 by mail. The NIDDM patients had a mean age of 58.4 years (±13.2), a mean age at onset of diabetes of 46.4 years (±12.1) and a mean duration of diabetes of 15.7 years (±8.1). The IDDM patient sample had a mean age of 35.4 years (±11.7), a mean age at onset of diabetes of 19.8 years (±9.1) and a mean duration of diabetes of 18.5 years (±10.7). The characteristics of each of the studies together with the main findings are summarised in Table 2.

Statistical Methods and Qualitative Judgements

Factor analysis was carried out on the pool of thirty-nine items generated during the initial design. The Scree Test (Cattell, 1966), an eigenvalue-based criterion, was used in the factor analyses to determine the likely number of factors present. The Scree Test involves plotting of eigenvalues against all potential factors to identify a point of inflection on the graph where the substantial factors are defined. Six factors were identified by this means. Rotation was used to achieve simple structure and define the final factor loadings. That is, the factor axes were rotated in the analyses to maximise the high loadings and minimise the low loadings. In this way, the simplest possible set of relationships can be found between the ATT39 items and the factors extracted. Orthogonal rotation was used in these analyses (as opposed to oblique rotation), although in practice this distinction is unimportant as the overall pattern of significant and non-significant loadings found using the two approaches is very similar.

Bott and his colleagues evaluated the factor structure and reliability of the ATT39 as part of their psychometric groundwork prior to using the measure to detect change in emotional adjustment over the course of a German diabetes intervention study. The factor analytic procedures of the original study of Dunn *et al.* (1986) were repeated (i.e. the Scree Test was used to identify the likely factors) resulting in the identification of six factors. The original "Diabetes stress" factor was well replicated, although different item combinations formed the other five factors and these were labelled "Deficient coping and isolation", "Relationship to medical practitioner", "Personal responsibility", "Self-competence conviction" and "Unrealistic optimism".

Gosselin & Bergeron (submitted for publication) translated the ATT39 into French, excluding six items on the basis of low item to total correlations and renamed the measure the "ATED", which they used with French-Canadian patients. Factor analyses were then conducted in which the eigenvalues greater than unity rule was applied. This procedure identified twelve factors, six of which were retained as being the substantial factors. These subscales were labelled "Diabetes-related stress", "Receptivity to treatment", "Confidence in the treatment", "Personal efficacy" Perception about health" and "Social acceptance".

Table 2 Summary of available findings from studies involving the ATT39 and the ATT19

Author(s)	N	Age, sex ratio	Type of diabetes	Description of study	Study setting	ATT39 findings
ATT39						
Bott et al. (1988)	546	26 yrs	IDDM	Evaluation of a diabetes education programme	Diabetes centres in 9 German cities	Significant improvement in ATT39 total score at 1 year. Convergence of 4 of 6 ATT39 subscales towards normal
Boulton et al. (submitted for publication)	33/32	Children mean age 11.2 yrs	IDDM	Comparison of adjustment of a group of children with parents' ratings	Diabetes Education Centre, Newcastle, NSW, Australian	Children score higher on Alienation (F4). Also, significant trend overall to report better adjustment
Dunn et al. (1990)	309	49 yrs	IDDM/ NIDDM	Evaluation of a diabetes education programme	Diabetes Centre, Royal Prince Alfred Hospital, Sydney, Australia	ATT39 total score and score change correlated significantly with HbA1$_c$ improvement
Maxwell et al. (1992)	38/62	20-81 yrs 93/111 M/F	IDDM/ NIDDM	Comparison of a diabetes education plus social support group with education only group	Intensive Diabetes Outpatient Training and Education Centre, Cedars-Sinai Medical Centre, Los Angeles, US	Both groups scored higher on the total test score of a modified version of the ATT39. No difference between groups
Northam (1992, personal communication)	79/59	Age range 14-16 yrs	IDDM	Comparison of a group of adolescent patients with with a group of adult patients	Department of Child Family Therapy, The Royal Childrens Hospital, Victoria, Australia	Similar ATT39 subscale scores except for Dependence (F6). Boys higher than girls on Illness conviction

Table 2 (continued)

Author(s)	N	Age, sex ratio	Type of diabetes	Description of study	Study setting	ATT39 or ATT19 findings
O'Driscoll et al. (1992, personal communication)	29/28	29.8 years 60% M	IDDM	Comparison of a "brittle diabetes" group with a group having good control	Manchester Diabetes Centre, UK	ATT39 total score lower in brittle group, but not significant (mean 138.7 vs 143.9)
ATT39						
Seal (1992, personal communication)	52/52	57 yrs 59% M	NIDDM	Comparison of a comprehensive diabetes education programme with a control group that was simply posted written material	Diabetes Association of Western Australia	ATT39 total score higher in Programme group than Control group at 4 weeks
ATT19						
Welch et al. (in preparation)	142/198 303/177	36/35 yrs 49/58 yrs	IDDM NIDDM	Re-analysis of ATT39 validation data for the ATT19	Diabetes education centres at 5 public hospitals in Sydney, Australia and the Wellington Diabetes Service, Wellington Hospital, New Zealand	ATT19 correlated significantly and positively with diabetes knowledge, signficantly and negatively with locus of control. Patient group with complications had significantly poorer (lower) scores than a group without complications

Welch *et al.* (1992) in a New Zealand study examined the factor structure of the ATT39 using two samples of insulin-users attending the Wellington Diabetes Service, Wellington Hospital and a mixed sample of 170 IDDM and NIDDM patients from the original study of Dunn *et al.* (1986). In this study, the authors drew attention to current criticism of traditional eigenvalue-based criteria such as the Scree Test used in the earlier Sydney, German and French-Canadian studies. Eigenvalue-based criteria typically produce overfactoring of the true structure of a given measure (see Boyle, 1985; Walkey & McCormick, 1985; Zwick & Velicer, 1986). Welch *et al.* argued for the need to demonstrate replicability of the ATT39 factor solution and employed a factor matching procedure (FACTOREP, Walkey & McCormick, 1983) to help compare the ATT39 factor loading matrices and determine the most replicable solution. FACTOREP provides a strict criterion of the replicability of a measure's factor structure. The results did not support a six-factor solution and instead showed a single subscale to be the best interpretation. The twenty-item scale used by Welch *et al.* was based largely on items from the original "Diabetes stress" subscale (F1) and the "Guilt" subscale (F3).

The most recent factor-analytic study of the ATT39 by Welch *et al.* (in preparation) is an Australian study which has extended the previous series by determining the replicated factor structure of the ATT39 for IDDM and NIDDM patient groups separately. This separation of the analyses into IDDM and NIDDM was considered important, given the known clinical differences between these two subclasses of diabetes in terms of age of illness onset, treatment demands and type and timing of diabetes complications. In this study four patient samples from two Metropolitan hospital districts in Australia and New Zealand were used (see Table 1). In addition to Sydney samples of IDDM and NIDDM patients, further Wellington IDDM and NIDDM samples were obtained to provide replication samples for the factor analyses. In the results described below, the Sydney samples will be labelled as IDDM-Syd and NIDDM-Syd and the Wellington samples as IDDM-Wn and NIDDM-Wn.

The results of the initial six-factor analyses conducted separately for IDDM and NIDDM patient samples in this study showed little support for a six-factor solution. Further analyses were conducted for 5, 4, 3, and 2 and lastly, a single-factor analysis. The most replicable interpretation was found for a single-factor for both IDDM and NIDDM patient samples with a large group of significant items found to be in common when the unrotated first-factor loadings were inspected. There were twenty-eight significant items loading at or above 0.30 (see Nunnally, 1967, p.357) on this single factor for IDDM-Wn and 25 for IDDM-Syd, with 23 in common. For the NIDDM samples, there were 23 loading significantly for NIDDM-Wn and 21 for NIDDM-S, with 20 in common. Furthermore, nineteen of these significant items were common to both IDDM and NIDDM (see Figure 2). This set of items was therefore identified as the replicable core of the ATT39 for both IDDM and NIDDM and was labelled "Diabetes Integration" on the basis of its item content. Patients low on the ATT19 would be resentful, embarrassed, anxious, helpless, isolated and poorly adjusted to their diabetes, while those scoring high would be accepting of their diabetes, comfortable with public awareness of their diabetes, be calm, have a sense of self-control and feel well adjusted to their diabetes.

Reliability

Internal consistency

Dunn *et al.* (1986) reported the internal reliability of the ATT39 total test as measured by Cronbach's alpha to be 0.78. Bott *et al.* (1988) reported 0.71 and Seal (1992, personal communication) found 0.80. Gosselin & Bergeron (submitted for publication) found 0.80 for the thirty-three item French version, the ATED. Internal reliability coefficients of 0.56, 0.59, and 0.62 respectively were reported for the three fourteen-item short forms, the ATTA, ATTB and ATTC (Dunn *et al.*, 1990). Maxwell *et al.* (1992) reported a shortened fifteen-item form of the ATT39 that had a modest coefficient alpha of 0.66.

The coefficient alphas for the twenty-item subscale found by Welch *et al.* (1992) for the two samples of insulin users were 0.83 and 0.84, demonstrating improved reliability for this scale compared to the original ATT39 despite being halved in length as a result of the analyses. Similarly, coefficient alphas for the ATT19 (Diabetes Integration) measure were 0.84 and 0.82 for the Wellington and Sydney IDDM groups respectively. For the NIDDM samples, they were 0.82 and 0.83 (Welch *et al.*, in preparation).

Test-retest reliability

Two-week test-retest reliability (n = 24) was 0.70 for the original total ATT39 (Dunn *et al.*, 1986) with values from 0.39 to 0.83 for the six subscales. Test-retest reliability at three months (n = 149) was 0.76 for the total test with factor score values ranging from 0.40 to 0.77. At six months test-retest reliability (n = 81) was 0.76 for the total test with factor score values ranging from 0.37 to 0.76.

Validity of the ATT39

Face validity

In our experience of administering the ATT39 in studies based in diabetes outpatient settings, diabetes education groups and patient postal surveys where the measure was completed in the patient's own home, the ATT39 has appeared to have good face validity to patients in terms of its acceptability, the completion rate of its items and the perceived relevance of the items to the impact and management of diabetes. Similarly, the measure was acceptable to health professionals administering the ATT39 in these situations.

Concurrent and construct validity

ATT39 factor scores for 134 IDDM and 166 NIDDM patients were found by Dunn *et al.* (1986) to correlate significantly with the Cattell 16PF personality measure (Cattell *et al.*, 1970) and a locus of control scale developed by Craig *et al.* (1984). Anxiety as measured by the 16PF was associated with significant diabetes-related stress (F1), regardless of treatment, and with poorer adaptation (F2) and guilt (F3) in NIDDM. An external locus of control on the Craig *et al.* measure was related to increased stress (F1) and guilt (F3). For IDDM patients, age was positively related to better adaptation (F2), increased feelings of guilt (F3) and a more co-operative attitude to staff and treatment (F4). In NIDDM, age was associated with increasing resignation to a conviction of chronic illness (F5) and less tolerance for the ambiguities involved in diabetes (F6).

Predictive validity

Dunn *et al.*(1990) evaluated the impact of a two day diabetes education programme over a fifteen month period on attitudes to diabetes as measured by the three ATT39 short forms. ATT39 scores showed a significant convergence towards normal during the intervention (p<0.05) for the 309 patients and remained stable in a subset of 177 patients at three months follow up. Mean HbA1 improvement (from 11.3% to 9.0%) for the group was significant (p<0.001)) and predicted by stepwise regression from initial diabetes control (57%) and psychosocial factors (17%) which were: male sex (5%), higher (i.e. more positive attitude) score on the ATT39 (5%) and lower compulsiveness, higher sensitivity and emotional stability (7%) based on the 16PF personality test.

A German multicentre diabetes intervention study (Bott *et al.*, 1988) reported a convergence of ATT39 factor scores towards the mean for "Diabetes-related stress", "Deficient coping", "Relationship to medical practitioners", and "self-competence conviction" one year after a five day structured education programme. The authors had reversed the scoring of the ATT39 so that a low score represented good adjustment and found the thirty-nine item total score had significantly improved (p<0.0001) from 99.4 (±14.7) to 94.3 (±12.8) 1 year after the intervention. Neither ATT39 total scores or subscales were related significantly to HbA1.

Gosselin and Bergeron applied a thirty-three item French version of the ATT39 (the ATED) in a Canadian study that drew on Janis' (1984) model of stages of psychological adaptation and applied it to diabetes (Gosselin & Bergeron, submitted for publication). The results of a multiple regression analysis showed that patients showing positive attitudes towards diabetes and its treatment (i.e. in the last two stages of the adaptation model, "Self-assessment and receptivity" or "Active acceptance") showed greater improvement in HbA$_{1C}$ values three months after a diabetes education programme than those with the negative attitudes of "Opposition and ventilation of feelings" and "Bargaining" (regression coefficient = .16, p<0.05). In a second study, two of their defined ATT39 subscales ("Confidence in the treatment" and "Social acceptance") were found to be predictive of HbA$_{1C}$ improvement of patients three months after their attendance at a diabetes education programme.

Discriminant validity

Other studies by Dunn and colleagues have explored aspects of the discriminant validity of the ATT39. A cross-sectional study of the stability of psychological adjustment to diabetes involved the use of multivariate analyses of variance and covariance to assess effects of treatment and duration of diabetes on the six ATT39 factor scores for three groups defined in terms of age at diagnosis (Dunn *et al.*, 1985). The age at diagnosis groups were: Early onset ($\leq$ 35 years), Middle onset (36 to 55 years) and Late onset (> 55 years). The results showed duration of diabetes was significantly related to changes in ATT39 subscale profiles in the Early ($p<0.05$) and Late ($p<0.01$) onset groups, but not the Middle group.

Seal (1992, personal communication) used the ATT39 total test in an evaluation of a four week community-based diabetes education programme conducted by the Diabetes Association of Western Australia. One hundred and four NIDDM patients took part in the study (mean age = 57 years, 59% male). Patients were allocated either to an education programme group (n = 52), receiving twelve hours of teaching in diabetes and its management, or to a minimal intervention group (n = 52) that simply received written material through the mail. Total ATT39 scores were obtained from summing unit weights. There was a significant increase in mean ATT39 total score for the full intervention group from 135.4 ($\pm$11.9) at baseline to 141.2 ($\pm$12.5) at follow up, but no difference for the minimal intervention group which scored 138.6 ($\pm$13.1) at baseline and 140.9 ($\pm$12.6) at follow-up.

O'Driscoll *et al.* (1992, personal communication) compared a group of twenty-nine insulin-dependent patients with brittle diabetes attending the Manchester Diabetes Centre, UK with twenty-nine well controlled patients on a range of personality, cognitive, psychiatric and social measures that included the ATT39. The two groups were matched for age, sex and length of illness. Interim findings showed that the control group scored higher on the ATT39 total test than the brittle diabetes group, indicating better psychological adjustment (mean scores = 152.0 versus 141.0) and lower on the Holmes-Rahe Life Stress Scale (mean scores = 89 versus 137) although these trends did not reach statistical significance. The control group also scored significantly lower on the General Health Questionnaire, a measure of probable psychiatric illness (mean score of 13 versus 22, $p<0.01$), and the Present State Examination, a rating of psychiatric symptomatology (mean scores = 0 versus 4, $p<0.001$). There was no difference between the two groups on a measure of social stress and support and a measure of memory performance.

Boulton *et al.* (submitted for publication) compared the psychological adjustment of thirty-three children (twenty-one girls, twelve boys) with IDDM attending a diabetes education centre in Newcastle, Australia with ratings given for the children by their parents. The children had a mean age of 11.2 years and diabetes duration ranging from 2 to 6.5 years. The authors reported that parent ratings of child adjustment were lower than those obtained from their children. There was a trend overall across all factors for parents to rate their child's adjustment as poorer, ranging in standardised difference scores from 0.04 for Alienation (F4) to 0.24 for Tolerance for Ambiguity (F6) and an overall mean of 0.15.

Maxwell *et al.* (1992) compared the ATT39 scores of a group of IDDM and NID-DM patients in Los Angeles, USA receiving diabetes education together with social support with a second group that received individual diabetes education only. ATT39 scores for a shortened fifteen-item version of the measure improved significantly for both groups at seven-months follow-up (p<0.002) although there was no difference between the two groups in mean score on this short form of the ATT39.

Other Studies Using the ATT39

Northam (1992, personal communication) compared ATT39 scores for seventy-nine adolescents with insulin-dependent diabetes attending the Department of Child and Family Psychiatry at the Royal Childrens' Hospital, Melbourne, with those of a sample of fifty-nine adult patients. Adolescents differed from adults only on Tolerance for Ambiguity (F6). Boys expressed significantly higher Illness conviction (F5) than girls (t = 3.6, p<0.001) but did not differ on the other sub-scales. ATT39 subscales were not related to metabolic control as measured by HbA_{1c}.

Validity of the ATT19

Concurrent and construct validity

Welch *et al.* (in preparation) in a recent joint study between Australia and New Zealand, explored the clinical usefulness of the nineteen-item subscale described above and labelled the ATT19 or "Diabetes Integration" scale. This study used the IDDM (n = 142) and NIDDM (n = 303) patient samples described above in the 1992 Sydney analyses. Also, further IDDM (n = 69) and NIDDM (n = 67) samples of attenders at the Wellington Diabetes Service were gathered prospectively to examine the relationship between ATT19 and blood glucose control (i.e. HbA_1). The response rate to the completion of the ATT39 by the latter patients was 73%. The two groups had mean HbA_1 values of 6.4% and 7.0% respectively.

The results showed the ATT19 to correlate significantly with diabetes knowledge as measured by the DKN scales (Dunn *et al.*, 1984; Beeney *et al.*, this volume) for the IDDM-S and NIDDM-S groups (r = 0.19, p<0.01), indicating that greater knowledge of diabetes was associated with better adjustment. Also, it correlated significantly and negatively with the Craig *et al.* (1984) locus of control measure for both IDDM (r = -0.52, p<0.001) and NIDDM (r = -0.29, p<0.001), indicating that an internal locus of control was related to better psychological adjustment. The ATT19 did not correlate significantly with glycosylated haemoglobin when adjustment was made for age of onset and duration of diabetes. Comparison of mean ATT19 scores across IDDM and NIDDM groups using non-parametric one-way analysis of variance showed that there was no overall difference between the 4 groups.

Seal (1992, personal communication) reanalysed the ATT39 data from her evaluation of a four-week community-based NIDDM diabetes education programme in Western Australia to calculate the changes in patient ATT19 scores (see above for details). ATT19 scores at baseline for the total group (n = 104) were not correlated with body mass index (r = -0.01, n.s.), HbA1$_C$ (r = -0.06, n.s.) or diabetes knowledge as measured by the DKN scales (p = -0.07, n.s.). Change in ATT19 score for the total group over the four-week intervention correlated non-significantly with body mass index (r = 0.11), HbA1$_C$ (r = -0.13) or DKN (r = 0.15).

Discriminant validity

Dunn & Beeney (1988, unpublished) examined the relationship between the ATT19 and diabetes complications status in a subset of outpatients for whom complications could be clearly established as either absent (n = 112) or present (n = 23) as determined from medical records. Patients were classified as having complications if there was at least one serious microvascular or macrovascular complication present and described in the patient notes (e.g., retinopathy, neuropathy, nephropathy). The results showed a significant difference (t = 3.54, p<0.001) between mean ATT19 scores for the Complications group (mean score = 67.9±8.0) and Non-complications group (72.4±5.6) indicating that patients who were experiencing the onset of complications were more resentful, embarrassed, anxious, helpless, isolated and poorly adjusted to their diabetes than those without complications.

Seal (1992, personal communication), in her evaluation of a four-week community-based diabetes education programme, found a significant increase in mean ATT19 total scores for the full intervention group (n = 52) from 68.2±9.4 to 72.2±8.4 (p<0.001) and the mininum intervention group (n = 52) from 69.8±10.0 to 71.9±8.2 (p<0.04).

DISCUSSION

The clinical utility of the ATT39 is now augmented by the development of the nineteen-item ATT19 scale which is applicable for both IDDM and NIDDM. The internal reliability of the ATT19 is high despite it being shortened by half compared to the original thirty-nine item measure. The simpler scoring of the ATT19 and its relative brevity should help make it more user-friendly for the clinician or researcher based in a busy diabetes clinic as it can be completed and scored in a few minutes.

The ATT19 appears, on face inspection, to measure the extent to which diabetes is integrated into the patient's lifestyle and personality. Anderson (1986), in discussing the importance of the personal meaning of diabetes for each patient, drew attention to the fact that patients "must learn to incorporate the disorder into the self-concept" and that "how well the diabetes and self-concept are integrated influences how much the disorder will become a psychological problem and what a person's behavioural response will be". From our reading of the current diabetes literature, Anderson's concept of integration comes closest to our perception of the characteristic measured by the ATT19. Hopefully, the original ATT39 will continue to be used by researchers interested in replicating and extending the detailed subscale analyses reported so far.

Despite encouraging early findings, the ATT19 remains at a relatively early stage of development and further information is needed both from reanalyses of data reported on the original ATT39 measure and from new studies. In particular, there is a need for further studies to evaluate the new measure's sensitivity to detect change in patient adjustment following clinical and educational interventions, to determine its discriminatory power with respect to clinically-relevant criterion groups (such as those with poor versus good adherence to diabetes treatment regimens) and its relationship to a range of salient clinical and demographic variables.

Interestingly, the more recent studies for the ATT19 and those for the original ATT39 show that the measure does not appear to be related in any simple way to glycosylated haemoglobin. On reflection, this may be predictable given the time frame assessed by this index of metabolic control. Psychological distress associated with fluctuating control is more likely to be related to blood glucose levels than to HbA_1 levels which average out blood glucose fluctuations. We look forward to continued collaboration with clinicians and researchers who use the ATT39 and ATT19 scales which are made available here to encourage further research.

SUMMARY AND CONCLUSION

The ATT39 is a self-report measure designed to help health professionals to assess patient psychological adjustment to diabetes and to measure change in this adjustment process over time, e.g. over the course of diabetes education programmes or treatment interventions. The measure appears acceptable to patients in terms of its face validity and ease of comprehension and its scoring has recently been simplified to involve the summation of unit weights rather than the use of factor scores.

Its psychometric properties have been examined in a number of studies, the more recent of which have applied rigorous factor analytic criteria to identify its replicable core. As part of the refinement of these analyses, the ATT39 internal structure has been examined separately for IDDM and NIDDM patient groups, based on the known clinical differences between these subclasses of diabetes. Factor analysis is an important component of the process of establishing the construct validity of a measure as it examines empirically the rationale for a total score and for any subscales that are described. It can provide strong evidence on the nature of the internal structure of a given measure, particularly if the findings can be replicated across several independent samples. The replicated factor analytic studies of the ATT39 using a factor matching technique have highlighted its unidimensional nature as an index of psychological adjustment to diabetes and identified a subscale comprising nineteen items as the central core (the ATT19 or Diabetes Integration) common to both IDDM and NIDDM patient groups.

The clinical utility of the original ATT39 has been assessed in several studies involving the total test and its six factor scores. These have focused on its relationship to selected demographic and clinical variables, the measurement of change in patient psychological adjustment following diabetes education programmes and on its ability to discriminate between criterion groups selected on the basis of clinical criteria.

The majority of studies reported to date on the clinical application of the ATT39 has focused on the earlier multidimensional forms of the measure and their predictive, concurrent and discriminant validity. Data are now appearing on the discriminant and construct validity of the ATT19. The latter studies have provided some encouraging support for the potential clinical usefulness of this new measure, including some evidence that it shows sensitivity to change over the course of Diabetes Education Programmes, that it correlates as predicted with diabetes knowledge and with locus of control.

REFERENCES

Anderson, B. (1986). The personal meaning of having diabetes: Implications for patient behaviour and education. *Diabetic Medicine*, **3**, 85–89

Boulton, J., Garrick, D., Dunn, S. and Mensch, M. (submitted for publication) Attitudes of children and their parents to diabetes: Focus on emotional adjustment. Submitted to *Journal of Paediatrics and Child Health*

Bott, U., Scholz, V., Grusser, M., Jorgens, V., Muhlhauser, I. and Berger, M. (1988) Emotional adjustment in 546 Type I Diabetic Patients using the ATT39 scale. *Diabetes Research and Clinical Practice, supplement 1*, **5**, S648

Boyle, G. (1985) Self report measures of depression. Some psychometric considerations. *British Journal of Clinical Psychology*, **124**, 45–59

Cattell, R.B. (1966) *Handbook of Multivariate Experimental Psychology*. Chicago, Rand-MacNally

Cattell, R.B., Eber, H. and Tatsuoka, M. (1970). *Handbook for the Sixteen Personality Factor Questionnaire (16PF)*. Champaign, Illinois: Institute for Personality and Ability Testing

Cohen, J. (1990). "Things I have learned so far". *American Psychologist*, (December) 1306

Craig, A.R., Franklin, J.A. and and Andrews, G. (1984). A scale to measure locus of control of behaviour. *British Journal of Medical Psychology*, **57**, 173–180

Dunn, S.M. (1984) *The Psychological Impact of Diabetes Education: Implications for Metabolic Control*. Doctoral Thesis, Faculty of Medicine, University of Sydney, Australia

Dunn, S.M. (1986) Reactions to educational techniques: coping strategies for diabetes and learning. *Diabetic Medicine* **3**(5), 419-429

Dunn, S.M. and Turtle, J. (1981) The myth of the diabetic personality. *Diabetes Care*, **4**, 640–646

Dunn, S.M., Bryson J.M., Hoskins P.L., Alford J.B., Handelsman D.J. and Turtle J.R. (1984) Development of the Diabetes Knowledge (DKN) Scales: Forms DKNA, DKNB, and DKNC. **7**(1), 36–41

Dunn, S.M., Hoskins P.L., Beeney L.J. and Turtle J.R. (1985) Knowledge and attitude change in diabetes education and their relation to metabolic control. Proceedings of the International Diabetes Federation, Madrid, 1985. *Diabetes Research & Clinical Practice* (suppl 1), 369

Dunn, S.M., Beeney, L. and Turtle, J. (1985a) The instability of adjustment in diabetes. *Proceedings of the Australian Diabetes Association/Australian Diabetes Educators Association*, 43

Dunn, S.M., Smartt, H., Beeney, L. and Turtle, J. (1986) Measurement of emotional adjustment in diabetic patients: Validity and reliability of ATT39. *Diabetes Care*, 9, 480–489

Dunn, S.M., Beeney, L. and Turtle, J. (1986a) Psychological adjustment and metabolic control in IDD. *Proceedings of the Australian Diabetes Association/Australian Diabetes Educators Association*, 13

Dunn, S.M., Beeney, L., Hoskins, P. and Turtle, J. (1990) Knowledge and attitude change as predictors of metabolic improvement in diabetes education. *Social Science and Medicine*, 31, 1135–1141

Eross, J., Kreutzman, D. and Jiminiz, M. (1984) Calorimetric measurement of glycosylated protein in whole blood, red blood cells, plasma and dried blood. *Annals of Clinical Biochemistry*, 21, 477–438

Gosselin, M. and Bergeron, J. (submitted for publication) Evaluative study of the diabetes stress adaptation model.

Janis, I. (1984) Patient as a decision maker. In W.D. Gentry, (ed.) *Handbook of behavioural medicine*. New York: Guilford Press

Maxwell, A., Hunt, I. and Bush, M. (1992) Effects of a social support group as an adjunct to diabetes training on metabolic control and psychosocial outcomes. *The Diabetes Educator* 18(4), 303–309

Nunnally, J. C. (1967) *Psychometric Theory*. McGraw-Hill: New York

Papadam, A., Dunn, S.M., Yue, D.K and Turtle, J. (1985). Ethnic differences in diabetes adjustment. *Proceedings of the Australian Diabetes Association/Australian Diabetes Educators Association*, 41

Simon, M. and Elssler, J. (1980) Critical factors in the chromatographic measurement of glycohaemoglobin (HbA_1). *Diabetes*, 28, 467–474

Simonds, J., Goldstein, D., Walker, B. and Rawlings, S. (1981) The relationship between psychological factors and blood glucose regulation in insulin-dependent diabetic adolescents. *Diabetes Care*, 4, 610–615

Walkey, F. and McCormick, I. (1983) *FACTOREP: A Pascal programme to examine factor replication*. Victoria University of Wellington publications in Psychology, No. 29, Victoria University of Wellington, Wellington, New Zealand

Walkey, F. and McCormick, I. (1985) Multiple replication of factor structure: a logical solution for a number of factors problem. *Multivariate Behavioural Research*, 20, 57–67

Welborn, T., Garcia-Webb, P., Bonser, A., McCann, V. and Constable, I. (1983) Clinical criteria that reflect C–peptide status in idiopathic diabetes. *Diabetes Care*, 6, 315–316

Welch, G., Beeney, L., Dunn, S. and Smith, R.B.W. (1994) The development of the Diabetes Integration scale: A psychometric study of the ATT39. *Multivariate Experimental Clinical Research*. 11(2) (In press)

Welch, G., Beeney, L., Dunn, S. and Smith, R.B.W. (in preparation) Psychological adjustment to diabetes: An exploration of differences between IDD and NIDD

Welch, G., Smith, R.B.W. and Walkey, F. (1992) Styles of psychological adjustment in diabetes: A focus on key psychometric issues and the ATT39. *Journal of Clinical Psychology*. 48(5), 648–658

Wilkinson, G. (1987) The influence of psychiatric, psychological and social factors on the control of insulin-dependent diabetes mellitus. *Journal of Psychosomatic Research*, 31, 277–286.

Zwick, W. and Velicer, W. (1986) Comparison of five rules for the number of components to retain. *Psychological Medicine*, 99, 432–442

CHAPTER 12

MEASURES OF DIABETES-SPECIFIC HEALTH BELIEFS

KATHRYN S. LEWIS[1] and CLARE BRADLEY[2]

[1]*Department of Psychology, University of Sheffield, South Yorkshire S10 2TN, UK.*
[2]*Department of Psychology, Royal Holloway, University of London, Egham Hill, Egham, Surrey TW20 0EX, UK*

INTRODUCTION

This chapter describes two sets of health belief scales which were developed respectively from the responses of insulin-treated and tablet-treated diabetic individuals who attended hospital outpatient clinics in Sheffield, UK. Measures specific to these different types of diabetic regimen were conceived because it has been noted that the psychological responses of individuals to their disorder will differ according to disease type and treatment mode (Davis *et al.,* 1987). The main purpose of the scales was to measure beliefs about diabetes and its complications in order to understand individual differences in preferences for different treatment regimens and to assess treatment efficacy. They are likely to be particularly useful in research which aims to assess the effectiveness of interventions such as education programmes seeking to modify health beliefs to achieve desired health outcomes. The scales may be useful also as instruments of audit if indicators about the suitability of possible interventions are sought. It is important to appreciate, however, that it is not appropriate to use the measures to specify a 'gold standard' pattern of beliefs recommended for all people with diabetes mellitus. Indeed, the scales provide measures of psychological processes rather than outcomes. As such, they may be used to understand how patients' beliefs are associated with their behaviour in the context of the treatment and education provided, and the particular health care system in which they find themselves. Health care practitioners should then be better informed in order to intervene more appropriately and organise their services to achieve greater effectiveness.

The two sets of scales described below have been employed in several types of research studies. The scales designed for insulin-treated individuals and described in Part 1 of this chapter, have been used in a feasibility study of continuous subcutaneous insulin infusion (CSII) pumps in order to assess their usefulness in understanding individual differences in treatment choice and perceived efficacy of treatment (Bradley *et al.,* 1987). They have also been used to predict the risk of diabetic ketoacidosis in patients using CSII pumps (Bradley *et al.,* 1986). In a study of Swedish patients, Sjoberg et al., (1988) employed the scales designed for insulin users in order to compare the health beliefs of individuals with and without residual insulin secretion and Gillespie (1989) has used them in a study which assessed the relationship between health beliefs, knowledge of diabetes, perceptions of control, and metabolic control. The health belief measures relating to tablet-treated diabetes, described in Part 2 of this chapter, have been developed more recently (Lewis *et al.*, 1990) and were based on the experience of developing and interpreting findings from the insulin users' scales (Bradley *et al.*, 1984). The newer measures have been employed in a diabetes education intervention study and were used to predict blood glucose control six months later (Lewis, 1992). They have also been included during the various phases of a study which compared CSII with conventional insulin therapy in patients with poorly controlled tablet-treated diabetes (Jennings *et al.*, 1991; Lewis, 1993).

The first set of scales described in this chapter are for insulin users and were developed because no diabetes-specific health beliefs scales were available that had been developed psychometrically. Previously researchers had employed versions of health belief scales with samples of diabetic patients (Alogna, 1980; Bloom Cerkoney et al., 1980; Harris *et al.*, 1982) but none had presented data on the reliability of the scales and few had provided sufficient detail about scale contents even to judge face validity. Although their results had looked promising, support for their hypotheses had been limited and inconsistent. We were not alone in recognising the need for scales of known reliability and some evidence of validity. Several research groups developed health belief scales psychometrically with various samples of people with diabetes. Given *et al.* (1983) developed health belief scales for a mixed sample of patients with Type 1 or Type 2 diabetes in the USA. Harris *et al.* (1987) went on to develop their previously undeveloped scales with a sample of male patients with Type 2 diabetes. Brownlee Duffolk *et al.* (1987) developed a scale with Type 1 patients. Davis *et al.*, (1987) have developed measures of health beliefs as part of a package of psychosocial measures called the 'The Diabetes Education Profile' (see Appendix). The Profile has been developed with Type 1 and Type 2 patients treated with insulin, tablets and/or diet. The present scales were developed with British samples of men and women with diabetes; insulin-treated patients were the sample for the first of the scales and tablet-treated patients were the sample for the second version. Thus, the scales presented here are offered as two of several available health belief scales which have varying levels of specificity to different sub-samples of the population of people with diabetes.

PART 1: HEALTH BELIEF SCALES FOR INSULIN-TREATED PATIENTS

Design

The psychosocial model underpinning the scales is the Health Belief Model (HBM) which was developed by four social psychologists: Hochbaum, Kegeles, Leventhal, and Rosenstock (Hochbaum, 1958; Rosenstock, 1966) to explain preventative health behaviour and was later modified by Becker and colleagues (1974, 1975) to explain sick role behaviours. According to the HBM, there are four important belief factors which determine whether or not an individual will follow the treatment recommended. These beliefs concern perceptions of (1) the severity of the disorder, (2) vulnerability to the disorder, (3) the benefits of treatment, and (4) the barriers to treatment. Thus, in relation to diabetes, an individual's readiness to follow the treatment regimen is highly dependent, on the one hand, upon the perceived desirability of avoiding the symptoms and complications of the disorder, and on the other, upon beliefs that the health action(s) necessary will be effective but not too costly in relation to other valued aspects of the individual's lifestyle. Beliefs about the degree of severity and vulnerability are hypothesized to provide the impetus to act, and the perceived 'cost-effectiveness' of treatment (benefits less barriers) to influence the preferred health action. The HBM also specifies that behaviour is triggered by 'cues to action' which make health threats more salient to the individual. Such stimuli might include the individual's internal symptoms, or they may be external prompts such as reminders from health care staff, family members or the media. As mentioned by Janz and Becker (1984), the HBM is limited to accounting for the proportion of variance in individuals' health-related behaviours that can be explained by their beliefs. Other mediating and enabling factors such as demographic variables, knowledge, perceived control and self-efficacy, and social support are also important in shaping health behaviour. Diabetes-specific scales which measure some of these variables can be found elsewhere in this book in other chapters (e.g. Bradley's chapter on measures of Perceived Control of Diabetes, and Beeney et al.'s chapter on measurement of diabetes knowledge and in the Appendix.

In accordance with the HBM, the present questionnaires were constructed to measure perceived Benefits of, and Barriers to, treatment, and perceived Severity of, and Vulnerability to, the complications of diabetes. The original scales designed were modified from unpublished scales designed for adults with diabetes by Shillitoe (1981, personal communication). The developed versions of the scales for insulin-treated patients are presented in Figures 1-3.

Perceived Benefits and Barriers

The measurement of perceived benefits of, and barriers to, treatment was achieved by creating a pool of twenty eight statements each with a seven point scale ranging from "strongly agree" to "strongly disagree". Statements were explicitly concerned with the respondents' views about themselves and their disorder and were designed in order to reflect the advantages and disadvantages of following the treatment recommendations for insulin users.

Perceived Severity and Vulnerability

In order to measure perceived severity, the questionnaire was designed to ask respondents to rate how serious they thought various disorders related and unrelated to diabetes would be if they were to develop them. Perceived vulnerability

was measured in a similar manner by asking respondents to rate how likely they
were to develop the disorders.

Scoring

Perceived Benefits and Barriers

Respondents rate their agreement or disagreement with each statement on the
seven-point scale from 6 (strongly agree) to 0 (strongly disagree). The developed
scales consist of six benefits items and six barriers items (see Figure 1). Ratings
for the benefits statements should be summed separately from ratings for the barriers statements in order to obtain:

   a) total score for perceived Benefits: items $1 + 4 + 7 + 8 + 10 + 12$
   b) total score for perceived Barriers: items $2 + 3 + 5 + 6 + 9 + 11$

   Scores on the Barriers and Benefits subscales range from 0 to 36 with higher
scores indicating more perceived Benefits or more perceived Barriers. A measure
of perceived "Cost-effectiveness" of treatment may be obtained by subtracting the
Barriers score from the Benefits score for each subject.

Perceived Severity and Vulnerability

On the respective questionnaires (see Figures 2 and 3), respondents rate the seriousness of various problems and the likelihood of having them on six-point scales
from 5 (extremely serious/very likely) to 0 (not serious at all/very unlikely). Fifteen of the problems are not specifically related to diabetes: Stomach ulcer, Bronchitis, Problems with hearing, Ingrowing toenail, Loss of bladder control, Flu,
Piles (haemorrhoids), Arthritis, Shortness of breath, Depression requiring treatment, Loss of appetite for more than one day, Cancer, Broken arm, Constipation,
and Gall stones. Eight of the problems are manifestations of the long-term complications of diabetes: High blood pressure, Deteriorating eyesight, Aching legs,
Heart trouble, Numbness in the feet, Blurred vision for more than one day, Circulatory problems in the feet, Kidney problems. Two short-term complications of
insulin-treated diabetes are included: Diabetic coma (high sugar coma) and
hypoglycaemic coma (low sugar coma). Three items are concerned with general
management problems: Insulin reaction (hypo), Very high sugar levels for more
than one day (blood sugars 17 mmol/L or more, or urine sugars 3% or more),
Excessive weight gain. Three of the items on the severity scale are about diabetes
and its complications in general: Your diabetes now, Your diabetes in twenty
years' time, and Complications arising from diabetes. Only the third item of these
last three, Complications arising from diabetes, was included in the vulnerability
scale as all the respondents will have diabetes already.

Figure 1

EXPERIENCE OF TREATMENT BENEFITS AND BARRIERS

In this section would you please circle one of the numbers on each of the scales to indicate how strongly you agree or disagree with each of the following statements.

On these scales   6   would indicate that you strongly agree
                      5 =   moderately agree
                      4 =   mildly agree
                      3 =   neither agree nor disagree
                      2 =   mildly disagree
                      1 =   moderately disagree
                      0 =   strongly disagree

	strongly disagree						strongly agree
1. Regular, controlled exercise helps in the management of my diabetes	0	1	2	3	4	5	6
2. Controlling my diabetes well imposes restrictions on my whole lifestyle	0	1	2	3	4	5	6
3. Controlling my diabetes well interferes with my work (housework or paid work)	0	1	2	3	4	5	6
4. The risk of insulin reactions (hypos) is reduced if I eat meals at regular intervals	0	1	2	3	4	5	6
5. It is just not possible to control my diabetes properly and live in a way that is acceptable to me	0	1	2	3	4	5	6
6. Controlling my diabetes well interferes with my leisure activities	0	1	2	3	4	5	6
7. It is important for me to visit the diabetic clinic regularly even in the absence of symptoms	0	1	2	3	4	5	6
8. High blood sugars can be prevented if I plan ahead	0	1	2	3	4	5	6
9. Sticking to my diet makes eating out difficult	0	1	2	3	4	5	6
10. Insulin reactions (hypos) can be prevented if I plan ahead	0	1	2	3	4	5	6
11. Controlling my diabetes when I am away from home often causes me embarrassment	0	1	2	3	4	5	6
12. By careful planning of diet, exercise and insulin, I can control my diabetes at least as well as most other people with diabetes	0	1	2	3	4	5	6

Please make sure that you have considered each of the 12 statements and have circled a number on each of the scales.

Figure 2

BELIEFS ABOUT SEVERITY

In this section would you please circle a number on each of the scales to indicate how serious you think the following problems would be if you were to develop them.

On these scales   5   would indicate that the problem is extremely serious
                    4 = very serious
                    3 = moderately serious
                    2 = mildly serious
                    1 = not serious enough to be worrying
                    0 = not serious at all

	not serious at all					extremely serious
1. Stomach ulcer	0	1	2	3	4	5
2. High blood pressure	0	1	2	3	4	5
3. Bronchitis	0	1	2	3	4	5
4. Problems with hearing	0	1	2	3	4	5
5. Deteriorating eyesight	0	1	2	3	4	5
6. Aching legs	0	1	2	3	4	5
7. Ingrowing toenail	0	1	2	3	4	5
8. Heart trouble	0	1	2	3	4	5
9. Numbness in the feet	0	1	2	3	4	5
10. Loss of bladder control	0	1	2	3	4	5
11. Diabetic coma (high sugar coma)	0	1	2	3	4	5
12. Flu	0	1	2	3	4	5
13. Blurred vision for more than one day	0	1	2	3	4	5
14. Your diabetes now	0	1	2	3	4	5
15. Your diabetes in 20 years' time	0	1	2	3	4	5
16. Hypoglycaemic coma (low sugar coma)	0	1	2	3	4	5
17. Piles (haemorrhoids)	0	1	2	3	4	5
18. Arthritis	0	1	2	3	4	5
19. Insulin reaction (hypo)	0	1	2	3	4	5
20. Very high sugar levels for more than one day (blood sugars 17mmol/L or more or urine sugars 3% or more)	0	1	2	3	4	5
21. Shortness of breath	0	1	2	3	4	5
22. Depression requiring treatment	0	1	2	3	4	5
23. Circulatory problems in the feet	0	1	2	3	4	5
24. Loss of appetite for more than one day	0	1	2	3	4	5
25. Cancer	0	1	2	3	4	5
26. Broken arm	0	1	2	3	4	5
27. Kidney problems	0	1	2	3	4	5
28. Excessive weight gain	0	1	2	3	4	5
29. Constipation	0	1	2	3	4	5
30. Gall stones	0	1	2	3	4	5
31. Complications arising from diabetes	0	1	2	3	4	5

Please make sure that you have circled one number on each of the 31 scales.

Figure 3

BELIEFS ABOUT VULNERABILITY

In this section would you please circle a number on each of the scales to indicate how likely you feel you are to develop the following problems.

Please answer according to how you feel personally rather than according to what you believe the frequency of each problem to be generally.

On these scales	5	would indicate that you are very likely to develop the problem
	4 =	quite likely
	3 =	probably
	2 =	probably not
	1 =	quite unlikely
	0 =	very unlikely

At any time in the future, how likely do you feel you are to develop the following problems?

	Very unlikely					Very likely
1. Gall stones	0	1	2	3	4	5
2. Arthritis	0	1	2	3	4	5
3. Deteriorating eyesight	0	1	2	3	4	5
4. Kidney problems	0	1	2	3	4	5
5. Diabetic coma (high sugar coma)	0	1	2	3	4	5
6. Stomach ulcer	0	1	2	3	4	5
7. Broken arm	0	1	2	3	4	5
8. Circulatory problems (of the feet)	0	1	2	3	4	5
9. High blood pressure	0	1	2	3	4	5
10. Numbness in the feet	0	1	2	3	4	5
11. Aching legs	0	1	2	3	4	5
12. Piles (haemorrhoids)	0	1	2	3	4	5
13. Blurred vision for more than one day	0	1	2	3	4	5
14. Bronchitis	0	1	2	3	4	5
15. Excessive weight gain	0	1	2	3	4	5
16. Insulin reaction (hypo)	0	1	2	3	4	5
17. Heart trouble	0	1	2	3	4	5
18. Problems with hearing	0	1	2	3	4	5
19. Complications arising from diabetes	0	1	2	3	4	5
20. Ingrowing toenail	0	1	2	3	4	5
21. Hypoglyaemic coma (low sugar coma)	0	1	2	3	4	5
22. Depression requiring treatment	0	1	2	3	4	5
23. Cancer	0	1	2	3	4	5
24. Loss of bladder control	0	1	2	3	4	5
25. Flu	0	1	2	3	4	5
26. Very high sugar levels for more than one day (blood sugars 17mmol/L or more or urine sugars 3% or more)	0	1	2	3	4	5

27. Constipation	0	1	2	3	4	5
28. Shortness of breath	0	1	2	3	4	5
29. Loss of appetite for more than one day	0	1	2	3	4	5

Please make sure that you have circled one number on each of the 29 scales.

Health Beliefs I/3.2: © Sept 93 Dr Clare Bradley, Royal Holloway, University of London, Egham, Surrey, TW20 0EX, UK

Scores for the individual items may be used in analyses. However, researchers may wish to sum the responses to the problems related and not specifically related to diabetes, respectively, in order to obtain composite variables. Bradley *et al.* (1984, 1986, 1987) did not include all of the items in the questionnaire for the purpose of analyses, and selected instead representative long term complications and equivalent disorders unrelated to diabetes. The Complications items selected were Deteriorating eyesight, Kidney problems, Circulatory problems in the feet, and Heart trouble. The General disorders items selected were Bronchitis, Cancer, Stomach ulcer, and Arthritis.

Scores for individual items range from 0 to 5 with higher scores indicating greater perceived Severity of, or Vulnerability to, the particular problem. (The earlier versions of the Severity and Vulnerability scales were scored from 1-6 but have now been changed to be consistent with the other scales.) Composite scores will depend on the number of items included but for the above selections of Complications and General disorders range from 0 to 20, in each case. Once again higher scores indicate greater perceived Severity or Vulnerability.

DEVELOPMENT OF THE SCALES FOR INSULIN-TREATED PATIENTS

Subject Samples and Procedures

Study 1:   Sheffield feasibility study of CSII: Bradley et al. (1984)

The sample in this study provided the original data from which the factor structure and internal reliability of the perceived Benefits and Barriers scales were obtained.

Three hundred and eighty-two insulin-requiring diabetic patients (195 men and 187 women) at the Royal Hallamshire Hospital, Sheffield, UK, involved in a feasibility study of CSII were included in the study. Patients aged between sixteen and fifty nine were considered for inclusion in this study unless CSII was considered to be impractical, disruptive or potentially dangerous. Individuals were excluded if they were using less than twenty four units of insulin per day, had been treated with insulin for fewer than six months, were blind or had undergone amputation of a lower limb, were currently pregnant, on a renal dialysis programme or were receiving psychiatric treatment. Questionnaires were completed and returned by

286 patients (146 men and 140 women) indicating a 75% response rate from the total population sample of 382 patients.

The patients were initially invited to an illustrated lecture on the treatments offered. The lecture emphasized that evidence suggested that poor blood glucose control was related to later development of complications in diabetes. CSII and intensified conventional treatment (ICT) were then presented as methods for improving glycaemic control in conjunction with home blood glucose monitoring. The patients could choose between CSII, ICT or to remain on their conventional treatment (CT). Patients were given the questionnaires when they attended a subsequent individual consultation. Following the consultation, patients chose one of the treatments offered. Questionnaires were completed at or shortly after the initial consultation before any change in treatment regimen and were returned in prepaid envelopes addressed to the Psychology Department, Sheffield University, UK. Data were available from 95 respondents who chose CSII, 122 who chose ICT and 69 who chose CT. The Diabetes-Specific Health Belief Scales and scales developed to measure perceived control of insulin-treated diabetes (see Chapter 13) were used in order to predict treatment choice and efficacy.

Study 2: Diabetic ketoacidosis (DKA) study: Bradley et al. (1986)

The subjects in this study were a subsample of the patients described in Study 1. The subsample consisted of twenty two patients. Eleven of them had been selected because they had experienced episodes of diabetic ketoacidosis over a period of two years and six months while using CSII. They were then matched for age, sex and duration of diabetes with eleven patients using the same treatment who had not experienced ketoacidosis. The rationale for the study was to assess whether various patient characteristics (including Health Beliefs), could predict occurrence of ketoacidosis in pump users.

Study 3: C-peptide study: Sjoberg et al. (1988)

The subjects of this study were outpatients in a Swedish hospital who had been invited by letter to participate. Selection criteria were: onset of Type 1 diabetes prior to age thirty years, duration of the disorder from nine to sixteen years; and body mass index <25 kg/m^2. Out of 108 patients invited, 97 agreed to participate. The participants provided urine samples for C-peptide analysis and 36% were positive (≥ 0.2 nmol/24 h). Each C-peptide-positive patient was matched with a C-peptide-negative patient for age at onset (≤ 5 years) and disease duration (≤ 2 years). Twenty nine pairs were obtained and twenty two of them completed the investigation. There were no significant differences between the C-peptide excretor and non-excretor groups in sex ratio, duration of diabetes, age at onset, body mass index, insulin dose, insulin type, or injection frequency. However, the non-excretor group did take significantly greater insulin doses (mean = 0.79 U/kg $\pm$ 0.06 vs 0.59 U/kg $\pm$ 0.07; p<0.05) and had significantly higher HbA$_{1c}$ levels (7.9% $\pm$ 0.3 vs 6.9% $\pm$ 0.3; p<0.05) than the excretor group.

This research group employed the health belief scales in order to see if they would discriminate patients with and without residual insulin secretion, reasoning that because individuals with residual insulin secretion tend to have better blood glucose control, this will be reflected in a more favourable pattern of health beliefs. The items in the perceived severity and vulnerability measures selected for analysis were the same as those suggested by Bradley *et al.* (1984) and described above in the section on scoring.

Study 4: Northampton study: Gillespie (1989)

Seventy two patients with insulin-requiring diabetes (thirty six men and thirty six women) were recruited when they attended an out-patient clinic in the UK for consulation. Selection criteria were: duration of insulin-requiring diabetes ≥ 1 year, and age >21 years. Pregnancy and disabling complications were exclusion criteria. Two thirds of the sample (fifty four patients) were included in the study because the physician involved in their care considered that they had diabetes management problems, reflected by $HbA_{1c} >10\%$. Eighteen additional patients from the sample were selected as representative of those with few problems with diabetes management, as reflected by $HbA_{1c} \leq 10\%$.

The two groups of patients completed the health belief scales for insulin users together with measures of Knowledge of Diabetes (Meadows *et al.*, 1988), Perceived Control of (insulin-treated) Diabetes (Bradley *et al.*, 1984; see also chapter by Bradley in this volume), and metabolic control. The purpose for the study was to investigate the relationships between these variables.

Statistical Methods

In studies 1 and 2, the original Sheffield work, all data were analysed using SPSS on a Prime mainframe computer. Study 1 employed a principal components analysis with varimax rotation to assess the structure of responses to the initial pool of twenty eight benefits and barriers items and a two factor solution was requested. The factor loadings were used to guide selection of six items for the Benefits and Barriers scales respectively. Internal reliability of these new scales was assessed using Cronbach's (1951) alpha coefficient. Psychometric analyses were not performed on the perceived severity and vulnerability data but responses to the individual problems were compared using paired scores *t*-tests in order to determine whether respondents discriminated between diabetes-related disorders and those not specifically related to diabetes. These analyses were also used to provide data about patterns of response to the individual short-term and long-term complications for this population. Multiple regression analyses were used in order to identify which patients would wish to intensify their treatment and which mode of treatment they would prefer. Further multiple regression analyses were conducted in order to predict efficacy of the treatments in terms of glycosylated haemoglobin levels twelve months later (Bradley *et al.*, 1987). In the

DKA study (study 2), independent group t-tests were used for comparisons between the two groups on all measures.

Study 3, Sjoberg *et al.*'s (1988) C-peptide study, used paired scores *t*-tests and chi-square to assess differences between the group with residual insulin secretion and the group without residual insulin secretion.

Study 4, Gillespie's Northampton study (1989), examined the relationships between the different variables using Pearson correlations which will be reported here. Gillespie's thesis includes a wealth of analyses exploring the value of the health belief variables together with variables from Bradley *et al.*'s Perceived Control of Diabetes Scales (Bradley *et al.*, 1984; see also Chapter 13) and other variables in attempting to predict patients' satisfaction with the consultation and concurrent and subsequent blood glucose control.

Structure of the Benefits and Barriers Scales

Factor analysis of the Sheffield data showed that the two factors accounted for 17.7% and 10.4% of the variance, respectively. Ten items had loadings greater than 0.4 on the first factor and all of these items were barrier statements. All the seven items with loadings greater than 0.4 on the second factor were benefits statements. From these high-loading items, twelve were selected to constitute the Benefits and Barriers scale (Bradley *et al.*, 1984). The loadings for the individual items in the final Benefits and Barriers scales are shown in Table 1.

Reliability

Cronbach's alpha indicated acceptable levels of reliability for the six-item Benefits and Barriers subscales with alphas of 0.67 and 0.79 respectively (Bradley *et al.*, 1984).

Validity

Face and content validity

Items in the Benefits and Barriers scale and the Severity and Vulnerability scales had been constructed in order to represent, unambiguously, the dimensions of the HBM in relation to insulin-requiring diabetes and are considered on these grounds to have face validity. In the original Sheffield work, when selecting items for inclusion in the scales from the high loading items in the factor analysis, those items included in the scales were chosen after detailed consideration and discussion about the breadth of inclusion and the suitability and representativeness of the items for this population.

Table 1: Factor loadings to Benefits and Barriers items for insulin-treated patients

	Benefit factor loading	Barrier factor loading
Benefits items		
Regular, controlled exercise helps in the management of my diabetes.	0.47	0.005
By careful planning of diet, exercise and insulin, I can control my diabetes at least as well as most other people with diabetes.	0.46	-0.14
The risk of insulin reactions (hypos) is reduced if I eat meals at regular intervals.	0.46	-0.09
High blood sugars can be prevented if I plan ahead.	0.46	-0.06
It is important for me to visit the diabetic clinic regularly even even in the absence of symptoms	0.44	-0.06
Insulin reactions (hypos) can be prevented if I plan ahead.	0.46	-0.06
Barrier items		
Controlling my diabetes well imposes restrictions on my whole life-style.	0.07	0.60
Controlling my diabetes well interferes with my work (housework or paid work).	-0.02	0.64
It is just not possible to control my diabetes properly and live in a way that is acceptable to me.	-0.12	0.60
Controlling my diabetes well interferes with my leisure activities.	-0.06	0.67
Sticking to my diet makes eating out difficult.	-0.03	0.58
Controlling my diabetes well when I am away from home often causes me embarrassment.	0.02	0.66

Reproduced by permission of John Wiley & Sons Ltd from Bradley et al. (1984)

Construct validity

Bradley *et al.* (1984) reported that the mean scores for the perceived Benefits and Barriers scales were 28.9 ($\pm$ 5.9) on the Benefits scale and 11.5 ($\pm$ 8.7) on the Barriers scale with higher scores indicating more perceived benefits or barriers. It is evident therefore that the perceived benefits of treatment were felt to be substantially greater than the perceived barriers to treatment (t = 26.0, p<0.0001). Thus the majority of respondents believed their treatment to be "Cost-effective". Construct validity of the perceived Severity and Vulnerability measures was indicated when comparisons were made between ratings for problems related and unrelated to diabetes. As predicted, respondents felt that the diabetes-related problems were more severe and, with the exception of heart disease, perceived themselves as more vulnerable to these disorders (see Table 2).

Table 2: Perceived vulnerability and severity of disorders related and unrelated to diabetes: mean scores for insulin users

	Vulnerability	Severity
Insulin reaction (hypo)	4.60	3.83
High sugar coma	3.15	5.44
Deterioting eyesight	4.23	5.36
Kidney problems	3.41	5.36
Circulatory problems in the feet	3.71	4.66
Heart trouble	2.92	5.56
Bronchitis	2.91	3.83
Cancer	2.71	5.84
Stomach ulcer	2.42	4.41
Arthritis	3.36	4.02

Reproduced by permission of John Wiley & Sons Ltd from Bradley et al. (1984)

N.B. Scoring of these items was on scale of 1 to 6 instead of the scoring of 0 to 5 now recommended

Sjoberg *et al.* (1988) noted a similar pattern of responses to disorders related and unrelated to diabetes and, in accordance with Bradley *et al.* (1984), observed that heart disease appears to be a less well-known complication of diabetes. When assessing group differences, however, they found that the scores for the group of insulin secretors were not significantly different from the scores for non-secretors for any of the composite measures. Nevertheless, they did note that the group without residual insulin secretion perceived themselves to be more vulnerable to kidney problems (3.8 ± 0.3 vs 4.5 ± 0.3, $p<0.025$) when compared with the insulin secretors (who had significantly better blood glucose control). No comparisons were reported for any composite vulnerability and severity scores for the two groups. In accordance with the predictions of the HBM, a significant association was found between better blood glucose control and greater perceived Vulnerability to Complications for the group of patients with residual insulin secretion ($r = -0.57$; $p<0.01$). For non-secretors, however, better metabolic control was associated with greater perceived Barriers to treatment ($r = -0.55$; $p<0.01$). Although this latter result is contrary to Health Belief Model predictions, Sjoberg *et al.* reasoned that these patients perceived more barriers in their efforts to obtain lower blood glucose levels because they had to impose greater restrictions on their lifestyle. This study indicates, therefore, how the health belief patterns of different groups of patients may vary as a result of their physiological status.

In Gillespie's work (Gillespie, 1989), construct validity was indicated when predicted and consistent patterns of correlations between the scales and other variables were obtained. Better blood glucose control was associated with more perceived Benefits of treatment ($r = -0.32$; $p<0.01$), fewer perceived Barriers to treatment ($r = 0.37$; $p<0.001$), and greater perceived "Cost-effectiveness" of treatment ($r = -0.49$; $p<0.001$). No significant associations were found between perceived Vulnerability or Severity and metabolic control. Greater knowledge about the general management of diabetes was significantly related to more perceived Benefits (r = 0.28; p<0.01). Finally, greater perceived External Control of diabetes was related to more perceived Barriers (r = 0.28; p<0.01) and lower perceived "Cost-effectiveness" of treatment (r = -0.29; p<0.01), while greater perceived Personal Control of diabetes was significantly related to greater perceived "Cost-effectiveness" of treatment (r = 0.30; p<0.01).

Predictive validity

Bradley *et al.* (1986) found that the group who had developed ketoacidosis while using CSII pumps, rated themselves (before starting to use the pump) to be more vulnerable to hyperglycaemic coma (*t* = -2.5, df 20, p<0.05). Prior experience of DKA was similar in both those who developed DKA on pumps and those who did not and it is unclear why those who developed DKA felt they were more vulnerable though future events showed their belief to be predictive.

Bradley *et al.* (1987) noted that patients who wished to intensify their regimen perceived their current treatment to be less "Cost-effective" (ß = -0.15; F = 4.76, df 1,223, p<0.05). "Cost-effectiveness" also contributed to the prediction of mode of treatment (CSII versus injections) along with three other variables; Personal Control, Medical Control and age (R^2 = 0.046; F = 2.71, df 4,223, p<0.05) though only the Personal Control variable contributed significantly in its own right. Surprisingly, the perceived Severity and Vulnerability measures (composite scores derived from summing the responses to the four common complications suggested earlier (see Scoring)) did not predict treatment intensification or mode. Indeed, the HBM would predict that feelings of vulnerability to severe complications is likely to intensify preventive health care behaviour.

Discussion

Results of the psychometric analyses and the various studies which have utilized the Diabetes-Specific Health Belief scales designed for insulin-requiring patients suggest that the Benefits and Barriers scales have good reliability and validity. The principal components analysis of the original twenty eight items indicated two independent benefits and barriers factors with high loadings for each item. Comparison of the loadings for the items on each scale suggests that the barriers items form the more coherent of the two scales although internal reliability was highly satisfactory for both of the measures. The resulting six-item scales contain a wide range of diverse items and they have not been inflated by reworded versions of single items which would artificially elevate the alpha coefficient of internal consistency (such as repetitive statements about diet adherence).

The studies which have employed the perceived Benefits and Barriers scales have provided evidence for the validity of these measures. Indeed, most of the findings from these studies have shown relationships consistent with the predictions of the HBM. Between-scale comparisons in the Sheffield data showed that the majority of patients perceived significantly more benefits than barriers to treatment and therefore perceived their treatment to be "Cost-effective". This pattern of results was also found when comparing the Benefits and Barriers scores from the version designed for tablet-treated patients, described in Part 2 of this chapter. Evidence for the construct validity of the Benefits and Barriers scales was shown by Gillespie (1989) where predicted and consistent patterns of correlations between the scales and other variables were obtained. In particular, good blood glucose control was found to be associated with more perceived Benefits, fewer perceived Barriers, and, overall, greater perceived "Cost-effectiveness" of treatment. Furthermore, greater knowledge about the general management of diabetes was significantly related to more perceived Benefits; greater perceived external control was associated with more perceived Barriers and lower perceived "Cost-effectiveness" of treatment; and greater perceived Personal Control was significantly related to greater perceived "Cost-effectiveness" of treatment. Predictive validity of the Benefits and Barriers scales was demonstrated by Bradley *et al.* (1987) which showed that low perceived treatment "Cost-effectiveness" significantly predicted which patients would wish to intensify their treatment regimen.

The scales relating to perceived Severity and Vulnerability were not developed to the same extent as the Benefits and Barriers scales because of the nature of the measures which required the participants to respond to a list of diverse disorders rather than a set of questions or statements designed to produce particular patterns of response. It was predicted, however, that respondents would rate themselves as more vulnerable to diabetes-related problems than to equivalent disorders unrelated to diabetes. Indeed, this prediction was confirmed in data reported by Bradley *et al.* (1984) and by Sjoberg *et al.* (1988). Evidence for the construct and predictive validity of the Severity and Vulnerability scales was patchy and inconsistent. In Gillespie's (1989) Northampton study, for example, poorer knowledge about the general management of diabetes and blood glucose monitoring was found to be associated with greater perceived Severity of Complications (composite measure), but no significant relationships were found between the Severity and Vulnerability measures and glycaemic control or Perceived Control of Diabetes despite predictions to the contrary. Furthermore, in Sjoberg et al.'s (1988) C-peptide study, the group of patients without residual insulin secretion perceived themselves as more vulnerable to kidney problems but not to any of the other complications. The single item measuring perceived Vulnerability to hyperglycaemic coma was a significant predictor of subsequent development of ketoacidosis in Bradley *et al.*'s (1986) study, but none of the composite Severity and Vulnerability scales were successful in predicting treatment choice or efficacy in the Sheffield feasibility study (Bradley *et al.*, 1987). A consistent finding in two of the studies (Bradley *et al.*, 1984; Sjoberg *et al.*, 1988) was that the risk of developing heart disease was less well known than the risk of developing the other complications. It is interesting to note that in a study by Lundman *et al.* (1990) which employed a different version of the vulnerability scales a similar pattern of results was also obtained.

Bradley *et al.* (1987) expressed dissatisfaction with the Severity and Vulnerability measures because of problems in interpretation. A low vulnerability score, for ex-

ample, may indicate that a person may be ignorant of, underestimating, or deny-
ing the risk of complications, but it may also be that, whilst being aware of the
general risks, these perceptions of vulnerability are mediated by personal risk-re-
ducing strategies. Such strategies might be the patient's efforts to improve blood
glucose or weight control, or they may feel that because they have regular checks
at the hospital this renders them less vulnerable. It is also possible that factors
such as a family history may make an individual feel more vulnerable to a particular disorder but he or she may be unaware that it is a complication of diabetes and
so behaviour related to diabetes management may be unaffected. The Severity
and Vulnerability measures were also criticised by Bradley *et al.* because they did
not take into account that some respondents already had one or more of the complications. The more recently developed scales for tablet-treated patients described in Part 2 of this chapter were radically altered during the design stage in
response to the problems just described. It is suggested, therefore, that researchers who wish to employ the scales for insulin-treated patients should consider using the new version of the Severity and Vulnerability measures. No validity data are
yet available for the insulin-treated population when using the new scales but
when employed in studies of tablet-treated patients they have produced promising
results. The reader should consult Part 2 of this chapter for more detailed information about these measures.

With respect to the scales designed for insulin users, a limitation of the validity
data presented above is that much of it is drawn from studies which have correlated the measures with outcome variables collected retrospectively or concurrently.
This leaves the direction of the relationship open to question as it is impossible to
say whether beliefs determine behaviour or whether people rationalize their beliefs to be consistent with their behaviour. The Sheffield feasibility study and the
DKA study, which provided predictive validity for some of the scales, are exceptions in that they employed outcome data which were collected at a later date. Prospective studies of this kind provide particularly valuable data on the validity of
such scales. Intervention studies which attempt to modify health beliefs and evaluate the success of the modification and the effects on health-related behaviour
and associated outcomes would also be valuable. No such studies have been conducted with insulin users, to our knowledge, though intervention studies with tablet-treated patients have been reported and are included in Part 2 of this chapter.

PART 2: HEALTH BELIEF SCALES FOR TABLET-TREATED PATIENTS

Design

The theoretical underpin of the Health Belief scales designed for tablet-treated
patients is the same as that described for the insulin users' scales, i.e. the HBM
(see Part 1: Design). Accordingly, measures of perceived Benefits of, and Barriers to, treatment, and perceived Severity of, and Vulnerability to, the complica-

tions, were adapted from the versions for insulin-treated individuals so that they were relevant to tablet-treated diabetes. As mentioned in Part 1, Bradley *et al.* (1987) were dissatisfied with the Severity and Vulnerability scales designed for insulin users because of problems in interpretation. These measures were therefore radically redesigned in response to these problems. The final versions of the scales for tablet-treated patients are presented in Figures 4–6.

Perceived Benefits and Barriers

The benefits of, and barriers to, treatment questionnaire initially consisted of twenty four adapted or newly-constructed statements with which respondents agreed or disagreed. This pool of statements included two items constructed in order to measure health value.

Perceived Severity and Vulnerability

Perceived severity was measured by asking patients to rate how serious various disorders would be if they were to develop them. Eight of the disorders were complications and eight were not specifically related to diabetes. In addition, two further items were included ('Your diabetes now' and 'Your diabetes in ten years' time') which focused respondents' attention on their diabetes as a whole. In order to avoid patients construing certain disorders in different ways, the items were made more specific than previously. Cancer, for example, covers a multitude of different types and stages with differing prognoses whereas leukaemia is more specific in type and prognosis. The questionnaires were also constructed so that if patients were unable to rate the seriousness of a problem because they did not know what the problem was, they could indicate this by ticking a box next to the disorder concerned.

The Perceived Vulnerability Questionnaire included the same disorders as those used in the measurement of Perceived Severity. It was not sensible to include the two items about patients' diabetes in general so they were substituted with a single item: 'Complications arising from diabetes'. If respondents thought they already had any of the problems listed, they could indicate this next to the disorder concerned. The measure was also designed so that respondents were asked to rate the vulnerability of an 'average person with your kind of diabetes' who is the same age, sex, follows the same kind of treatment, and has 'average control over his/her diabetes'. It was reasoned that ratings of an 'average person' would provide an estimate of vulnerability which is less influenced by mediating factors such as perceived personal-risk-reducing strategies.

The measures of perceived Severity and Vulnerability designed for insulin-requiring patients employed six-point scales. The present measures of perceived Severity and Vulnerability were redesigned with five-point scales because of the similarity of two of the points on the previous scales and to create a mid-point.

Figure 4

EXPERIENCE OF TREATMENT BENEFITS AND BARRIERS

In this section would you please circle one of the numbers on each of the scales to indicate how strongly you agree or disagree with each of the following statements.

On these scales   0   would indicate that you strongly disagree
               1 = moderately disagree
               2 = mildly disagree
               3 = neither agree nor disagree
               4 = mildly agree
               5 = moderately agree
               6 = strongly agree

	strongly disagree						strongly agree
1. By careful planning of diet and exercise, I can control my diabetes at least as well as most other people with diabetes	0	1	2	3	4	5	6
2. Sticking to my diet makes eating out difficult	0	1	2	3	4	5	6
3. High blood sugars can be prevented if I plan ahead	0	1	2	3	4	5	6
4. It is just not possible to control my diabetes properly and live in a way that is acceptable to me	0	1	2	3	4	5	6
5. Sticking to my diet causes inconvenience to other people	0	1	2	3	4	5	6
6. Controlling my diabetes well interferes with my social life	0	1	2	3	4	5	6
7. Good control of my diabetes reduces the possibility of developing complications	0	1	2	3	4	5	6
8. It is important to take all my tablets at the times recommended by the doctor if I am to achieve good control of my diabetes	0	1	2	3	4	5	6
9. The diet I am supposed to follow is rather dull and uninteresting	0	1	2	3	4	5	6
10. I find that keeping to a diet is helpful in controlling my diabetes	0	1	2	3	4	5	6

Please make sure that you have considered each of the 10 statements and have circled a number on each of the scales.

Figure 5

BELIEFS ABOUT SEVERITY

In this section would you please circle a number on each of the scales to indicate how serious you think the following problems would be if you were to develop them.

On these scales   0   would indicate that the problem is not serious at all
                                1   =   not serious enough to be worrying
                                  2   =   moderately serious
                                  3   =   very serious
                                  4   =   extremely serious

If you are unable to rate the seriousness of a problem because you are not sure what the problem is, please tick the box on the right-hand side.

	not serious at all				extremely serious	not sure what the problem is
1. High blood pressure	0	1	2	3	4	☐
2. Stomach ulcer	0	1	2	3	4	☐
3. Blindness	0	1	2	3	4	☐
4. Ear infection	0	1	2	3	4	☐
5. Kidney disease	0	1	2	3	4	☐
6. Aching legs	0	1	2	3	4	☐
7. Leukaemia (cancer of the blood)	0	1	2	3	4	☐
8. Gum disease	0	1	2	3	4	☐
9. Bronchitis	0	1	2	3	4	☐
10. Deafness (complete loss of hearing)	0	1	2	3	4	☐
11. Numbness in the feet	0	1	2	3	4	☐
12. Heart disease	0	1	2	3	4	☐
13. Asthma	0	1	2	3	4	☐
14. Failing eyesight	0	1	2	3	4	☐
15. Loss of hearing (partly deaf)	0	1	2	3	4	☐
16. Gangrene	0	1	2	3	4	☐
17. Your diabetes now	0	1	2	3	4	☐
18. Your diabetes in 10 years' time	0	1	2	3	4	☐

Please make sure that you have circled one number on each of the 18 scales.

Figure 6

BELIEFS ABOUT VULNERABILITY

In this section we are asking you to make two ratings for each of the problems listed.

First: Consider an **average person** with your kind of diabetes who is
              - your age
              - your sex
              - follows the same kind of treatment as yourself
              - has average control over his or her diabetes
              and indicate how likely you feel it is that this person
              will develop the following problems.

Second: Indicate how likely you feel it is that **you** will develop the following problems.

On these scales   0   would indicate that you feel that the development of the problem is
                  very unlikely
              1 =   quite unlikely
              2 =   neither likely nor unlikely
              3 =   quite likely
              4 =   very likely

If you already have or think you may have any of these problems, please tick the box on the
right-hand side.

		very unlikely				very likely	I already have this problem
1.	**High blood pressure**						
	Average person with your kind of diabetes	0	1	2	3	4	
	Yourself	0	1	2	3	4	☐
2.	**Stomach ulcer**						
	Average person with your kind of diabetes	0	1	2	3	4	
	Yourself	0	1	2	3	4	☐
3.	**Blindness**						
	Average person with your kind of diabetes	0	1	2	3	4	
	Yourself	0	1	2	3	4	☐
4.	**Ear infection**						
	Average person with your kind of diabetes	0	1	2	3	4	
	Yourself	0	1	2	3	4	☐
5.	**Kidney disease**						
	Average person with your kind of diabetes	0	1	2	3	4	
	Yourself	0	1	2	3	4	☐
6.	**Aching legs**						
	Average person with your kind of diabetes	0	1	2	3	4	
	Yourself	0	1	2	3	4	☐

	very unlikely				very likely	I already have this problem
7. Leukaemia (cancer of blood)						
Average person with your kind of diabetes	0	1	2	3	4	
Yourself	0	1	2	3	4	☐
8. Gum disease						
Average person with your kind of diabetes	0	1	2	3	4	
Yourself	0	1	2	3	4	☐
9. Bronchitis						
Average person with your kind of diabetes	0	1	2	3	4	
Yourself	0	1	2	3	4	☐
10. Deafness (complete loss of hearing)						
Average person with your kind of diabetes	0	1	2	3	4	
Yourself	0	1	2	3	4	☐
11. Numbness in the feet						
Average person with your kind of diabetes	0	1	2	3	4	
Yourself	0	1	2	3	4	☐
12. Heart disease						
Average person with your kind of diabetes	0	1	2	3	4	
Yourself	0	1	2	3	4	☐
13. Asthma						
Average person with your kind of diabetes	0	1	2	3	4	
Yourself	0	1	2	3	4	☐
14. Failing eyesight						
Average person with your kind of diabetes	0	1	2	3	4	
Yourself	0	1	2	3	4	☐
15. Loss of hearing (partly deaf)						
Average person with your kind of diabetes	0	1	2	3	4	
Yourself	0	1	2	3	4	☐
16. Gangrene						
Average person with your kind of diabetes	0	1	2	3	4	
Yourself	0	1	2	3	4	☐
17. Complications arising from diabetes						
Average person with your kind of diabetes	0	1	2	3	4	
Yourself	0	1	2	3	4	☐

Please make sure that you have circled one number on each of the 17 scales.

Scoring

Perceived Benefits and Barriers

Respondents to the questionnaire rate their agreement or disagreement with each statement on a seven-point scale from 0 (strongly disagree) to 6 (strongly agree). The final scales comprise five benefits items and five barriers items (see Table 3). Similar to the scales for insulin users, the ratings for the benefits statements should be summed separately from ratings for the barriers statements to obtain:

a) a total score for perceived Benefits: items 1+ 3 + 7 + 8 + 10
b) a total score for perceived Barriers: items 2 + 4 + 5 + 6 + 9

The range of scores possible for each of the Benefits and Barriers scales is 0 to 30, higher scores indicating greater perceived benefits or barriers. A measure of perceived treatment "Cost-effectiveness" can also be calculated by subtracting the Barriers score from the Benefits score for each subject.

Perceived Severity and Vulnerability

In order to measure perceived severity, respondents are asked to rate on five-point scales from 0 (not serious at all) to 4 (extremely serious) the severity of the various disorders. If respondents tick the box next to a particular problem in order to indicate that they are not sure about it (what it is or how serious it is), this enables the researcher to exclude potentially unreliable data.

Perceived vulnerability is measured in a similar manner by asking respondents to rate the likelihood of developing the various disorders on five-point scales from 0 (extremely unlikely) to 4 (extremely likely). Separate ratings are requested for the respondents themselves and for the 'average person'.

Scores relating to the eight complications items and eight disorders not specifically related to diabetes are summed separately to form the following measures:

a) Perceived Severity of Complications: items 1 + 3 + 5 + 6 + 11 + 12 + 14 + 16
b) Perceived Severity of General Disorders: items 2 + 4 + 7 + 8 + 9 + 10 + 13 + 15
c) Perceived Vulnerability to Complications: items 1 + 3 + 5 + 6 + 11 + 12 + 14 + 16
d) Perceived Vulnerability to General Disorders: items 2 + 4 + 7 + 8 + 9 + 10 + 13 + 15.

The perceived vulnerability scores for the 'average person' can be similarly summed to form further separate measures and labelled:

e) Perceived Vulnerability of the Average Person to Complications: item numbers as for (c)
f) Perceived Vulnerability of the Average Person to General Disorders: item numbers as for (d).

Table 3: Factor loadings for perceived benefits of, and barriers to treatment items: data from patients with tablets-treated diabetes

	Factor loadings	
	Factor 1	Factor 2
Perceived Benefits		
By careful planning of diet and exercise, I can control my diabetes at least as well as most other people with diabetes.	-0.04	**0.80**
High blood sugars can be prevented if I plan ahead.	-0.05	**0.60**
Good control of my diabetes reduces the possibility of developing complications.	0.09	**0.54**
It is important to take all my tablets at the times recommended by the doctor if I am to achieve good control of my diebetes.	-0.09	**0.52**
I find that keeping to a diet is helpful in controlling my diabetes	-0.07	**0.81**
Perceived Barriers		
Sticking to my diet makes eating out difficult.	**0.73**	0.07
It is just not possible to control my diabetes properly and live in a way that is acceptable to me.	**0.72**	-0.08
Sticking to my diet causes inconvenience to other people.	**0.79**	0.07
Controlling my diabetes well interferes with my social life.	**0.84**	-0.05
The diet I am supposed to follow is rather dull and uninteresting.	**0.65**	-0.29

Reproduced by permission of John Wiley & Sons Ltd from Lewis et al. (1990)

The magnitude of the factor loading indicates degree of relationship to each factor

The scores relating to perceived severity of the patient's diabetes now and in ten years' time may be treated separately or summed to form a measure labelled:

g) Perceived Severity of Diabetes: items 17 + 18.

During the development of the health belief measures it was noted that a substantial proportion of the respondents (50%) indicated that they believed they already had one or more of the complications. If the method of listwise deletion of cases is employed when analysing total perceived Vulnerability to Complications scores this creates a large amount of missing data. In order to utilize data from the maximum number of respondents, therefore, the mean of the available perceived vulnerability scores for the individual complications can be calculated for each respondent.

The range of scores possible for each of the Benefits and Barriers scales is 0 to 30, and for each of the eight item perceived Severity and Vulnerability scales is 0 to 32 with higher scores indicating greater perceived benefits, barriers, severity, or vulnerability. Scores possible for the two-item perceived Severity of Diabetes measure range from 0 to 8 and once again, higher scores indicate greater perceived severity.

DEVELOPMENT OF THE SCALES FOR TABLET-TREATED PATIENTS

Subject Samples and Procedures

Study A: Main Sheffield sample of tablet-treated patients: Lewis et al. (1990)

Two hundred and thirty nine patients (141 men and 98 women) with Type 2 diabetes, treated with oral hypoglycaemic agents and attending two outpatient clinics at the Royal Hallamshire Hospital, Sheffield, UK, were invited to take part in a study evaluating the management of Type 2 diabetes (Jennings *et al.*, 1988, 1991). Age range was 40 to 65 years. Those who were blind or partially sighted were not included. Two hundred and nineteen (92%) patients (130 men and 89 women) agreed to take part and were screened by a physician in order to establish their health status. There were no significant differences between participants and those who refused to take part for any of the available measures, including sex, age, duration of diabetes and glycosylated haemoglobin (HbA$_1$) levels. The patients were given a booklet of questionnaires, including the health belief scales, to complete at home and were asked to return them within two days in a prepaid envelope addressed to the Psychology Department, Sheffield University. Anyone who did not return a booklet within one month of their appointment received a reminder. One hundred and eighty seven (85%) patients (110 men and 77 women) returned completed booklets of questionnaires. This final sample provided the data for the psychometric analyses reported here. There were no significant differences between responders and non-responders to the questionnaires in sex, age, duration of diabetes, HbA$_1$ or percent ideal body weight.

Study B: Education study: Sheffield subsample: Lewis (1994)

The subjects in this study were a self-selected subsample of the patients described in Study A, all of whom were invited by one of the physicians in the research team to attend an education session (with the exception of those subjects with particularly inadequate control who were recruited for the insulin intervention (study C below)). The rationale for the study was to assess the effects of an education intervention on health beliefs and to investigate whether post-education beliefs would predict HbA_1 approximately six months later. All patients were encouraged to bring a spouse, partner or friend if they desired. Altogether, 81 (47%) of the 173 patients who were invited attended one of thirteen education sessions. The attenders were found to have experienced their diabetes for significantly fewer years than those who did not attend (mean = 5.7 years ± 5.5 vs 7.9 ± 5.1; p<0.01) and they had previously reported (Study A) significantly greater perceived Severity of Complications when compared with non-attenders (z = -2.0; p<0.05).

The education intervention was designed so that benefits of treatment were emphasised and any difficulties with the regimen could be addressed. Information about severity and vulnerability was given at the beginning of each session but this was followed immediately by positive information about how to improve diabetes control with a view to arresting/preventing the short- and long-term complications. Accordingly, it was predicted that the education intervention would increase the perceived Benefits of treatment, reduce the perceived Barriers to treatment and, overall, increase perceived treatment 'Cost-effectiveness'. Since attenders' ratings of Severity of Complications were significantly greater than non-attenders, no significant changes in perceived Severity were predicted. Furthermore, any increases in perceived Vulnerability to Complications were predicted to be offset by the preventative information provided during the session.

Patients' knowledge about diabetes was measured by questionnaire (designed and developed for the study by Lewis, 1994) immediately before and immediately after the education sessions and a similar booklet of questionnaires to that employed in Study A was given to them for completion at home. They were asked to complete the booklet of questionnaires within the next two days and return them in the prepaid envelope provided (addressed to the Psychology Department, Sheffield University). Those who did not return a booklet within two weeks were sent a reminder. Seventy nine (97.5%) patients returned a completed booklet of questionnaires.

Approximately six months after each education session, fifty seven of the eighty one people who had attended were followed up in relation to their HbA_1. The selection of those who were followed up was determined by routine attendance at the two clinics from which they were drawn. These individuals had experienced their diabetes for significantly fewer years when compared to those who were not followed up (mean = 5.0 years ± 5.5 vs 7.3 years ± 5.2; p<0.05).

Study C: Insulin treatment for poorly controlled Sheffield subsample with Type 2 diabetes: Jennings et al.(1991), Lewis (1994)

The aim of this study was to assess the impact on health beliefs of information, education, feedback about control, and the introduction of two types of insulin delivery. The subjects in the study had Type 2 diabetes which was progressively inadequately controlled with oral hypoglycaemic agents and diet. Insulin treatment would have been routinely prescribed at a particular threshold of hyperglycaemia but these patients were approached before they reached this threshold in order to ascertain whether they would volunteer to take part in the insulin study, whether they could improve their diabetes control prior to insulin therapy after an educational input and improved feedback about control, and to assess the efficacy of insulin injections and CSII pump therapy. Health Beliefs and other psychological variables were measured by questionnaires prior to, and after each intervention of the study.

The thirty two patients approached for the study were aged forty to sixty five years, treated with maximum doses of sulphonylureas, had HbA_1 concentrations above 55 mmol HMF/mol Hb (Sheffield measure of HbA_1 can be divided by five to produce the more usual percentage figure), had an ideal body weight of <160%, were free from severe diabetic complications, and had been satisfactorily treated with sulphonylureas for at least one year. Twenty six of the subjects were a subsample of the patients described in Study A so they had completed a baseline questionnaire prior to being approached. In order to increase the number of subjects in the study, six patients were approached when they attended the outpatient clinics so baseline psychological data were not obtained from these individuals.

This study consisted of three interventions. Intervention 1 involved giving feedback and information to thirty two patients about their poor diabetes control and the increased risk of complications. They were then informed about the study and asked if they would participate. Twenty five (78%) of those approached agreed to participate in the insulin study. Of those who declined to take part, three subsequently achieved improved glycaemic control (HbA_1< 55 mmol HMF/mol Hb or 11%), two failed to attend for appointments, one died following a myocardial infarction, and one received insulin therapy according to the usual clinic regimen. Intervention 2 involved the patients in a preliminary three month run-in phase in which treatment with diet and tablets was optimized through home blood glucose monitoring and dietary advice. At the end of the three months, five of the participants improved their blood glucose control, achieving an HbA_1 level of less than the criterion set (<50 mmol HMF/mol Hb or 10%) and, as a result, continued with sulphonylurea therapy. The twenty patients (eight men and twelve women) who were unable to lower their HbA_1 sufficiently were entered into the four month insulin phase of the study. This final intervention involved insulin treatment using twice-daily injections or CSII pumps. Prior to, and during the insulin phase of the study, patients were provided with dietary advice and given instruction about insulin therapy. After randomisation, each treatment group consisted of four men and six women.

Study D: American study of older adults treated with insulin, tablets and/or diet: Polly (1992)

This American study employed the scales for tablet-treated patients in order to examine the relationships between health beliefs and adherence to the diabetes regimen in older adults. The sample included patients who were treated with insulin and with diet only as well as individuals treated with oral hypoglycaemic agents, so the scales were modified to make the questions relevant to the sample as a whole. Polly did not give details of these modifications and psychometric analysis of the responses to the modified scales was not reported.

The sample consisted of 102 adults (54 women and 48 men) aged 60 to 98 years (mean 69 ± 6.98). Eighty two per cent of them were aged 60 to 74 years. Ninety three of the subjects were white and nine were Afro-American. Seven of the subjects were treated with diet only, 46 were treated with diet and tablets, and 49 were treated with diet and insulin. Mean duration of diabetes was 10.6 years ± 7.4. Patients were not considered for the study if they could not speak English, had anaemia, consumed ≥ 3 measures of alcohol daily, or if they had been hospitalized during the previous three months. All the participants attended a diabetes clinic located in a state teaching hospital in Billings, Montana.

Potential subjects were approached to participate in the study by the clinic nurse educator. During the clinic visit those who agreed to participate filled in a Diabetes Self-Care Behaviours Questionnaire (to measure self-reported adherence to the recommended treatment regimen) and the Diabetes-Specific Health Belief scales. Subjects who had visual difficulties were assisted by the author of the study who read the items from the questionnaire to them. In addition to the questionnaires, blood samples were obtained from the subjects during the clinic visit in order to measure glycosylated haemoglobin (HbA_{1c}).

Statistical Methods

All data from the three Sheffield studies (A, B and C) were analysed using SPSS[X] on an IBM mainframe computer. The structure of the perceived Benefits of, and Barriers to, treatment scales was explored using a principal components factor analysis with varimax rotation. Reliability of all the scales was assessed using Cronbach's (1951) alpha coefficient of internal consistency and item-total correlations. The distributions of scores for the perceived Benefits and perceived Severity scales were skewed, indicating the need for non-parametric statistical tests in subsequent analyses of these measures. Between-scale comparisons were therefore explored using the Wilcoxon matched pairs signed ranks test and their relationships to other variables were examined using Spearman rank correlations. The distributions of the perceived Vulnerability scores satisfied the assumptions of parametric statistical tests, so between-scale comparisons were explored using Student's t-tests (paired scores), and relationships to other variables were examined using Pearson's correlation coefficient.

Analysis of data from the education study demonstrated marked skewness in the distribution of the scores for the post-education perceived Benefits of, and Barriers to treatment measures and in the measure of perceived Severity of Complications, indicating the need for non-parametric statistical tests in subsequent analyses. All the other post-education measures satisfied the assumptions of parametric statistical tests. Between-scale comparisons were made using the Wilcoxon matched pairs signed ranks test or the Student's t-test (paired scores), as appropriate, and relationships to other variables were examined using either Spearman rank correlations or Pearson's correlations. Hierarchical multiple regression analyses were also employed in order to ascertain whether multiplicative combinations of some of the health belief variables and a measure of perceived Personal control/Self efficacy could predict a greater proportion of the variance in HbA_1 six months later. Interactions were calculated by converting the component variables to z scores and obtaining their product.

In the third of the Sheffield studies, the distribution of scores for the health belief variables at all stages of the study met the assumptions of parametric statistical tests with the exception of perceived Severity of General Disorders at baseline, and perceived Severity of Complications after deciding whether or not to take part in the study. Both of the exceptions were negatively skewed. Between-stage comparisons were made using the Wilcoxon matched pairs signed ranks test and the Student's t-test (paired scores), as appropriate.

Polly's American study of older adults used Spearman's correlations to assess relationships between self-reported adherence to the treatment regimen, glycaemic control, and health beliefs. Multiple regression analyses were also performed in order to assess whether the health belief variables could predict reported adherence or HbA_1.

Structure of the Benefits and Barriers Scales

The initial principal components analysis conducted on the undeveloped twenty-four item questionnaire produced six factors; therefore a forced two-factor solution was tried in order to check that the perceived benefits and barriers items would load separately. This solution provided distinct factors characterized by items with loadings >0.4 relating to perceived benefits and barriers respectively. Eleven of the items loaded on the perceived barriers factor and nine loaded on the perceived benefits factor. Each of the items in the scales was examined for item-total correlations and contribution to internal consistency. Within each scale, items were dropped if they inflated the internal reliability coefficient because of their similarity to other items and/or had the lowest item-total correlations. Items were also dropped if they reduced internal reliability or, qualitatively, restricted the measure to a subgroup of patients such as those testing for urinary glucose rather than blood glucose. The two health items were dropped because they did not load together in any of the unforced and forced solutions. An equal number of items in each scale was sought, and the final perceived Benefits and Barriers scales comprised five items each. A confirmatory, unforced factor analysis was carried out on the responses to the final items which produced two factors comprising the barriers and benefits items separately (Table 3) and accounted for a total of 52% of the variance (30% and 22% respectively).

Reliability

The internal reliability of each of the health belief scales was calculated using the Sheffield data in study A and a satisfactory alpha coefficient was found in each case (Table 4). Once again, because listwise deletion methods would have reduced the number of cases to be analysed, calculation of the reliability of the personal perceived Vulnerability to Complications scale was carried out including available data from missing cases. This increased the number of cases analysed to a satisfactory level for internal reliability analysis (Kline, 1986).

Validity

Face and content validity

When constructing or adapting items for the health belief scales, face validity was achieved by ensuring that all items unambiguously represented the various dimensions of the HBM within the context of tablet-treated diabetes. Content validity was established by making sure that each item was relevant to, and representative of, the experience of having tablet-treated diabetes and covered the breadth of experience typical of this patient group.

Construct validity and sensitivity to change

In order to assess construct validity the scales were correlated with other variables collected at the time of completion of the questionnaires in the three Sheffield studies. Construct validity was established when associations between appropriate variables and the scales were significant and consistent. A correlation matrix is presented in Table 5.

Glycosylated haemoglobin (HbA$_1$): Patients who had higher HbA1 levels perceived themselves ($r = 0.16$; $p<0.05$) and the 'average person' ($r = 0.15$; $p<0.05$) to be more vulnerable to Complications.

Percent ideal body weight: Individuals who were more overweight perceived more Barriers to ($r = 0.14$; $p<0.05$), and fewer Benefits of treatment ($r = -0.19$; $p<0.01$). Overall, their treatment was felt to be less "Cost-effective" ($r = -0.20$; $p<0.01$). More overweight respondents also perceived their Diabetes ($r = 0.24$; $p<0.001$) and Complications ($r = 0.16$; $p<0.05$) to be more severe, and they felt that the 'average person' was more vulnerable to Complications than did less overweight respondents ($r = 0.15$; $p<0.05$). The expected association between perceived personal Vulnerability to Complications and percent ideal body weight was not significant ($r = 0.09$).

Table 4 Mean (SD), minimum and maximum scores, reliability (alpha) coefficient, and range of item-total correlations for each scale: data from tablet-treated patients reported by Lewis et al. (1990)[+]

	Mean	(SD)	Minimum found	Maximum found	Possible range	Alpha coefficient	Range of item-total correlations
Perceived							
Benefits	27.2	(3.4)	9	30	0-30	0.67	0.32-0.59
Barriers	13.5	(8.2)	0	30	0-30	0.80	0.51-0.69
Perceived Severity							
Complications	28.3	(3.5)	8	32	0-32	0.77	0.30-0.64
General Disorders	23.8	(5.8)	0	32	0-32	0.88	0.40-0.72
Diabetes (2 items)	4.9	(1.9)	0	8	0-8	—	—
Perceived Vulnerability							
Complications	13.5	(7.6)	0	31	0-32	0.84	0.46-0.68
Complications (averaged)	1.9	(1.0)	0	4	0-4	—	—
General Disorders	9.3	(6.6)	0	32	0-32	0.89	0.53-0.70
'Complications arising from diabetes' (single item)	2.3	(1.2)	0	4	0-4	—	—
Perceived Vulnerability of the 'average person'							
Complications	16.6	(6.8)	0	32	0-32	0.87	0.49-0.75
General Disorders	10.8	(6.9)	0	32	0-32	0.89	0.61-0.78
'Complications arising from diabetes' (single item)	2.3	(1.2)	0	4	0-4	—	—

Higher scores indicate more perceived Benefits and Barriers, and greater perceived Severity and Vulnerability
+ Reproduced by permission of John Wiley & Sons Ltd from Lewis et al. (1990)

Table 5 Correlation of the health belief measures with other variables: Data from tablet-treated patients reported by Lewis et al. (1990)[+]

	HbA$_1$	%Ideal body weight	Subjective estimates of diabetes control	Depression	Anxiety	Positive Well-being	Satisfaction
Perceived							
Benefits	-0.02	-0.19**	-0.18*	-0.10	-0.14*	0.19**	0.31***
Barrier	0.11	0.14*	0.22**	0.27***	0.34***	-0.34***	-0.27***
Treatment 'Cost-effectiveness'	-0.11	-0.20**	-0.29***	-0.27***	-0.33***	0.36***	0.35***
Perceived Severity							
Complications	0.06	0.16*	0.08	-0.01	0.01	0.05	-0.01
General Disorders	-0.01	0.15*	0.00	-0.09	0.00	0.08	-0.04
Diabetes	0.10	0.24***	0.19**	0.20**	0.14*	-0.13	-0.22**
Perceived Vulnerability							
Complications (n=83)	0.15	-0.08	0.27**	0.39***	0.25*	-0.27	-0.34***
Complications (averaged)	0.16*	0.09	0.24***	0.34***	0.26***	-0.29***	-0.29***
General Disorders	0.13	-0.06	0.21**	0.28***	0.20**	-0.37***	-0.27***
'Complications arising from diabetes' (single item)	0.24***	0.07	0.33***	0.25***	0.14*	-0.23**	-0.27***
Perceived Vulnerability of 'average person'							
Complications	0.15*	0.15*	0.22**	0.37***	0.33***	-0.32***	-0.31***
General Disorders	0.16*	-0.03	0.16*	0.27***	0.19**	-0.26***	-0.23**
'Complications arising from diabetes' (single item)	0.23***	0.11	0.31***	0.27***	0.17*	-0.24***	-0.24***

*** p<0.001; **p<0.01; *p<0.05

Higher scores indicate subjective estimates of poorer control, more perceived Benefits, Barriers, and treatment 'Cost-effectiveness' and greater perceived Severity, Vulnerability, Depression, Anxiety, and Positive Well-being.
[+]*Reproduced by permission of John Wiley & Sons Ltd from Lewis et al. (1990)*

Subjective estimates of control: Participants were asked to estimate how well their diabetes had been controlled over the previous few weeks on a seven point scale from 1 (very well controlled) to 7 (very poorly controlled). Subjective estimates of poorer diabetes control were significantly associated with more perceived Barriers to treatment (r = 0.22; p<0.01), fewer perceived Benefits of treatment (r = -0.18; p<0.05), and lower perceived treatment 'Cost-effectiveness' (r = -0.29; p<0.001). Patients who estimated their diabetes control to be worse also felt that their diabetes was more severe (r = 0.19; p<0.01) and reported greater Vulnerability to Complications for themselves (r = 0.24; p<0.001) and the 'average person' (r = 0.22; p<0.01).

Psychological well-being: The measures of Well-being are described by Bradley in Chapter 6. Patients with higher Depression scores perceived more Barriers to treatment (r = 0.27; p<0.001), lower treatment 'Cost-effectiveness" (r = -0.27; p<0.001), greater Severity of Diabetes (r = 0.20; p<0.01), and greater Vulnerability to Complications for themselves (r = 0.34; p<0.001) and the 'average person' (r = 0.37; p<0.001). Higher Anxiety scores were associated with more perceived Barriers to treatment (r = 0.34; p<0.001), fewer perceived Benefits of treatment (r = -0.14; p<0.05), lower perceived treatment 'Cost-effectiveness' (r = -0.33; p<0.001), greater perceived Severity of Diabetes (r = 0.14; p<0.05) and greater perceived Vulnerability to Complications for the patients themselves (r = 0.26; p<0.001) and for the 'average person' (r = 0.33; p<0.001). Respondents who reported greater Positive Well-being, however, perceived fewer Barriers (r = -0.34; p<0.001), more Benefits (r = 0.19; p<0.01), greater treatment 'Cost-effectiveness' (r = 0.36; p<0.001), and less Vulnerability to Complications for themselves (r = -0.29; p<0.001) and the 'average person' (r = -0.32; p<0.001).

Treatment satisfaction: The Treatment Satisfaction measure is described by Bradley in Chapter 7. Greater Treatment Satisfaction was related to fewer perceived Barriers (r = -0.27; p<0.001), more perceived Benefits (r = 0.31; p<0.001), greater perceived 'Cost-effectiveness' of treatment (r = 0.35; p<0.001), lower perceived Severity of Diabetes (r = -0.22; p<0.01), and less perceived Vulnerability for the patients themselves (r = -0.29; p<0.001) and the 'average person' (r = -0.31; p<0.001).

Further evidence of construct validity was provided when a Wilcoxon test indicated that respondents gave higher ratings to perceived Benefits of treatment than to perceived Barriers to treatment and therefore considered their treatment to be 'Cost-effective'. Similar results were obtained with the scales for insulin users, indicating a consistent response to the measures. It was also noted that, as would be expected, respondents felt that Complications were significantly more severe than General Disorders (z = -9.5; p<0.001). Furthermore, in accordance with Weinstein's findings (1982, 1984, 1987) when compared with the 'average person', participants saw themselves as less vulnerable to both Complications (z = -4.0; p<0.001) and General Disorders (z = -2.9; p<0.01).

Further evidence of the construct validity of the scales was provided in the Sheffield education study when the post-education health belief measures were correlated with other variables collected immediately after the education intervention. These data were reported by Lewis (1993) and are summarised below.

Subjective estimates of diabetes control (post education): More optimistic subjective estimates of control were significantly associated with lower perceived Vulnerability (r = -0.30; p<0.01).

Psychological well-being (post education): Greater Depression scores were significantly associated with fewer perceived Benefits of treatment (r = -0.29; p<0.01), lower perceived treatment 'Cost-effectiveness' (r = -0.23; p<0.05), greater perceived Vulnerability to Complications for themselves (r = 0.30; p<0.01) and the 'average person' (r = 0.30; p<0.01), and greater perceived Vulnerability to General Disorders (r = 0.27; p<0.05). Greater Anxiety scores were significantly associated with more perceived Barriers to treatment (r = 0.32; p<0.01), fewer perceived Benefits of treatment (r = -0.35; p<0.01), lower perceived treatment 'Cost-effectiveness' (r = -0.40; p<0.001), greater perceived personal Vulnerability to Complications (r = 0.26; p<0.05), and greater perceived Vulnerability to General Disorders (r = 0.33; p<0.01). Greater Positive Well-being scores were significantly associated with fewer perceived Barriers to treatment (r = -0.20; p<0.05), more perceived Benefits of Treatment (r = 0.28; p<0.01), greater perceived treatment 'Cost-effectiveness' (r = 0.25; p<0.05), and lower perceived Vulnerability to Complications for themselves (r = -0.23; p<0.05) and the 'average person' (r = -0.26; p<0.05).

Treatment satisfaction (post education): Greater Treatment Satisfaction was significantly related to fewer perceived Barriers (r = -0.23; p<0.05), more perceived Benefits (r = 0.31; p<0.01), greater perceived treatment 'Cost-effectiveness' (r = 0.29; p<0.01), and lower perceived Vulnerability to Complications for themselves (r = -0.22; p<0.05) and the 'average person' (r = -0.24; p<0.05).

Percent knowledge improvement: Given that some of the patients who attended an education session already had a good knowledge of diabetes with relatively little scope for improvement, a measure of Knowledge Improvement was calculated which took into account pre-education scores. This measure was computed by expressing the difference scores as a percentage of the pre-education score. In correlations, greater percent of Knowledge Improvement was significantly associated with fewer perceived Benefits (r = -0.24; p<0.05) and lower perceived treatment 'Cost-effectiveness' (r = -0.24; p<0.05). Contrary to expectations, therefore, the pattern of correlations between these Health Beliefs and Knowledge scores indicated that those who increased their knowledge the most were more negative about their diabetes management after education. However, inspection of correlations between Knowledge scores and baseline Health Beliefs revealed a fairly similar pattern of associations, indicating that these patients were predisposed to negative perceptions about their diabetes.

Additional evidence of construct validity and sensitivity: Further evidence of construct validity and sensitivity of the scales was provided when predicted changes in health beliefs were achieved after the education intervention. In comparison with the baseline measures, patients perceived significantly more Benefits of treatment ($z = -2.52$; $p<0.05$), fewer Barriers to treatment ($z = -2.85$; $p<0.01$), and overall, perceived their treatment to be significantly more 'Cost-effective' ($t = -3.88$; $p<0.001$).

In the third Sheffield study where insulin therapy and other interventions were introduced, construct validity and sensitivity to change was established when health beliefs changed significantly in the predicted direction after certain interventions. Further details of the findings summarised below can be found in Lewis (1994). In particular, it was noted that, overall, participants perceived significantly fewer Barriers to treatment ($t = 2.2$; $p<0.05$) and significantly greater treatment 'Cost-effectiveness' ($t = -2.6$; $p<0.05$) after the run-in (treatment optimization) phase of the study. When data from nine patients who managed to improve their blood glucose control during this phase were compared with those who were unable to improve their glycaemic control, it was noted that those who improved reported their treatment to be significantly more 'Cost-effective' ($z = -2.3$; $p<0.05$). After the insulin treatment phase of the study, HbA_1 improved significantly for both groups of patients (CSII: $z = -2.74$, $p<0.01$; CIT: $z = -2.67$, $p<0.01$). Accordingly, when compared with the previous study phase, patients reported significantly fewer Barriers to treatment ($t = 2.2$; $p<0.05$) and perceived their new treatment to be significantly more 'Cost-effective' ($t = -2.6$; $p<0.02$). Although not statistically significant, there was an apparent tendency for patients overall to report reduced Severity of Diabetes ratings ($t = 1.9$; $p<0.08$) when compared to the previous study phase. This difference was significant, however, for the group using CSII ($t = 4.6$; $p<0.01$).

It was predicted that after Intervention 1 (approached for study and given feedback about control and information about risk of complications) patients would perceive their treatment to be less 'Cost-effective' and they would indicate significantly greater perceived Severity of Diabetes and Complications, and greater perceived Vulnerability to Complications. No significant changes in these beliefs were noted but there was an apparent tendency to report greater perceived Severity of Complications ($z = -1.8$; $p<0.09$) and Vulnerability to Complications ($t = -2.1$; $p<0.06$). The effect of the first intervention on health beliefs was probably mediated by expectations about the proposed treatments.

There was some evidence of construct validity from the American study of older patients (Polly, 1992). When the modified health belief scales were correlated with self-reported adherence scores and HbA_{1c}, greater self-reported adherence was significantly associated with fewer perceived Barriers ($r = -0.24$; $p<0.05$), and, in accordance with the first two Sheffield studies, better blood glucose control was significantly related to lower perceived Severity of Diabetes ($r = 0.21$; $p<0.05$). No other significant associations were found. Although no details of the analyses were reported, Polly reported that she attempted various regression analyses in which demographic and clinical variables were also entered into the regression equation but was unable to obtain improved predictions of the variance in self-reported adherence or HbA_{1c}. An attempt was also made to combine some of the variables in the regression analyses (no details reported) but this was similarly unsuccessful.

Predictive validity

Evidence of predictive validity was provided in the education study when health belief measures immediately after education were used to predict HbA_1 approximately six months later. In bivariate correlations, lower HbA_1 concentrations were significantly associated with more perceived Benefits of treatment ($r = -0.30$; $p<0.01$). The correlation between perceived Vulnerability to Complications (single item) and follow-up HbA_1 did not reach significance ($r = 0.22$; $p<0.07$) but the direction of the relationship was the same as that found with the baseline data (Study A). The greater the Vulnerability score, the higher the HbA_1 indicating poorer metabolic control.

It appears that most research using the HBM to date has assumed implicitly that the HBM components combine additively. However, value-expectancy theories imply that the theoretical components of perceived Severity and Vulnerability combine in a multiplicative fashion. Hierarchical multiple regression analyses were employed by Lewis (1994) using the Sheffield data, in order to ascertain whether multiplicative combinations of the present HBM variables together with a measure of Personal Control/Self-efficacy, would predict additional amounts of the variance in follow-up HbA_1. (The Personal Control/Self-efficacy measure was a composite variable from the Perceived Control of Diabetes Scales described by Bradley *et al.* (1990) and presented in Chapter 14 in this volume. The composite measure used by Lewis combined the three variables labelled Internality, Personal control and Foreseeability.) Initially, treatment 'Cost-effectiveness', perceived Severity of Diabetes, perceived Vulnerability to Complications (single item), and perceived Personal Control/Self-efficacy were entered on the first step, and Severity multiplied by Vulnerability (z scores) were entered on the second step. In a similar manner, multiplicative composites of Severity x Vulnerability x treatment 'Cost-effectiveness', and Severity x Vulnerability x treatment 'Cost-effectiveness' x Personal Control/Self-efficacy, were entered on the third and fourth steps. A total of 35% (22% adjusted) was explained by the variables but only perceived Personal Control/Self-efficacy and the multiplicative composite of Severity x Vulnerability x treatment 'Cost-effectiveness' x Personal Control/Self-efficacy, accounted for significant amounts of unique variance [11% ($p<0.05$) and 10% ($p<0.05$) respectively].

Prior analyses had indicated that post-education Well-being was significantly associated with perceptions about Vulnerability, treatment 'Cost-effectiveness', and

Personal Control/Self-efficacy, yet the association between General Well-being and follow-up HbA_1 was relatively weak and not statistically significant ($r = 0.12$; $p>0.05$). In view of this pattern of associations which suggested that General Well-being might act as a suppressor variable, a second regression analysis was conducted in which General Well-being entered the equation on the first step, the individual HBM variables and the measure of perceived Personal Control/Self-efficacy were entered on the second step, and the multiplicative composites were entered on the third and subsequent steps. The results of this analysis are summarized in Table 6. It can be seen that when the variance associated with General Well-being was partialled out on the first step, the prediction of follow-up HbA_1 from the HBM and Personal Control/Self-efficacy variables substantially improved. When all the variables had been entered into the equation a total of 47% (33% adjusted) of the variance in HbA1 was explained. Perceived Vulnerability to Complications, perceived Personal Control/Self-efficacy, and the multiplicative composite of Severity x Vulnerability all contributed unique amounts of explained variance [16% ($p<0.01$); 16% ($p<0.01$); and 12% ($p<0.02$) respectively]. When the multiplicative composite of Severity x Vulnerability was entered on the third step, the R^2 increased by 0.19 ($p<0.01$) indicating that there is a significant multiplicative relationship between perceived Severity of Diabetes and perceived Vulnerability to Complications. None of the other multiplicative composites significantly increased the overall amount of variance explained.

Discussion

The Diabetes-Specific Health Belief scales for tablet-treated patients reported above have been shown to have satisfactory alpha coefficients of reliability. Similar to the scales for insulin-requiring patients, the principal components analysis of the benefits and barriers items indicated two independent factors with high loadings for each item.

The improvements to the format of the perceived Severity and Vulnerability questionnaires since the design of the scales for insulin-treated patients allow the researcher to gain more information about the perceptions of respondents. Patients now report which complication they believe they already have, and these reports can be compared with information from their medical records. Discrepancies between actual and perceived occurrence of Complications are likely to be reflected in the patient's health beliefs. Perceived Vulnerability to Complications may also be examined in relation to both the patient personally, and his or her estimate for the 'average person'. Study A demonstrated that patients perceived the 'average person' to be significantly more vulnerable than themselves to both Complications and General Disorders. Weinstein (1982, 1984, 1987) found a similar optimistic bias when assessing the perceived susceptibility of individuals to a variety of environmental hazards. If this optimism is unrealistic, it is likely to constitute a barrier to preventive action and, therefore, measurement of this

Table 6 Hierarchical multiple regression analysis including General Well-being, the HBM variables, perceived Personal Control/Self-efficacy, and some multiplication combinations. Data from tablet-treated patients reported by Lewis (1994)

B		β	sr^{2a}
General Well-being	0.391	0.35	0.06
Treatment 'Cost-effectiveness'	-0.481	-0.26	0.05
Severity of Diabetes	0.747	0.12	0.01
Vulnerability to Complications	4.584	0.45	0.16**
Personal Control/Self-efficacy	-0.602	-0.55	0.16**
Severity x Vulnerability	6.295	0.47	0.12*
Severity x Vulnerability x Treatment 'Cost effectiveness'	-3.482	-0.20	0.03
Personal Control/Self-efficacy	-0.049	-0.00	0.00

Statistics for each step in the Regression Analysis

	Step	R	R^2	$AdjR^2$	ΔR^2	F
General Well-being	1	0.10	0.01	-0.02	0.01	0.43
Personal Control/Self-efficacy Vulnerability to Complications Severity of Diabetes Treatment 'Cost-effectiveness'	2	0.49	0.24	0.12	0.23	2.04
Severity x Vulnerability	3	0.66	0.43	0.33	0.19**	4.07**
Severity x Vulnerability x Treatment 'Cost-effectiveness'	4	0.69	0.47	0.35	0.03	3.94**
Severity x Vulnerability x Treatment 'Cost-effectiveness' x Personal Control/Self-efficacy	5	0.69	0.47	0.33	0.00	3.33**

[a]sr^2= squared semipartial correlation using Type III sums of squares to indicate the unique variance accounted for by the variable.

*p<0.05 **p<0.01

attitude may provide additional explanation of the variance in health outcomes. Lewis (1994) noted, however, that this optimistic bias disappeared when comparisons were made between the respondents' vulnerability ratings for themselves and for the 'average person' in relation to the single item, 'Complications arising from diabetes'. This is probably explained, on the one hand, by lack of knowledge regarding which disorders are complications, and on the other, by a restricted or idiosyncratic interpretation of the single complications item. Indeed, Lewis *et al.* (1990) noted that frequency counts for 'I already have this problem' were much lower for the single item than for most of the individual complications, suggesting that respondents in the Sheffield sample were not aware of all the complications, or perceived 'Complications arising from diabetes' as something other than the disorders listed in the questionnaire. It may be that optimistic biases will only prevail if the disorder in question is perceived to be irrelevant to current health status. Thus, the general tendency to assume that 'it won't happen to me', may diminish when a risk appears to be more salient.

Patients' beliefs about severity and vulnerability are likely to be influenced by their knowledge of diabetes and its complications, which is largely determined by the type of education received. For this reason, the single perceived vulnerability item 'Complications arising from diabetes' was more strongly correlated with HbA_1 levels and subjective estimates of diabetes control than the composite perceived Vulnerability to Complications scale. It is evident, however, that scores contributing to the composite measure are artificially reduced by lack of knowledge about which health problems are complications of diabetes. The single item therefore measures perceived vulnerability to what are understood to be complications of diabetes. This distinction should be borne in mind particularly when inspecting relationships between health beliefs and behaviour. If, for example, a patient is unaware that heart disease is a complication of diabetes then he or she may make less effort to reduce fat intake, consume fewer calories or take more exercise than if the risks were known. Perceived vulnerability to 'Complications arising from diabetes' may be high, therefore, but perceived vulnerability to heart disease may be relatively low. This distinction between scores for the scale and scores for the single item allow researchers to identify discrepancies in beliefs about Vulnerability to Complications which may benefit from intervention.

Evidence for the sensitivity and validity of the scales has been demonstrated in the various studies described above. Construct validity was indicated by consistent and predicted patterns of correlations between the scales and outcome variables such as glycaemic control, percent ideal body weight, subjective estimates of control, well-being and treatment satisfaction, and by predicted changes in health beliefs after different interventions. Although associations between the perceived Benefits and Barriers scales and the clinical outcome measures were as expected, the direction of the associations between the perceived Severity and Vulnerability scales and these outcome variables was contrary to that which the original HBM would have predicted. However, other researchers who have correlated diabetes control with different measures of perceived susceptibility to complications have noted relationships between these variables of a similar direction to those found here (Harris *et al.*, 1987; Brownlee-Duffeck *et al.*, 1987). Moreover, similar results were obtained in Study B, the education study, when using a prospective measure of HbA_1. It appears, therefore, that higher levels of perceived Severity and Vulnerability not only reflect current health status but also predict continuing poor control.

Predictive validity was demonstrated when selected health belief measures in combination with other variables were used prospectively to predict a subsequent measure of HbA_1 in Study B. The results of this latter study were interesting because introduction of General Well-being on the first step of the regression analysis resulted in the suppression of irrelevant variance and improved the prediction of glycaemic control from the selected HBM variables and the measure of Personal Control/Self-efficacy. Furthermore, the multiplicative combination of Severity x Vulnerability (Severity of Diabetes x Vulnerability to 'Complications arising from diabetes') explained an additional significant proportion of the variance in HbA_1. However, the number of cases analysed in the regression analyses was small (N = 44) and therefore the amount of variance in health outcome explained may have been inflated, despite adjustments to R^2. Further studies involving larger samples of patients are needed in order to ascertain whether these results can be replicated. It is worthy of note that in this study, the education intervention itself probably made health threats more salient than previously and thus provided the cue to action specified by the HBM as necessary for triggering preventive health behaviours.

Study D by Polly (1992) assessed whether a modified version of the health belief scales could predict self-reported adherence to treatment and glycosylated haemoglobin in a sample of older patients following a variety of treatment regimens. Evidence of validity of the scales was very limited given the small number of associations obtained. This may have been due to the nature of the sample and/or the changed format of the scales. As mentioned at the beginning of this chapter, measures specific to the different types of treatment regimen were conceived because research has indicated that the psychological responses of individuals to their diabetes will differ according to the type of treatment and the nature of the treatment involved (Davis *et al.*, 1987). The sample in Study D consisted of patients who were treated with diet only, diet and oral hypoglycaemic agents, and diet and insulin. The responses of these patients are likely, therefore, to have been influenced by very different experiences of diabetes management which are, in turn, determined by physiological status. Since Polly did not report details of how the scales were modified, it is not possible to judge whether validity might have been compromised by the construction of items or important omissions. It is important to note, however, that following modification of developed scales, psychometric evaluation of internal reliability and factor structure is needed, in addition to tests of validity, to facilitate interpretation particularly when findings run contrary to predictions. When no such assessments are carried out, firm conclusions about experimental hypotheses are hard to justify because of doubts about the measure involved.

The scales developed for use with tablet-treated patients appear, on the face of it, to be appropriate for use with patients treated by diet alone with the exception of one benefits item "It is important to take all my tablets at the times recommended by the doctor if I am to achieve good control of my diabetes". The Sheffield analyses indicated that the alpha coefficient of 0.67 would have been reduced to 0.66 if this item had been deleted. Thus the reliability of the scales will not be adversely affected if this item is excluded.

In summary, the Diabetes-Specific Health Belief scales for tablet-treated patients have been shown to be internally reliable and sensitive to change. Furthermore, construct and predictive validity have been demonstrated by consistent patterns of associations with other variables, predicted changes after interventions, and the prospective prediction of subsequent glycaemic control.

OVERVIEW DISCUSSION

The perceived Benefits and Barriers scales provide two sets of beliefs specific to the experience of having insulin-treated and tablet-treated diabetes, respectively. Future users of the scales may wish to add to the questionnaires additional belief items to address issues of particular interest in their research. However, any such additional items should be scored separately unless there are sufficient patients in the study to permit psychometric assessment of the newly-extended measure.

The perceived Severity and Vulnerability scales were modified before use with tablet-treated patients partly to make the scales appropriate for tablet-treated patients (some items relating to comas, hypoglycaemic reactions and other short-term complications were removed and 'your diabetes in twenty years' time' was modified to ten years). However, the scales were also modified in order to aid interpretation. The findings reviewed in this chapter do suggest that interpretation is facilitated by the revisions made though at the expense of substantially increasing the length of the questionnaire. Where questionnaire overload is not a major concern it is recommended that the version of the Severity and Vulnerability scales shown in Figures 5 and 6 be used in preference to those shown in Figures 2 and 3, retyping the scales to include the extra items for insulin users and changing the reference to ten years back to twenty. As the wording of certain items has been changed it is important that the relevant Severity measure is paired with the matching Vulnerability measure (i.e. Figure 5 with Figure 6 or Figure 2 with Figure 3 but not 2 with 6 nor 3 with 5). Where shorter questionnaires are necessary for a study of people with tablets/or diet treated diabetes, the Vulnerability scales in Figure 6 may be modified to exclude the average person ratings. (For further discussion of the issue of scale modifications see the final chapter by Bradley in this volume.)

The HBM has provided an important framework for conceptualising the beliefs measured by the present scales and the findings obtained using the scales have provided some support for predictions derived from the model. However, it is clear that the relationship between perceptions of Severity and Vulnerability and measures of diabetes control are far from straightforward. Although beliefs may affect self-care behaviour which in turn affects diabetes control, perceptions of diabetes control can also affect beliefs. Thus feelings of vulnerability to complications may lead to improved diabetes control via greater attention to self-care, and in turn awareness of that improved diabetes control may lead to a reduction in feelings of vulnerability. However, if diabetes control is not improved, (e.g. because of competing priorities or lack of knowledge) this may lead to greater feelings of vulnerability, reduced self-efficacy and perceptions of control, and more perceived barriers to treatment, possibly resulting in a downward spiral of diminishing self-care. The dynamic nature of health beliefs has implications for the kinds of interventions used in health services. For example, an education programme or consultation with a physician may promote factual information at the expense of emphasising perceived self-efficacy and perceived control which may exacerbate a pre-existing lack of confidence or growing cynicism. Over time, therefore, it may be more difficult to modify patients' negative or inaccurate beliefs and attempted interventions could become increasingly ineffective. It has been noted by Lewis (1994) that patients with poor diabetes control who have lived with diabetes for a number of years are less likely than their counterparts with better diabetes control, or those more recently-diagnosed, to attend an education session. To complicate matters further, diabetes control may be influenced via the direct psychophysiological effects of stress-related catecholamine and corticosteroid activity which may link into the negative feedback loop described above.

Despite the complex range of possible pathways, consistencies in the relationships between beliefs and diabetes control have emerged although it cannot be assumed that such patterns of beliefs are universal. Not only are there likely to be differences between clinic populations as a result of variations in patient education, physicians' beliefs and other factors, there may be substantial differences in beliefs between individuals. This implies, therefore, that a systematic approach (which, at one level, places patients' beliefs in the context of their particular health care organisation and, at another level, within their individual life experiences) is desirable. In this way, investigation of health beliefs may reveal the causes of diabetes management problems and help to guide appropriate interventions. Investigation of health beliefs may also point to a need for changes in the education programme or some other aspect of the diabetes care service provided, with a view to encouraging the development of patterns or health beliefs which have constructive effects on self-management.

SUMMARY

The diabetes-specific Health Belief scales include scales to measure perceived Benefits of and Barriers to treatment, perceived Severity of diabetes and associated complications and perceived Vulnerability to the complications. Two versions of the scales are available; one for insulin users and one for people with tablet-treated diabetes. The version of the Vulnerability and Severity questionnaire for people with tablet-treated diabetes allows the option of measuring perceptions of vulnerability of the "average person with your kind of diabetes" as well as perceptions of personal vulnerability. Extensive data are summarised concerning the internal consistency and construct validity of the scales and their sensitivity to change as well as some limited data providing support for predictive validity.

REFERENCES

Alogna, M. (1980) Perception of severity of disease and health locus of control in compliant and non-compliant diabetic patients. *Diabetes Care*, **3**, 533-534

Becker, M.H. (1974) The health belief model and personal health behaviour. *Health Education Monographs*, **2**, 324-473

Becker, M.H. and Maiman, L.A. (1975) Sociobehavioural determinants of compliance with health and medical care recommendations. *Medical Care*, **13**, 10-24

Bloom Cerkoney, K.A. and Hart, L.A. (1980) The relationship between the health belief model and compliance of patients with diabetes mellitus. *Diabetes Care*, **3**, 594-598

Bradley, C., Brewin, C.R., Gamsu, D.S. and Moses, J.L. (1984) Development of scales to measure perceived control of diabetes mellitus and diabetes-related health beliefs. *Diabetic Medicine*, **1**, 213-218

Bradley, C., Gamsu, D.S., Knight, G., Boulton, A.M.J. and Ward, J.D. (1986) Predicting risk of diabetic ketoacidosis in patients using continuous subcutaneous insulin infusion. *British Medical Journal*, **293**, 242-243

Bradley, C., Gamsu, D.S., Moses, J.L., Knight, G., Boulton, A.M.J., Drury, J. and Ward, J.D. (1987) The use of diabetes specific perceived control and health belief measures to predict treatment choice and efficacy in a feasibility study of continuous subcutaneous insulin infusion pumps. *Psychology and Health*, **1**, 133-146

Brownlee-Duffeck, M., Peterson, L., Simonds, J.F., Goldstein, D., Kilo, C. and Hoette, S. (1987) The role of health beliefs in the regimen adherence and metabolic control of adolescents and adults with diabetes mellitus. *Journal of Consulting and Clinical Psychology*, **55**, 139-144

Cronbach, L.J. (1951) Coefficient alpha and the internal structure of tests. *Psychometrika*, **16**, 297-334

Davis, W.K., Hess, G.E. and Van Harrison, R. (1987) Psychosocial adjustment to and control of diabetes mellitus: differences by disease type and treatment. *Health Psychology*, **6**, 1-14

Gillespie, C.R. (1989) *Psychological variables in the self-regulation of diabetes mellitus*, Unpublished Ph.D. thesis, University of Sheffield

Given, C.W., Given, B.A., Gallin, R.S. and Condon, J.W. (1983) Development of scales to measure beliefs of diabetic patients. *Research in Nursing and Health*, **6**, 127-141

Harris, R., Skyler, J.S., Linn, M.W., Pollack, L. and Tewksbury, D. (1982) Relationship between the health belief model and compliance as a basis for intervention in diabetes mellitus. *Pediatric and Adolescent Endocrinology*, **10**, 123-132

Harris, R., Linn, M.W., Skyler, J.S. and Sandifer, R. (1987) Development of the diabetes health belief scale. *Diabetes Educator*, **13**, 292-297

Hochbaum, G. (1958) *Public participation in medical screening programs: a sociopsychological study*, Public Health Service Publication No. 572, Washington, D.C., Superintendent of Public Documents

Janz, N.K. and Becker, M.H. (1984) The health belief model: a decade later. *Health Education Quarterly*, **11**, 1-47

Jennings, A.M., Lewis, K.S., Bradley, C., Wilson, R.M. and Ward, J.D. (1988) Symptomatic hypoglycaemia in non-insulin dependent diabetic patients treated with oral hypoglycaemic agents, (Abstract). *Diabetic Medicine,* **5** (suppl. 1), 3

Jennings, A.M., Lewis K.S., Murdoch, S., Talbot, J.F., Bradley, C. and Ward, J.D. (1991) Randomised trial comparing continuous subcutaneous insulin infusion and conventional insulin therapy in type II diabetic patients poorly controlled with sulfonylureas. *Diabetes Care,* **14**, 738–744

Kline, P. (1986) *A handbook of test construction: introduction to psychometric design.* London: Methuen

Lewis, K.S. (1994) *An examination of the health belief model when applied to diabetes mellitus,* Unpublished Ph.D. thesis, University of Sheffield

Lewis, K.S., Jennings, A.M., Ward, J.D. and Bradley, C. (1990) Health belief scales developed specifically for people with tablet-treated type 2 diabetes. *Diabetic Medicine,* **7**, 148–155

Lundman, B., Asplund, K. and Norberg, A. (1990) Living with diabetes: perceptions of well-being. *Research in Nursing and Health,* **13**, 255–262

Meadows, K.A., Fromson, B., Gillespie, C., Brewer, A., Carter, C., Lockington, T., Clark, G. and Wise, P.H. (1988) Development, Validation and Application of Computer-linked Knowledge Questionnaires in Diabetes Education. *Diabetic Medicine,* **5**, 61–67

Polly, R.K. (1992) Diabetes health beliefs, self-care behaviours, and glycemic control among older adults with non-insulin-dependent diabetes mellitus. *Diabetes Educator,* **18**, 321-327

Rosenstock, I.M. (1966) Why people use health services. *Milbank Memorial Fund Quarterly,* **44**, 94–124

Sjoberg, S., Carlson, A., Rosenqvist, U. and Ostman, J. (1988) Health attitudes, self-monitoring of blood glucose, metabolic control, and residual insulin secretion in type 1 diabetic patients. *Diabetic Medicine,* **5**, 449–453

Weinstein, N.D. (1982) Unrealistic optimism about susceptibility to health problems. *Journal of Behavioural Medicine,* **5**, 441–460

Weinstein, N.D. (1984) Why it won't happen to me: perceptions of risk factors and susceptibility. *Health Psychology,* **3**, 431–457

Weinstein, N.D. (1987) Unrealistic optimism about susceptibility to health problems: conclusions from a community-wide sample. *Journal of Behavioural Medicine,* **10**, 481–500

CHAPTER 13

MEASURES OF PERCEIVED CONTROL OF DIABETES

CLARE BRADLEY

Department of Psychology, Royal Holloway, University of London, Egham, Surrey TW20 0EX, UK

INTRODUCTION

The Perceived Control of Diabetes Scales were originally designed in the early 1980s to be used alongside measures of health beliefs described elsewhere in this *Handbook* by Lewis and Bradley. The scales were included in a Sheffield based prospective study of insulin-requiring patients who were involved in a feasibility study of continuous subcutaneous insulin infusion (CSII) pumps. Patients were given a choice between two different intensities of injection regimen or CSII pumps (Bradley *et al.*, 1984). The new scales proved useful in understanding patients' preferences for the treatment options and individual differences between patients in the efficacy of the various treatments after twelve months on the chosen treatment regimen (Bradley *et al.*, 1987). The scales also proved useful in understanding the reasons for the marked increase in diabetic ketoacidosis (DKA) among users of CSII pumps (Bradley *et al.*, 1986). The scales have since been modified for use with patients treated with tablets rather than insulin (Bradley *et al.*, 1990) and for use by health care professionals (Gamsu and Bradley, 1987). Comparison of the perceptions of control over diabetes made by health care professionals and patients has highlighted predicted biases in professionals' perceptions that differ from those of patients in a way that is likely to be damaging to the therapeutic relationship (Gamsu and Bradley, 1987, 1992). Subsequent studies have evaluated interventions aimed to help professionals to appreciate patients' perceptions (Gillespie and Bradley, 1988; Gillespie, 1989) and recommendations have been made for improving therapeutic collaboration between professionals and their patients (Gillespie and Bradley, 1985; Bradley, 1989). Applying a speculative typology suggested by Wallston and Wallston (1982), the Perceived Control of Diabetes Scales were found to be significantly associated with HbA$_1$, percentage ideal body weight, well-being and satisfaction with treatment for patients with tablet-treated diabetes (Bradley *et al.*, 1990).

The Perceived Control of Diabetes Scales were influenced by earlier work on locus of control measurement (Rotter, 1966; Wallston *et al.*, 1976, 1978) and more recent developments of measures of attributional style (Peterson *et al.*, 1982). Measures of attributional style derive from attribution theory which is concerned with the attributions, or explanations that people use to account for events including their own behaviour and that of other people. Attributional theories predict that peoples' attributions or explanations for past events are likely to influence their expectations for the future and their future behaviour. A person's motivation to attempt a task can be viewed as a function of past experience of a similar nature and their attributions for previous successful or unsuccessful outcomes (Weiner, 1979). The concept of locus of control derives from social learning theory rather than from attribution theory and while attributional measures are concerned to measure attributions for hypothetical or real events in the past, locus of control refers to expectations of control over future events. Early measures of locus of control provided scores on a single dimension ranging from internal locus of control, where the individual expects to be able to control events, to external locus of control, where the individual has no expectation of personal control (Rotter, 1966). Later measures followed Levenson (1972) in distinguishing between different kinds of external locus of control; chance locus of control and control by powerful others. Among researchers in health-related fields the best known of the multidimensional locus of control scales is the Multidimensional Health Locus of Control (MHLC) scale developed by the Wallstons and their colleagues (Wallston *et al.*, 1978).

The Perceived Control of Diabetes Scales were developed because the concept was so clearly relevant to diabetes, non-specific locus of control scales appeared to be insensitive, and no diabetes-specific perceived control or locus of control scales were available at that time (Lowery and DuCette, 1976; Dickens, 1979; Alogna, 1980). There was reason to believe that patients' expectations of control over their diabetes bears little relationship to their generalised expectations of control measured by generic or health locus of control scales and diabetes-specific measures will be more useful in understanding behaviour and predicting outcomes.

Despite the disappointing performance of more general locus of control scales, many diabetes researchers have recognised that notions of perceived control over diabetes are likely to be important in understanding patients' motivation to manage their diabetes (see Bradley, 1985 for review). A person with diabetes who attributes diabetes control to good or bad luck favours a chance locus of control. Such a person would not be expected to be as well motivated to follow a demanding treatment regimen as a person who favours an internal locus of control and attributes good diabetes control to his or her own efforts. The Perceived Control of Diabetes Scales were designed to measure the way people explain short- and long-term outcomes specifically associated with their diabetes. In common with measures of attributional style, the present scales measure attributions for past events and are concerned not only with the locus of perceived control but also with perceptions of responsibility and foreseeability. In common with the MHLC and other locus of control measures, the present scales are concerned not only with patients' perceptions of their own control but also with their perceptions of control by their doctor and others. Evidence to suggest the importance of determining separately the perceptions of control for positive and negative outcomes (Brewin and Shapiro, 1984) influenced the design of the scales.

Wallston and Wallston (1982) offered a speculative health locus of control typology as a way of improving our understanding of the relationships between locus of control and health behaviour by looking at patterns of locus of control beliefs (measured by the MHLC scale) and their adaptiveness for specific situations. The MHLC includes three subscales for which separate scores are obtained; Internality, Powerful Others, and Chance. These subscale scores may be regarded as equivalent to the present questionnaire's scores for Personal Control, Medical Control and Situational Control. The type that was predicted to be the most adaptive and beneficial to a person who has to cope with a chronic illness such as diabetes was the type who scores high on Internality and Powerful Others and low on Chance which would be equivalent to high on Personal Control, high on Medical Control and low on Situational Control. People categorised in this type were labelled "Believers in Control" and would be expected to make the best use of their own personal resources and those of the health professionals advising them on diabetes management. Seven further types were identified and are described in Table 1. Bradley *et al.* (1990) applied the Wallstons' typology to the responses of tablet-treated patients completing the Perceived Control of Diabetes Scales and the data provide support for the value of the typology as well as support for the validity of the scales.

Table 1 Summary of Wallston and Wallston's typology and predicted consequences for diabetes management. (Modified from the original typology applied to diabetes management by Bradley *et al.* (1990) Diabetic Medicine, 7, 685-694, and reproduced (with minor amendments) by permission of John Wiley & Sons Ltd).

	Scale Scores			Predicted
Label	Personal Control	Medical Control	Situational Control	consequences for diabetes management
Believers in Control	High	High	Low	Good use of personal resources and health service resources
'Pure' Personal Control	High	Low	Low	Good use of personal resources but may not recognise when these are inadequate
'Pure' Medical Control Externals	Low	High	Low	Poor use of personal resources and unrealistic expectations of health service resources
'Pure' Situational Control Externals	Low	Low	High	Fatalistic: Poor use of all resources
Double Externals	Low	High	High	Poor use of personal resources, unrealistic expectations of health service resources and element of fatalism
Type VI	High	Low	High	The Wallstons suggested that this type would be non-existent or rare
Yea-sayers	High	High	High	Response bias? No clear predictions
Nay-sayers	Low	Low	Low	Response bias? No clear predictions

Other researchers have since developed measures of locus of control over dia-betes (Ferraro *et al.*, 1987; Kohlmann *et al.*, 1991). Ferraro *et al.* (1987) in Ohio, USA have published details of the development of a diabetes-specific locus of con-trol scale designed to measure three dimensions; Internality, Powerful Others, and Chance. The face and content validity of Ferraro *et al.*'s measure suggest that it may have promise. However, it should be noted that Powerful Others was defined very broadly by Ferraro *et al.* to include friends and family and even "other people who have diabetes" rather than limiting the concept to health professionals as do the scales presented here. Ferraro *et al.* did not appear to have attempted to bal-ance the presentations of positive versus negative outcomes in their items: the In-ternality and Powerful Others items are predominantly concerned with control over positive outcomes though the Chance items have more of a balance. It should be noted that the MHLC designed by the Wallstons and their colleagues (1978) also contained an imbalance of positive and negative outcomes. Experience of constructing a smoking locus of control scale where efforts were made to balance statements describing positive and negative outcomes and statements with which respondents agree versus disagree, illustrated the impossibility of achieving a bal-ance without sacrificing reliability to an unacceptable degree. Positively worded items and those with which respondents agreed in order to score higher on a sub-scale tended to be the more reliable items (Georgiou and Bradley, 1992). Kohl-mann *et al.*'s 1991 measure is designed and written in German specifically for insulin users. The questionnaire was constructed to elicit four subscale scores to indicate Internality, Powerful Others, Chance and Unpredictability. The Unpre-dictability subscale is an unusual feature for a locus of control scale though it is a common feature of attributional measures. Expectations of unpredictability are undoubtedly important in diabetes and this subscale is likely to be useful. In the present Perceived Control of Diabetes Scales, the Foreseeability subscale provides an equivalent measure. The psychometric properties of the German scale were summarised by Kohlmann *et al.* (1993) (high alpha coefficients for the four sub-scales, ranging from 0.84 to 0.89) in a paper describing the use of the scales to study differences in locus of control beliefs in patients using one of three forms of insulin treatment regimen.

The present chapter describes measures of perceived control for insulin users together with modified scales for tablet-treated patients. The main purpose of the scales was to measure perceived control over diabetes and its complications in or-der to understand individual differences in preferences for different treatment regimens and differences in the degree of diabetes control achieved. They are likely to be particularly useful in research which aims to assess the effectiveness of interventions such as education programmes seeking to modify perceptions of control to achieve desired health outcomes. The scales provide measures of psy-chological processes rather than outcomes. As such, they may be used to under-stand how patients' perceptions of control are associated with their behaviour in the context of their particular diabetes (which may be more or less difficult to con-trol), the treatment and education provided, and the particular health care system in which they find themselves. Health care practitioners should then be better informed in order to intervene more appropriately and organise their services to achieve greater effectiveness.

Design

The scales were designed to have a similar format to Peterson *et al.*'s (1982) Attributional Style Questionnaire. That is, a scenario was described followed by a space for the respondent to specify the most likely cause of such a scenario followed by a series of scales for rating the cause. The rating scales were influenced by, though differed from, those used by Peterson *et al.* in having separate scales for rating internality and externality. Rather than Peterson *et al.*'s single dimension from "totally due to me" through to "totally due to other people and circumstances", two separate scales were used thereby allowing for the possibility of ratings on these scales that are not interdependent. With this modification it becomes possible for a respondent to indicate a belief that an outcome was not due to themselves nor due to other people or circumstances but due, perhaps, to chance factors. Following developments in measurement of multidimensional locus of control, scales were included to measure attributions to the doctor and to the treatment. The scales for insulin users were balanced to include equal numbers of scenarios describing positive and negative outcomes following work suggesting that attributions differ according to the desirability of the outcome (Brewin and Shapiro, 1984). It was anticipated that the same attribution to, say, chance factors would have very different implications for future expectations of success in managing diabetes and future self-care behaviour if it was used to account for a positive outcome scenario compared with the implications if it was used to account for a negative outcome scenario. Thus a person who attributes positive outcomes of diabetes management to chance might be expected to expend less energy in achieving diabetes control than would be implied by an attribution of chance for a negative outcome. Thus three of the six scenarios for insulin users were concerned with positive outcomes while three described negative outcomes associated with diabetes management.

The first six scenarios presented in Figure 1 constitute the questionnaire for insulin users. Three of these scenarios for insulin users are also included in the version for tablet-treated patients which includes only five scenarios in total. Two scenarios which referred to hypoglycaemic reactions were ommitted from the version for tablet-treated patients as many of these latter patients would not have experienced hypoglycaemic reactions. Three new scenarios were designed but only two of these were included in the final version. The two new scenarios included are to be found in the scales in Figure 1 and are labelled "Perceived control II/4" and "Perceived control II/5" at the foot of the page. All other scenarios are labelled to indicate in which of the questionnaires they are included and the order in which they should appear in the questionnaire. Table 2 presents the scenarios grouped by positive and negative outcomes and indicates the version(s) of the questionnaire each scenario appears in.

Figure 1 Perceived Control of Diabetes Scales

INSTRUCTIONS FOR COMPLETION OF THE PERCEIVED
CONTROL OF DIABETES SCALES

The following questions are about the causes of situations which might happen to you.

We ask you to imagine that the events described have happened to you recently.

While events may have many causes, we want you to pick only one - the *major* cause of the situation as you see it.

Please write this cause in the space provided after each event.

Next, we want you to answer some questions about the cause by circling the most appropriate number of a sliding scale from 6 to 0.

Imagine that you have recently experienced a hypo

Write down the single most likely cause of the hypo in the space below

Now rate this cause on the following scales:

1. To what extent was the cause due to something about you?

   Totally due to me   6   5   4   3   2   1   0   Not at all due to me

2. To what extent was the cause due to the treatment recommended by your doctor?

   Totally due   6   5   4   3   2   1   0   Not at all due to
   to treatment   treatment
   recommended   recommended

3. To what extent was the cause something to do with other people or circumstances?

   Totally due   6   5   4   3   2   1   0   Not at all due
   to other people   to other people
   or circumstances   or circumstances

4. To what extent was the cause due to chance?

   Totally due   6   5   4   3   2   1   0   Not at all due
   to chance   to chance

5. To what extent was the cause controllable by you?

   Totally   6   5   4   3   2   1   0   Totally
   controllable by me   uncontrollable by me

6. To what extent was the cause controllable by your doctor?

   Totally   6   5   4   3   2   1   0   Totally
   controllable   uncontrollable
   by my doctor   by my doctor

7. To what extent do you think you could have foreseen the cause of the hypo?

   Totally   6   5   4   3   2   1   0   Totally
   foreseeable   unforeseeable
   by me   by me

Imagine that your diabetes has been well controlled for a period of several weeks during which time there has been little fluctuation in blood glucose, no reactions and you have felt fit and well

Write down the single most likely cause of this period of good control in the space below

---

Now rate this cause on the following scales:

1. To what extent was the cause due to something about you?

   Totally due to me   6   5   4   3   2   1   0   Not at all due to me

2. To what extent was the cause due to the treatment recommended by your doctor?

   Totally due   6   5   4   3   2   1   0   Not at all due
   to treatment   to treatment
   recommended   recommended

3. To what extent was the cause something to do with other people or circumstances?

   Totally due   6   5   4   3   2   1   0   Not at all due
   to other people   to other people
   or circumstances   or circumstances

4. To what extent was the cause due to chance?

   Totally due   6   5   4   3   2   1   0   Not at all due
   to chance   to chance

5. To what extent was the cause controllable by you?

   Totally   6   5   4   3   2   1   0   Totally
   controllable by me   uncontrollable by me

6. To what extent was the cause controllable by your doctor?

   Totally   6   5   4   3   2   1   0   Totally
   controllable   uncontrollable
   by my doctor   by my doctor

7. To what extent do you think you could have foreseen the cause of the period of good diabetes control?

   Totally   6   5   4   3   2   1   0   Totally
   foreseeable   unforeseeable
   by me   by me

Imagine that for several days you have found high levels of sugar when you tested your blood or urine

Write down the single most likely cause of the high sugar levels in the space below

_____

_____

Now rate this cause on the following scales:

1. To what extent was the cause due to something about you?
   Totally due to me   6   5   4   3   2   1   0   Not at all due to me

2. To what extent was the cause due to the treatment recommended by your doctor?

   Totally due   6   5   4   3   2   1   0   Not at all due
   to treatment   to treatment
   recommended   recommended

3. To what extent was the cause something to do with other people or circumstances?

   Totally due   6   5   4   3   2   1   0   Not at all due
   to other people   to other people
   or circumstances   or circumstances

4. To what extent was the cause due to chance?

   Totally due   6   5   4   3   2   1   0   Not at all due
   to chance   to chance

5. To what extent was the cause controllable by you?

   Totally   6   5   4   3   2   1   0   Totally
   controllable by me   uncontrollable by me

6. To what extent was the cause controllable by your doctor?

   Totally   6   5   4   3   2   1   0   Totally
   controllable   uncontrollable
   by my doctor   by my doctor

7. To what extent do you think you could have foreseen the cause of the high sugar levels?

   Totally   6   5   4   3   2   1   0   Totally
   foreseeable   unforeseeable
   by me   by me

Imagine that good control of your diabetes is restored after a period of poor control

Write down, in the space below, the single most likely cause of good control being restored

_____

_____

Now rate this cause on the following scales:

1. To what extent was the cause due to something about you?

   Totally due to me   6   5   4   3   2   1   0   Not at all due to me

2. To what extent was the cause due to the treatment recommended by your doctor?

   Totally due   6   5   4   3   2   1   0   Not at all due
   to treatment   to treatment
   recommended   recommended

3. To what extent was the cause something to do with other people or circumstances?

   Totally due   6   5   4   3   2   1   0   Not at all due
   to other people   to other people
   or circumstances   or circumstances

4. To what extent was the cause due to chance?

   Totally due   6   5   4   3   2   1   0   Not at all due
   to chance   to chance

5. To what extent was the cause controllable by you?

   Totally   6   5   4   3   2   1   0   Totally
   controllable by me   uncontrollable by me

6. To what extent was the cause controllable by your doctor?

   Totally   6   5   4   3   2   1   0   Totally
   controllable   uncontrollable
   by my doctor   by my doctor

7. To what extent do you think you could have foreseen the cause of good control being restored?

   Totally   6   5   4   3   2   1   0   Totally
   foreseeable   unforeseeable
   by me   by me

Imagine that you have successfully avoided the complications of diabetes such as problems with your feet

Write down, in the space below, the single most likely cause of the successful avoidance of diabetic complications such as problems with your feet

---

Now rate this cause on the following scales:
1. To what extent was the cause due to something about you?

| Totally due to me | 6 | 5 | 4 | 3 | 2 | 1 | 0 | Not at all due to me |

2. To what extent was the cause due to the treatment recommended by your doctor?

| Totally due to treatment recommended | 6 | 5 | 4 | 3 | 2 | 1 | 0 | Not at all due to treatment recommended |

3. To what extent was the cause something to do with other people or circumstances?

| Totally due to other people or circumstances | 6 | 5 | 4 | 3 | 2 | 1 | 0 | Not at all due to other people or circumstances |

4. To what extent was the cause due to chance?

| Totally due to chance | 6 | 5 | 4 | 3 | 2 | 1 | 0 | Not at all due to chance |

5. To what extent was the cause controllable by you?

| Totally controllable by me | 6 | 5 | 4 | 3 | 2 | 1 | 0 | Totally uncontrollable by me |

6. To what extent was the cause controllable by your doctor?

| Totally controllable by my doctor | 6 | 5 | 4 | 3 | 2 | 1 | 0 | Totally uncontrollable by my doctor |

7. To what extent do you think you could have foreseen the cause of successfully avoiding complications?

| Totally foreseeable by me | 6 | 5 | 4 | 3 | 2 | 1 | 0 | Totally unforeseeable by me |

Imagine that you have recently become unacceptably overweight

Write down, in the space below, the single most likely cause of becoming overweight

---

Now rate this cause on the following scales:

1. To what extent was the cause due to something about you?

   Totally due to me   6   5   4   3   2   1   0   Not at all due to me

2. To what extent was the cause due to the treatment recommended by your doctor?

   Totally due   6   5   4   3   2   1   0   Not at all due
   to treatment   to treatment
   recommended   recommended

3. To what extent was the cause something to do with other people or circumstances?

   Totally due   6   5   4   3   2   1   0   Not at all due
   to other people   to other people
   or circumstances   or circumstances

4. To what extent was the cause due to chance?

   Totally due   6   5   4   3   2   1   0   Not at all due
   to chance   to chance

5. To what extent was the cause controllable by you?

   Totally   6   5   4   3   2   1   0   Totally
   controllable by me   uncontrollable by me

6. To what extent was the cause controllable by your doctor?

   Totally   6   5   4   3   2   1   0   Totally
   controllable   uncontrollable
   by my doctor   by my doctor

7. To what extent do you think you could have foreseen the cause of becoming overweight?

   Totally   6   5   4   3   2   1   0   Totally
   foreseeable   unforeseeable
   by me   by me

Imagine that you have been able to keep your weight at an acceptable level for a period of several weeks and you have felt fit and well

Write down, in the space below, the single most likely cause of this period of good weight control and sense of general well-being

---

Now rate this cause on the following scales:

1. To what extent was the cause due to something about you?

   Totally due to me   6   5   4   3   2   1   0   Not at all due to me

2. To what extent was the cause due to the treatment recommended by your doctor?

   Totally due   6   5   4   3   2   1   0   Not at all due
   to treatment   to treatment
   recommended   recommended

3. To what extent was the cause something to do with other people or circumstances?

   Totally due   6   5   4   3   2   1   0   Not at all due
   to other people   to other people
   or circumstances   or circumstances

4. To what extent was the cause due to chance?

   Totally due   6   5   4   3   2   1   0   Not at all due
   to chance   to chance

5. To what extent was the cause controllable by you?

   Totally   6   5   4   3   2   1   0   Totally
   controllable by me   uncontrollable by me

6. To what extent was the cause controllable by your doctor?

   Totally   6   5   4   3   2   1   0   Totally
   controllable   uncontrollable
   by my doctor   by my doctor

7. To what extent do you think you could have foreseen the cause of the period of good weight control?

   Totally   6   5   4   3   2   1   0   Totally
   foreseeable   unforeseeable
   by me   by me

Imagine that you have reduced your weight to a satisfactory level after a period when you gained too much weight

Write down the single most likely cause of this weight reduction in the space below

---

Now rate this cause on the following scales:

1. To what extent was the cause due to something about you?

   Totally due to me   6   5   4   3   2   1   0   Not at all due to me

2. To what extent was the cause due to the treatment recommended by your doctor?

   Totally due   6   5   4   3   2   1   0   Not at all due
   to treatment   to treatment
   recommended   recommended

3. To what extent was the cause something to do with other people or circumstances?

   Totally due   6   5   4   3   2   1   0   Not at all due
   to other people   to other people
   or circumstances   or circumstances

4. To what extent was the cause due to chance?

   Totally due   6   5   4   3   2   1   0   Not at all due
   to chance   to chance

5. To what extent was the cause controllable by you?

   Totally   6   5   4   3   2   1   0   Totally
   controllable by me   uncontrollable by me

6. To what extent was the cause controllable by your doctor?

   Totally   6   5   4   3   2   1   0   Totally
   controllable   uncontrollable
   by my doctor   by my doctor

7. To what extent do you think you could have foreseen the cause of the weight reduction?

   Totally   6   5   4   3   2   1   0   Totally
   foreseeable   unforeseeable
   by me   by me

Table 2 Perceived Control of Diabetes Scales scenarios categorised by positive or negative outcomes. The version(s) of the questionnaire in which each scenario appears is indicated.

Questionnaire	Version of Perceived Control	
	I insulin-treated patients	*II* tablet-treated patients
Positive outcomes		
"Imagine that your diabetes has been well controlled for a period of several weeks during which time there has been little fluctuation in blood glucose, no reations and you have felt fit and well"	Yes	No
"Imagine that good control of your diabetes is restored after a period of poor control"	Yes	No
"Imagine that you have been able to keep your weight at an acceptable level for a period of several weeks and you have felt fit and well"	No	Yes
"Imagine that you have successfully avoided the complications of diabetes such as problems with your feet"	Yes	Yes
"Imagine that you have reduced your weight to a satisfactory level after a period when you gained too much weight"	No	Yes
Negative outcomes		
"Imagine that you have recently experienced a hypo"	Yes	No
"Imagine that for several days you have found high levels of sugar when you tested your blood or urine"	Yes	Yes
"Imagine that you have recently become unacceptably overweight"	Yes	Yes

For each hypothetical event, patients are asked to imagine that they have recently experienced the particular outcome, and to write down its single most likely cause. They then rate this cause on seven separate seven-point scales which are labelled as follows:

Internality	"To what extent was the cause due to something about you?"
Treatment	"To what extent was the cause due to the treatment recommended by your doctor?"
Externality	"To what extent was the cause something to do with other people or circumstances?"

Chance	"To what extent was the cause due to chance?"
Patient Control	"To what extent was the cause controllable by you?"
Doctor Control	"To what extent was the cause controllable by your doctor?"
Foreseeability	"To what extent do you think you could have foreseen the cause of *event x*?" (where *event x* is specified in the form of a short description of the scenario as shown in each page of Figure 1).

It should be noted that the subscales here labelled "Patient Control" and "Doctor Control" have in previous publications been labelled "Personal Control" and "Medical Control". The subscales have here been relabelled in order to preserve the terms "Personal Control" and "Medical Control" for labelling the composite scales as described below.

Scoring

Subscale scores

Ratings for each subscale may be summed across all the scenarios to obtain subscale total scores e.g. *Internality* (Scenario 1) + *Internality* (Scenario 2) + *Internality* (Scenario 3) ....etc. The six scores from the six scenarios in the insulin users' version of the questionnaire provide a possible range of scores from 0 to 36 where higher scores indicate greater weight being given to Internality, Treatment, Externality, Chance, Patient Control, Doctor Control, Foreseeability. The five scores from the five scenarios in the version of the questionnaire for patients with tablet-treated diabetes give a possible range of scores from 0 to 30. Where the differential effects of positive and negative outcomes are of interest, subscale scores may be computed separately for the positive and negative outcomes leading to ranges of scores of 0 to 18 for the positive and negative outcomes of the insulin-users' questionnaire and for the positive outcomes of the questionnaire for patients treated with tablets and a range of 0 to 12 for negative outcomes for tablet-treated patients.

Composite scale scores

The subscale scores can be used to compute composite scores labelled Personal Control, Medical Control and Situational Control as shown in Table 3.

If researchers wish to use only the composite scale scores and will not be using the separate subscale scores, then they may wish to consider reducing the length of the questionnaire by omitting a scenario. The particular scenarios that may be omitted with the least risk of unwanted consequences for the reliability of the instrument are considered in the sections on reliability and short forms of the measure.

Table 3 Scoring of composite Perceived Control of Diabetes Scales

Composite Scale label	Subscales included	Possible range of scores	
		Version I for insulin-treated patients	Version II for tablet-treated patients
Personal Control	Internality, Patient Control, Foreseeability: add scores on available items (18 for version I and 15 for version II) and divide by 3	0–36	0–30
Medical Control	Treatment, Doctor Control: add scores on available items (12 for version I and 10 for version II) and divide by 2	0–36	0–30
Situational Control	Externality, Chance: add scores on available items (12 for version I and 10 for version II) and divide by 2	0–36	0–30

SCALE DEVELOPMENT

Subject Samples and Procedures

Study 1: Sheffield feasibility study of CSII: Bradley et al. (1984)

The sample in this study provided the original data from which the factor structure and internal reliability of Version I of the Perceived Control of Diabetes Scales for insulin users were obtained. Three hundred and eighty-two insulin-requiring diabetic patients (195 men and 187 women) at the Royal Hallamshire Hospital, Sheffield, UK, involved in a feasibility study of CSII were included in the study. Patients aged between 16 and 59 were considered for inclusion in this study unless CSII was thought to be impractical, disruptive or potentially dangerous. Individuals were excluded if they were using fewer than twenty-four units of insulin per day, had been treated with insulin for fewer than six months, were blind or had undergone amputation of a lower limb, were currently pregnant, on a renal dialysis programme or were receiving psychiatric treatment. Questionnaires were completed and returned by 286 patients (146 men and 140 women) indicating a 75% response rate from the total population sample of 382 patients.

The patients were initially invited to an illustrated lecture on the treatments offered. The lecture emphasized the association between poor blood glucose control and development of later complications such as retinopathy, neuropathy and nephropathy. CSII and intensified conventional treatment (ICT) were then presented as methods for improving blood glucose control in conjunction with home blood glucose monitoring. The patients could choose between CSII or ICT or could remain on their conventional treatment (CT). Patients were given the questionnaires when they attended a subsequent individual consultation. Following the consultation, patients chose one of the treatments offered. Questionnaires were completed at or shortly after the initial consultation before any change in treatment regimen and were returned in pre-paid envelopes addressed to the university psychology department. Data were available from 95 respondents who chose CSII, 122 who chose ICT and 69 who chose CT. The Perceived Control of Diabetes Scales together with scales developed to measure health beliefs concerning insulin-requiring diabetes, described in the Chapter by Lewis and Bradley, were used in order to predict treatment choice and efficacy.

Study 2: Diabetic ketoacidosis (DKA) study: Bradley et al. (1986)

The subjects in this study were a sub-sample of the patients described in Study 1. The sub-sample consisted of twenty two patients. Eleven of them had been selected because they had experienced episodes of diabetic ketoacidosis over a period of two years and six months while using CSII. They were then matched for age, sex and duration of diabetes with eleven patients using the same treatment who had not experienced ketoacidosis. The rationale for the study was to assess whether various patient characteristics (including perceived control of diabetes), could help to account for occurrence of ketoacidosis in pump users.

Study 3: Northampton cross-sectional study: Gillespie (1989)

Seventy-two patients with insulin-requiring diabetes (thirty six men and thirty six women) were recruited when they attended an out-patient clinic in the UK for consultation. Selection criteria were: duration of insulin-requiring diabetes ≥ 1 year, and age ≥ 21 years. Pregnancy and disabling complications were exclusion criteria. Two thirds of the sample (fifty-four patients) were included in the study because the physician involved in their care considered that they had diabetes management problems, and/or they had HbA_{1c} levels greater than 10%. Eighteen additional patients from the sample were selected as representative of those with few problems with diabetes control, as reflected by $HbA_{1c} \leq 10\%$.

The two groups of patients completed the Perceived Control of Diabetes Scales for insulin users together with measures of knowledge of diabetes (Meadows *et al.*, 1988), Diabetes-Specific Health Belief Scales for insulin users described by Lewis and Bradley elsewhere in this volume, and metabolic control. The rationale for the study was to investigate the interrelationships between these variables with a view to understanding reasons for high HbA_{1c} levels.

Study 4: Northampton consultation intervention study with insulin users and their doctor: Gillespie and Bradley (1988) and Gillespie (1989).

The fifty-four patients in Study 3 who were judged to have diabetes management problems, were assigned to one of three forms of consultation: 1) routine consultation, 2) a consultation where doctor and patient explicitly negotiated and agreed the nature of the problem(s) to be discussed, 3) consultation as in (2) but doctor and patient also negotiated and agreed their causal attributions for the problems discussed. One doctor (an experienced general practitioner acting as a clinical assistant in a diabetes out-patient clinic) was involved in all fifty four consultations. The study was designed with a view to increasing congruence between doctor and patient in their views of the problems (groups 2 and 3) and in their attributions for those problems (group 3) and to investigate associated differences between doctor and patient in their perceptions of control over diabetes.

Study 5: Main Sheffield sample of tablet-treated patients: Bradley et al. (1990) and Lewis (1994).

Two hundred and thirty-nine patients (141 men and 98 women) with Type 2 diabetes, treated with oral hypoglycaemic agents and attending two outpatient clinics at the Royal Hallamshire Hospital, Sheffield, UK, were invited to take part in a study evaluating the management of Type 2 diabetes (Jennings *et al.*, 1988, 1991). Age range was forty to sixty five years. Those who were blind or partially sighted were not included. Two hundred and nineteen (92%) patients (130 men and 89 women) agreed to take part and were screened by a physician in order to establish their health status. There were no significant differences between participants and those who refused to take part, for any of the available measures, including sex, age, duration of diabetes and glycosylated hæmoglobin (HbA_1) levels. The patients were given a booklet of questionnaires, including the Perceived Control of Diabetes Scales, to complete at home and were asked to return them within two days in a pre-paid envelope addressed to the university psychology department. Anyone who did not return a booklet within one month of their appointment received a reminder. One hundred and eighty-seven (85%) patients (110 men and 77 women) returned completed booklets of questionnaires. This final sample provided the data for psychometric analyses reported here for tablet-treated patients and for the application of the Wallstons' typology. There were no significant differences between responders and non-responders to the questionnaires in sex, age, duration of diabetes, HbA_1 or percent ideal body weight.

Study 6: Education study: Sheffield subsample: Lewis (1993)

The subjects in this study were a self-selected subsample of the patients described in Study 5, all of whom were invited by one of the physicians in the research team to attend an education session (with the exception of those subjects with particularly inadequate control who were recruited for an insulin intervention study). The study included an assessment of the effects of an education intervention on perceived control and other measures of health beliefs (see Chapter by Lewis and Bradley). Altogether, 81 (47%) of the 173 patients who were invited attended one of thirteen education sessions. The attenders were found to have experienced their diabetes for significantly fewer years than those who did not attend (mean = 5.7 years ± 5.5 vs 7.9 ± 5.1; p<0.01) and they had previously reported (Study 5) significantly greater perceived Severity of Complications when compared with non-attenders (z = -2.0; p<0.05).

The education intervention was designed so that benefits of treatment were emphasised and any difficulties with the regimen could be addressed. Information about complications was given at the beginning of each session but this was followed immediately by positive information about how to improve diabetes control with a view to arresting/preventing the short- and long-term complications. Accordingly, it was predicted that the education intervention would increase perceived Personal Control while decreasing perceptions of Situational Control.

Patients' knowledge about diabetes was measured by questionnaire (designed and developed for the study by Lewis (1994) immediately before and immediately after the education sessions and a similar booklet of questionnaires to that employed in Study 5 was given to them for completion at home. They were asked to complete the booklet of questionnaires within the next two days and return them in the pre-paid envelope provided. Those who did not return a booklet within two weeks were sent a reminder. Seventy nine (97.5%) patients returned a completed booklet of questionnaires.

Statistical Methods and Qualitative Judgements

In Studies 1 and 2, the original Sheffield work, all data were analysed using SPSS on a Prime mainframe computer. Study 1 employed correlation matrices to examine responses within and between subscales and a principal components analysis with varimax rotation to assess the factor structure of the seven subscales. Internal reliability of the scales was assessed using Cronbach's (1951) alpha coefficient. Gillespie and Bradley (1988), repeated the principal components analysis and assessed Cronbach's alpha for the composite measures used as well as the individual scales. Bradley et al. (1987) used multiple regression analyses with the perceived control and other variables, including health beliefs, in order to identify which patients would wish to intensify their treatment and which mode of treatment they would prefer. Further multiple regression analyses were conducted in order to predict efficacy of the treatments in terms of glycosylated hæmoglobin levels twelve months later (Bradley et al., 1987). In the DKA study (Study 2), independent group t-tests were used for comparisons between the two groups on all measures.

Gillespie's thesis includes a wealth of analyses on the cross-sectional study and on the subsequent consultation intervention study, Study 4, including path analysis (Asher, 1983) to estimate the magnitude of linkages between the perceived control variables, the health belief variables described in the Chapter by Lewis and Bradley and other variables in attempting to develop a model of health actions in diabetes management. Findings will be mentioned only briefly here and the interested reader is referred to Gillespie (1989) for a detailed acount of the statistical procedures and variables involved in the process of developing a model that may help in generating hypotheses for future studies.

Data from the Sheffield study of patients with tablet-treated diabetes were analysed using SPSS^X on an IBM mainframe computer. The structure of the scales was explored using a principal components factor analysis with varimax rotation. Reliability was assessed using Cronbach's (1951) alpha coefficient of internal consistency and item-total correlations. The distribution of scores for two of the measures's subscales was skewed and required non-parametric tests in analyses. Between-scale differences were therefore explored using Friedman's Chi-square test, differences between ratings for positive and negative outcomes with Wilcoxon matched pairs signed ranks tests and the relationships of the scale scores to other variables using Spearman rank correlations. The Wallstons' speculative health locus of control typology was explored in relation to HbA_1, percent ideal body weight, the Well-being measure described in Chapter 6 and the Treatment Satisfaction measure described in Chapter 7 using Kruskal-Wallis H tests. Lewis (1994) employed hierarchical multiple regression analyses in order to investigate whether multiplicative combinations of a measure of "Perceived Personal Control/Self-efficacy" (here called the Personal Control composite measure) together with some of the health belief variables could predict a greater proportion of the variance in HbA_1 six months later. These analyses are described in detail in the Chapter on health beliefs by Lewis and Bradley.

Qualitative judgements were required in item selection. Observation of the data collected in Study 5 indicated that the responses of the tablet-treated patients to one of the hypothetical events were not always related to having diabetes. The scenario in question was "Imagine that you are very thirsty and have passed unusually large amounts of urine recently". Examples of the causes given for this scenario included "Hot weather", "Steroid tablets", "Eating salty food", "Exercise", and "Taking water tablets". Lack of knowledge about the typical symptoms of diabetes and the fact that not all patients with Type 2 diabetes experience such symptoms were thought to be responsible for many of these responses. Quantitative evidence from preliminary psychometric analyses supported the view that this scenario should be excluded from the final measure.

Structure of Scale

Principal components analysis on data collected from insulin users in the first Sheffield study indicated two independent factors. One factor was characterised by internality/externality and accounted for 37% of the variance. The subscales labelled Internality, Patient Control, Foreseeability loaded highly together with the Externality and Chance subscales which loaded highly in the opposite direction. The Treatment and Doctor Control subscales loaded highly together on Factor 2 (which accounted for 22% of the variance). Subsequent studies which have used principal components analysis on different patient samples have found similar patterns of relationships between the subscales though three factors have emerged rather than two. Internality, Patient Control and Foreseeability loaded highly on Factor 1 as before but Externality and Chance loaded separately on Factor 3. Gillespie and Bradley (1988) reported such a three-factor solution with Personal Control, Medical Control and Situational control accounting for 32%, 22% and 19% of the variance respectively while Bradley *et al.* (1990) reported 35%, 22% and 15% of the variance accounted for by an identical pattern of sub-scales from the version of the questionnaire for tablet-treated patients.

Because three-factor solutions were obtained in some of the samples studied, it is recommended that the distinction between Personal Control (Internality, Patient Control and Foreseeability subscales) and Situational Control (Externality and Chance subscales) be retained in scoring the composite scales.

Reliability

Cronbach's alpha coefficients of internal consistency were measured using responses from the original Sheffield sample of insulin users for each of the seven six-item subscales and values ranged from a rather low 0.42 for the Treatment subscale to a highly satisfactory 0.68 for the Externality subscale (Bradley *et al.*, 1984). Alpha coefficients for the composite scales were not reported for the original Sheffield sample though, given the pattern of intercorrelations reported between subscales, would be expected to show improved internal consistency for the composite scales compared with the separate subscales. Gillespie and Bradley (1988) did compute the alpha coefficients for the composite scales and reported values of 0.75 for Patient Control, 0.75 for Medical Control and 0.86 for Situational Control (or External Control as this measure was labelled at that time).

Bradley *et al.* (1990) reported alpha coefficients for the separate subscales and for composite scales for the tablet-treated sample. Subscale alphas for the five-item subscales ranged from a low of 0.49 for the Treatment subscale to a high of 0.79 for the Externality subscale. Composite scale alphas were 0.81 for the Personal Control composite scale, 0.75 for the Medical Control scale and 0.79 for the Situational Control scale. Alphas for the composite scales for the three positive scenarios and for the two negative scenarios were also reported and ranged from 0.70 for Medical Control over negative outcomes to 0.91 for Situational Control over negative outcomes.

The effects on reliability of specific scenarios

Version I for insulin users: The possibility of reducing the length of the questionnaire for insulin users by dropping one or more of the scenarios has been considered. None of the scenarios can be omitted without a reduction in alpha for at least one of the seven subscales and the levels of alpha are such that a reduction would be undesirable. The least damage is done to the alpha coefficients by dropping the complications scenario "Imagine that you have successfully avoided the complications of diabetes such as problems with your feet". The reliability analyses suggested that the alphas shown in Table 4 would be obtained for the five-item subscales if the complications scenario, restoration of good control, or overweight scenarios were dropped. In the case of the complications scenario, while reliability may not be substantially reduced, content validity would be. The complication item broadens the content considerably and it's omission might be felt to narrow the content to an unacceptable degree. Content validity might be least compromised by omission of the restoration of good control scenario "Imagine that good control of your diabetes is restored after a period of poor control". Table 4 shows that several of the five-item alphas are unacceptably low. Alphas would, however, be improved if the subscales were summed into composite scales. The scenario concerned with becoming unacceptably overweight could be dropped with less damage to the alpha coefficients, though loss of this item might be felt to reduce content validity rather more than the restoration of good control item. The issue of shortening the scales is considered further in the section on short forms below.

Table 4 Alpha coefficients of internal consistency for each of the 7 subscales for all 6 scenarios in Version I for Insulin users and following exclusion of specific scenarios

Scenarios Dropped (& scenario number)	No. Items	Internality	Treatment	Externality	Chance	Patient Control	Doctor Control	Foreseeability
None	6	0.49	0.42	0.68	0.62	0.49	0.62	0.57
Restoration of good control (I/4)	5	0.37	0.26	0.64	0.55	0.35	0.55	0.47
Complications (I/5)	5	0.46	0.42	0.65	0.59	0.47	0.62	0.53
Overweight (I/6)	5	0.45	0.40	0.64	0.57	0.49	0.62	0.54

Version II for tablet-treated patients: In the data from the tablet-treated sample, only two of the thirty-five item-total correlations were less than the minimum ideal coefficient of 0.2 (Kline, 1986). One of these arose with the Treatment subscale and the scenario "Imagine that you have recently become unacceptably overweight". This reflected the most extreme instance of a general reluctance to attribute negative outcomes to Treatment while readily attributing positive outcomes to Treatment. This general reluctance could be observed in data from insulin users as well.

The second low item-total correlation (0.16) found in the tablet-treated sample's responses was on the Patient Control subscale and was obtained with the scenario "Imagine that you have successfully avoided the complications of diabetes such as problems with your feet". Mean scores indicated that patients did not generally report feeling more or less personal control over complications of diabetes than over other aspects of diabetes. However, the low item-total correlation showed that the degree of personal control patients felt they have over complications bore little relation to the degree of personal control they felt they have over other aspects of management of their diabetes. The 'avoiding complications' scenario was associated with the lowest item-total correlation for the Foreseeability subscale and for the Internality subscale although in both cases the level of these correlations was acceptable. This scenario presented no problem where the other subscales were concerned (Bradley et al., 1990). Comparable details were not reported with respect to the insulin-users data. The impression gained was that the insulin users were better informed about the likely association between diabetes control and complications than were the tablet-treated patients resulting in notably low item-total correlations for the tablet-treated patients that did not appear to arise with insulin users.

Despite the inconsistencies noted above, Bradley et al. (1990) could not identify any of the five scenarios used that could be omitted without seriously reducing the alpha coefficient of at least one of the subscales. It was recommended that all five scenarios be used.

Validity

Face and content validity

The six scenarios for the insulin users were designed by Bradley and her psychologist co-authors (Bradley et al., 1984) in consultation with physicians involved in diabetes care. The three positive and three negative scenarios were designed to be of relevance to, and commonly experienced by insulin users and pilot work indicated that the questionnaires were acceptable and could be completed quite easily by most patients. It should be noted however that this questionnaire is more complex and lengthy than other questionnaires described in this book. A small minority of patients in the main sample reported difficulty in responding to scenarios which described events which they had not experienced. For example, some patients with chronically high blood glucose levels had never experienced a hypo (the first scenario), others could not imagine being unacceptably overweight (the sixth scenario). Such patients did not complete one or more pages of the questionnaire. When adapting the questionnaire for tablet-treated patients, scenarios mentioning hypos or reactions were excluded because hypoglycaemic episodes were believed to affect relatively few of the patients. Most of the tablet-treated patients at that time monitored urine glucose rather than blood glucose and would be much less aware of fluctuations in blood glucose than their insulin-treated counterparts. Weight control was, for tablet-treated patients, a more salient concern than blood glucose control and the scenarios were modified accordingly.

The content of the questionnaires for insulin users has elicited strong feelings which were voiced by a small minority of individuals. One patient's husband telephoned to complain that the questionnaire encouraged patients to consider the possibility that something or someone other than themselves was responsible when problems arose. On another occasion when the questionnaires were given out in a group session, one young patient who was having great difficulty in managing her diabetes started weeping while completing the questionnaire. The questionnaire had brought into focus her increasing despair in feeling unable to control her diabetes. Discussions with patients suggest that feelings of responsibility and control or the lack of control are highly salient to the way patients regard their diabetes mangement.

The only problems reported concerning the acceptability of the questionnaires for tablet-treated patients, have arisen when interviewers have been employed in pilot work to administer the questionnaire by reading the items to the patients (Naji, personal communication, 1991). Under these circumstances it takes much longer to complete the questionnaire and it can seem longwinded and irritating. It is recommended that wherever possible the instructions are explained but then patients are allowed to complete the questionnaires on their own with help being offered when needed.

Construct validity

Positive vs negative outcomes: As predicted, patients were more likely to see positive outcomes as due to treatment recommended, as under their own and their doctor's control, and as more foreseeable, than negative outcomes. They were more likely to see negative outcomes as caused by other people or circumstances, and by chance. This finding has been described as a form of predictable self-serving bias (Bradley *et al.*, 1984). In subsequent work by Gamsu and Bradley (1987) diabetes health professionals were more likely to rate patients as having less personal control over positive outcomes than did patients (t = 2.94, d.f. 338; p<0.01) and rated chance as more important for positive outcomes than did patients (t = -4.32, d.f. 338, p<0.001). Staff rated negative outcomes as being more foreseeable by patients than patients did themselves (t = -3.11, d.f. 346, p<0.01). Although health professionals were just as inclined to attribute positive outcomes to Treatment and Doctor Control as were the patients, they showed less disinclination to attribute negative outcomes to medical factors. Thus they were significantly less reluctant than patients to attribute negative outcomes to Treatment (t = -8.91, d.f. 347, p<0.0001) or Doctor Control (t = -4.99, d.f. 344, p<0.0001) (Gamsu and Bradley, 1987). Gillespie has reported broadly similar patterns of differences between positive and negative outcomes rated by patients and doctor from doctor-patient dyads in real-life consultations (Gillespie, 1989, p.208). Gillespie and Bradley (1988) investigated the effects of structuring consultations to improve communication between doctor and patient about the problems to be discussed in the consultation and their attributions for those problems. Differences in composite perceived control scores between the three groups of consultations were investigated for the doctor and patients separately. The doctor's ratings of Medical Control differed significantly across groups when differences between groups in age and knowledge were controlled for using analysis of covariance. However, it was only when the composite scores for the doctor's attributions to Medical Control were split by negative and positive outcomes that the differences across groups became fully visible. In Group 1 (unstructured consultation), the self-serving bias was visible. The initially significant difference with higher ratings on Medical Control made by the doctor for positive outcomes than for negative outcomes was erased by structuring the consultations (Gillespie and Bradley, 1988).

Despite these and other interesting differences between ratings of positive and negative outcomes there were, nevertheless, positive correlations between the responses to positive outcomes and responses to negative outcomes for the seven subscales. As a result, it was considered reasonable to combine the positive and negative outcomes for the purposes of many analyses.

Relationships among the perceived control scales: In insulin-treated and tablet-treated patients, attributions for their diabetes management were more likely to be made to Personal Control than to Medical or Situational Control. Attributions to Medical Control could be seen to have been made in preference to attributions to Situational Control when subscale scores summed across positive and negative outcomes were compared (Bradley *et al.*, 1984, 1990). Patients tended to see the positive outcomes as due more to Personal Control and Medical Control than they did the negative outcomes, and this pattern of differences was highly significant in both insulin and tablet-treated patient groups. For negative outcomes, the tendency for Medical Control to be rated as more important than Situational Control was reversed and Situational Control was rated more highly than Medical Control. The difference between positive and negative outcome ratings of Situational Control was significant for the insulin users with greater weight being given to situational explanations of negative outcomes than positive outcomes. There was a similar pattern of differences for tablet-treated patients though these did not reach significance.

Relationships between the perceived control scores and knowledge of diabetes: Gillespie (1989) in his work with insulin-requiring patients, measured knowledge of diabetes using the Charing Cross Scale (Meadows *et al.*, 1988). He looked for correlations between knowledge and perceived control using the three composite perceived control variables and the total and subscale scores of the knowledge measure and found no significant relationships. This suggests that for insulin users, perceptions of control were not systematically related to knowledge of diabetes. Lewis, with her sample of tablet-treated patients who participated in a diabetes education programme also reported no significant correlations between knowledge (measured with a questionnaire designed and developed for this clinic population) and the three composite perceived control scores obtained pre-education (Lewis, 1994, p.147). However, perceived control measured after the education session was significantly associated with pre- and post-education knowledge levels (Lewis, 1994, p.145). Higher post-education Personal Control scores were associated with significantly higher levels of knowledge pre-education ($r = 0.30$, $p<0.01$) but not significantly post-education ($r = 0.13$, n.s.). Where the Medical Control and Situational Control scores were concerned, higher post-education scores were associated with lower levels of knowledge pre-education ($r = -0.32$, $p<0.01$ and $r = -0.25$, $p<0.05$ respectively) and post-education ($r = -0.32$, $p<0.01$ and $r = -0.33$, $p<0.01$ respectively). Following the one-day education session, knowledge levels increased significantly along with levels of Personal Control. Medical Control and Situational Control scores did not change significantly (see section below on sensitivity to change). The expected relationships between knowledge and the perceived control composite measures were only apparent when perceived control was measured following an education session, not before. Prior to education, there were patients who had very low levels of knowledge who may have had perceptions of control that were illusory but were tenable in the absence of feedback about diabetes control. Prior to education there may also have been patients who knew a good deal about diabetes and its complications but did not feel that the outcomes were controllable. This particular education programme served to increase both Knowledge and Personal Control and increased the association between knowledge and the three measures of perceived control.

Relationships between the Perceived Control of Diabetes Scales and other variables: Evidence for the construct validity of the Perceived Control of Diabetes Scales is available in terms of expected relationships between perceived control and other variables measured. Gillespie (1989), in his cross-sectional study of insulin-treated patients, examined the correlations between the perceived control composite measures and HbA_{1c} levels. He reported that Personal Control and Medical Control were not significantly associated with HbA_{1c}. However, the predicted association between Situational Control and HbA_{1c} levels was significant ($r = 0.40$, $p<0.01$), showing that poorer metabolic control was associated with a stronger belief in situational factors. Bradley *et al.* (1990) reported a similar association between HbA_1 and Situational Control for tablet-treated patients and also reported a predicted significant association between Personal Control and HbA_1 ($r = -0.14$, $p<0.05$). Patients scoring higher on the Personal Control scale had significantly better glycaemic control and they also had lower weight and more favourable subjective estimates of diabetes control than patients scoring low on Personal Control. High scoring patients also showed significantly better General Well-being and greater Treatment Satisfaction than did low scoring patients. High scores on Situational Control among the tablet-treated patients were, in addition to being associated with significantly poorer HbA_1 levels, also associated with poorer subjective estimates of diabetes control and less Treatment Satisfaction though relationships with the Well-being variables and percentage ideal body weight did not reach significance. Not unexpectedly there were no significant relationships between the Medical Control scale and other variables. None were predicted for this scale considered independently from the other scales. The Medical Control variable has proved useful in combination with other variables as a predictor of choice and efficacy of treatment as described in the section on predictive validity below. Predictions involving the Medical Control scale in combination with the Personal Control and Situational Control scales were made using the Wallstons' typology as a guide.

Relationships between the Wallstons' typology and other variables: Bradley *et al.* (1990) applied the Wallstons' typology to understanding individual differences in HbA_1 and percentage ideal body weight in their tablet-treated sample. "Type VI", "Yea-sayers" and "Nay-sayers" were excluded from analyses as no predictions were made about these types (see Table 1) and response bias was likely to have influenced the typing of these respondents. As predicted, "Believers in Control" (who scored high on Personal Control and Medical Control and low on Situational Control) had the best glycaemic control of the five remaining types and most closely approximated their ideal body weight (see Table 5). "Double Externals" (who scored high on Medical Control and Situational Control and low on Personal Control) fared badly in terms of both HbA_1 and weight. The ordering of the types in relation to the outcomes of HbA_1 and weight, fitted predictions very well. Believers in control had the best measures of HbA_1 and weight followed closely by those with 'Pure' Personal Control (cf. the Wallstons' "Pure Internals"). At the other extreme, the Double Externals had the worst measures of HbA_1 and, together with the "Pure Medical Control Externals" (cf. Wallstons' "Pure Powerful Others Externals"), also fared badly in terms of weight. The "Pure Situational Control Externals" did rather better than the Pure Medical Control Externals or the Double Externals in terms of weight with a mean percentage ideal body weight of 127.2 (s.d. 22.2) compared with means of 134.9 (26.5) and 133.7 (25.7) for the other two External groups respectively. The HbA_1 levels of the Pure Situational Control Externals was no worse than that obtained by the Pure Medical Control Externals and better than those of the Double Externals. Kruskal-Wallis tests for significance showed significant differences between the five types for percentage ideal body weight ($p < 0.02$) and HbA_1 levels ($p < 0.05$). When subjects' well-being scores (from the questionnaire described by Bradley in Chapter 6) were examined in relation to the Wallstons' typology, no significant differences were found between the groups. However, there were significant differences in Treatment Satisfaction ($p < 0.001$) and, as expected, the pattern of scores was similar to those found for HbA_1 and percentage ideal body weight. The most satisfied patients were the Believers in Control and Pure Personal Control patients. The least satisfied patients were the Double Externals. Inclusion of the types for which no predictions were made, clouded the picture somewhat although Kruskal Wallis tests still reached or approached significance (HbA_1: $p < 0.051$; percent ideal body weight: $p < 0.02$; Treatment Satisfaction: $p < 0.001$) indicating the robustness of the predictions made.

Table 5 Numbers of subjects, Mean, SD, and range of HbA$_1$, percentage ideal body weight, Well-being, and Treatment Satisfaction scores by the Wallstons' MHLC typology (Reproduced by permission of John Wiley & Sons Ltd from Bradley *et al.*, 1990)

	Believers in Control	Pure Internals	Pure Powerful Others Externals	Pure Chance Externals	Double Externals	Type VI	Yea-sayer	Nay-sayer
Number of subjects	19	32	16	17	23	14	14	15
HbA1*								
Mean	49.3	50.1	53.4	53.4	59.5	55.1	59.9	54.7
SD	10.4	12.2	9.8	10.6	13.6	14.6	12.8	12.8
Range	41–75	29–75	34–70	34–72	34–83	30–81	38–77	32–83
% ideal body weight								
Mean	110.3	123.3	134.9	127.2	133.7	129.6	115.2	125.9
SD	13.7	21.7	26.5	22.2	25.7	18.2	25.4	27.3
Range	83–130	90–178	94–172	101–177	92–210	102–176	80–175	79–178
General Well-being								
Mean	41.2	43.2	40.1	36.8	38.9	44.1	38.7	42.6
SD	11.0	8.1	9.4	9.1	11.7	8.3	8.5	8.5
Range	25–54	17–54	20–51	18–51	13–54	26–54	23–54	29–54
Treatment Satisfaction								
Mean	32.9	31.7	27.5	28.5	25.3	29.1	29.4	28.9
SD	3.0	4.6	7.8	6.3	6.4	6.6	5.8	5.4
Range	26–36	20–36	11–36	16–36	6–34	11–36	14–36	19–36

Higher scores indicate greater General Well-being, and Treatment Satisfaction
*The Normal reference range for HbA$_1$ is 29.0 to 39-0 mmol/HMF

Predictive validity

The most clearcut evidence of predictive validity was provided by the studies of insulin-treated patients where the scales were used to predict choice and efficacy of treatments (Bradley *et al.*, 1986, 1987). As predicted, there were significant differences in the composite variable of Medical Control between patients choosing the different treatment options (F=3.26, df 2,241, p<0.04). Tukey tests of significance indicated that patients choosing CSII pumps had significantly higher Medical Control scores than patients choosing the minimal conventional treatment (CT). Patients choosing intensified conventional treatment (ICT) had produced mean Medical Control scores that fell between the other two groups but were, as expected, closer to the CSII group than to the CT group. Personal Control scores also differed significantly between the groups (F= 4.64, df 2,236, P<0.01). Patients choosing CSII had significantly lower scores than the other two groups on the composite Personal Control variable which in this case included reversed scores from the Chance and Externality subscales as well as the Internality, Personal Control and Foreseeability subscales. Multiple regression analyses were conducted using variables for which at least two of the three treatment group means differed significantly in analysis of variance; Personal Control, Medical Control, Cost effectiveness (a measure derived by subtracting perceived Barriers to treatment from perceived Benefits of treatment as described by Lewis and Bradley in Chapter 12) and Age and successfully predicted both intensity and mode of treatment chosen. Medical Control, Cost-effectiveness and Age, all contributed significantly to the equation predicting intensity of treatment ($R^2 = 0.074$; F = 4.48; df 4, 223, p<0.01). Patients who wished to intensify their treatment were younger, more likely to attribute responsibility for and control of their diabetes to medical factors and were less satisfied that their treatment was cost-effective. In predicting mode of treatment, the Personal Control variable used was the one variable of the four which significantly contributed to the equation ($R^2 = 0.046$; F = 2.71; df 4, 223, p<0.05). Patients choosing CSII pumps perceived less personal control over their diabetes than did patients choosing injection regimens (Bradley et al., 1987).

The perceived control variables measured at the start of the study were also useful predictors of the glycosylated haemoglobin (GHb) indicator of diabetes control twelve months later. Using the same four variables together with initial levels of GHb, diabetes control following twelve months of treatment with CSII pumps was succesfully predicted by multiple regression ($R^2 = 0.38$; F = 4.14; df 5, 34, p<0.01). Initial GHb level was the major predictor but Medical Control was also a significant predictor. Those patients who had better blood glucose control to start with and who perceived Medical Control to be *less* important in determining outcomes of diabetes management were the ones for whom CSII proved most effective in terms of improved diabetes control. The CSII group as a whole showed significantly improved diabetes control. The effectiveness of ICT was significantly predicted by multiple regression but initial GHb was the only significant predictor with those who initially had better diabetes control maintaining that advantage twelve months later when the group as a whole showed improved diabetes control. The Personal Control variable together with Age were the two variables of the five used to predict efficacy of CT significantly ($R^2 = 0.37$; F = 3.88; df 5,33, p<0.01). Those patients who had lower GHb levels, indicating better diabetes control, after twelve months of the minimum CT regimen were likely to be older patients who felt less of a sense of personal control over their diabetes. GHb levels did not improve significantly in the CT group during the year.

The above findings relating to efficacy of treatment were not predicted in advance. The association of less Personal Control with better levels of GHb in patients continuing with CT was not readily understood. Bradley et al. (1987) suggested that "Since patients in this group were less likely to be monitoring their blood glucose levels, there was more scope for an illusory sense of personal control". Those few CT patients who started monitoring blood glucose levels would be more likely to achieve lower levels of GHb and less likely to retain an illusory sense of Personal Control. However, as the patients with lower GHb levels were also significantly older, it is possible that these patients may have been insulin-requiring Type 2 patients who were secreting endogenous insulin which helped in the control of their blood glucose and led to feelings of greater personal control and less of a sense of chance factors and other situational factors affecting the success of diabetes management.

The association of greater perceptions of Medical Control with worse blood glucose control using CSII pump treatment, though not anticipated in advance, was readily understandable in the context of the circumstances of patient recruitment into this particular study. The kinds of beliefs that led patients to choose CSII in the first place included greater perceived Medical Control and less perceived Personal Control over their diabetes. These were the patients that were attracted to CSII pumps by the introductory lecture from which they received the impression that CSII pumps would control their diabetes for them. They did not expect to need to take more personal control over their diabetes, though, as it turned out, the reality of CSII pumps required more rather than less active involvement of patients. This form of pump is an open-loop system which cannot detect the patient's blood glucose levels or respond to those levels on its own. The patients need to monitor their blood glucose levels and decide how much insulin to administer. The pump automatically provides a background level of insulin according to instructions pre-programmed by the doctor but the patient has to decide how much extra insulin to instruct the pump to administer prior to each meal. Furthermore, it was found during the course of the study that, because the levels of blood glucose were substantially lower in some patients when they were using CSII than had been the case with their injection regimens, ketoacidosis could occur at much lower levels of blood glucose than would have previously have given these patients any cause for concern.

Several early studies evaluating CSII pumps in the management of diabetes, reported an increased incidence of diabetic ketoacidosis (DKA) during pump use compared with injections. The Sheffield feasibility study was no exception. Eleven patients experienced episodes of DKA over a period of two years and six months while using CSII. These patients were matched for age, sex and duration of diabetes with eleven patients using CSII who had not experienced DKA. All the patients had, before starting CSII treatment, completed the Perceived Control of Diabetes Scales and the measures of health beliefs described in Chapter 12. The groups did not differ on a variety of clinical and biochemical measures including daily insulin dosage, carbohydrate intake, duration of insulin use, and GHb levels measured at the start of the study and twelve months later. The only measures to differ significantly between the groups were psychological variables and one demographic measure - age at leaving full-time education. Patients who developed DKA had significantly fewer years of education than those who did not experience DKA. One of the health belief variables "perceived vulnerability to hyperglycaemic coma" differed significantly between the groups with the DKA group perceiving greater vulnerability at the start of the study despite prior experience of DKA being similar in both groups (see Chapter 12); section on predictive validity for further comment). The most useful information was obtained from the pattern of differences seen in the seven perceived control subscales (composite scores had not been computed at this time). The pattern of results indicated that those who developed DKA had, at the start of the study, less sense of personal control over their diabetes and were more likely to attribute outcomes to medical factors. This pattern of differences was apparent across all the scales with t-tests indicating significant differences between the groups for Patient Control ($t = 2.98$, df 16, $p<0.001$) and approximating significance for Foreseeability ($t = 1.92$, df 17, $p<0.071$) and for Treatment ($t = -2.09$, df 17, $p<0.052$). It appeared that these DKA patients were looking for a medical solution to their diabetes and considered that they personally had little control over their condition. Such patients would be expected to be less likely to detect metabolic problems and to take emergency action when needed. Bradley *et al.* (1986) suggested that over-optimistic expectations of CSII pumps may have encouraged patients to assume that they would have less need to take personal responsibility for their diabetes when they changed from injection treatment to CSII, though in reality they needed to take greater care.

Sensitivity to Change

Mention has already been made (see section on positive versus negative outcomes) of changes in the doctor's ratings of perceived control which followed the introduction of structured consultations in the Gillespie and Bradley (1988) study. These findings indicate that doctors' views about who or what is the cause of diabetes management outcomes in their patients can be influenced by the patients' views. Patients frequently construed their problems very differently from the doctor or used different explanations to account for problems. When doctor and patient were encouraged to share their views and negotiate an agreed view, the doctor's view was the one which changed the most (Gillespie and Bradley, 1988; Gillespie, 1989).

There is evidence for the Perceived Control of Diabetes Scales' sensitivity to change following diabetes education in the sub-sample of Sheffield tablet-treated patients who participated in diabetes education. Lewis (1994) reported that, as predicted, the composite score of Personal Control increased significantly ($z = -2.48$; $p<0.05$) from a baseline mean (s.d.) of 70.1 (14.5) to a post-education mean (s.d.) of 74.5 (11.6). The Medical Control and Situational Control composite scores did not change significantly (Lewis, 1994, pp142–143).

Norms and Data on Specific Comparison Groups

Bradley *et al.* (1984) provided means and standard deviations for their substantial sample of insulin users showing each of the seven perceived control subscale means with all six scenarios combined and the positive and negative outcomes scored separately. It should be noted, however, that glycosylated haemoglobin measures and self-monitoring of blood glucose levels were recent innovations in

1982 when the study started. Only a small minority of patients received feedback about their blood glucose levels other than blood glucose measurements taken at infrequent clinic visits and the indirect and often misleading feedback from urine glucose testing at home. It is now rare for insulin users not to be monitoring their own blood glucose levels as a matter of course and increasingly patients treated with tablets or diet alone are using blood glucose monitoring and learning more about their diabetes and its management as a result. Thus it might be expected that perceptions of control of blood glucose-testing patients in 1994 would relate more closely to their GHb and blood glucose levels than was the case in data published in 1984 and an illusory sense of personal control would be less likely to influence behaviour now than it was in 1984. Bradley *et al.* (1987) reported means and standard deviations for the composite Personal Control score (which here included the reversed Chance and Externality subscales) and the Medical Control composite score for each of the three treatment groups using pumps or one of the two injection regimens. Bradley *et al.* (1986) provided means and standard deviations for each of the seven subscales for pump users who experienced DKA and for a matched group who did not experience DKA. Gillespie provided means and standard deviations for the small sample of the patients in the unstructured consultation group for each of the seven subscales (Gillespie, 1989, p. 208).

Means and standard deviations are available for the large sample of tablet-treated patients for each of the seven subscales, the total composite scales and the composite scales for positive and negative items scored separately (Bradley *et al.*, 1990).

Means and standard deviations for health professionals' perceived control ratings for a typical insulin-treated patient are provided by Gamsu and Bradley 1987, while Gillespie (1989, p.208) provides similar data for a single doctor rating a series of individual patients. Sowden (1992, p.79) provides means and standard deviations for health professionals' ratings of elderly tablet-treated patients.

Short Forms

The Perceived Control of Diabetes Scales involve five or six pages of questionnaire and there is a demand for a shorter form. The section on reliability, above, provides information about the consequences for reliability of excluding one of the subscales from the version of the scales for insulin users in order to reduce the questionnaire from six pages to five. An alternative strategy for shortening the questionnaire might be to cut subscales rather than scenarios. For example, the Patient Control, Doctor Control and Chance subscales might be used and summed across the six scenarios while the other four subscales are omitted from the questionnaire which might then be presented with two scenarios on each page. What cannot be recommended is the use of a single scenario which will give rise to seven scores from 0 to 6. Though it is possible that when combining these into composite scores of Personal Control, Medical Control and Situational Control, sufficient reliability and sensitivity to change will be obtained, the risk that reliability would be unacceptably reduced and the measure become insensitive to change is judged to be high.

In sum, if researchers wish to use separate subscale scores, they are advised to include all scenarios. Though it might be reasonable to omit some of the subscales, comparability with existing published data may be affected and the option of combining subscales into more reliable composite measures will be lost. If composite scores will provide sufficient information and subscale scores are not required, then one scenario may be dropped without undue loss of reliability. It is possible that two scenarios could be dropped without excessive loss of reliability to the composite scores which would include a minimum of eight items though the effects on reliability of dropping two items would need to be investigated.

Modified Scales for Completion by Health Professionals and Others

Gamsu and Bradley (1987) modified the scales for completion by health professionals. Respondents were first asked to describe a typical insulin-requiring patient in their clinic. They were then asked to complete the scales with that patient in mind. The wording of each item was changed as appropriate so that, for example, "To what extent was the cause due to something about you?" became "To what extent was the cause due to something about the patient?" The psychometric properties of the modified scales were presented by Gamsu and Bradley (1987) together with comparisons with earlier data collected from patients. Gillespie further modified the Gamsu and Bradley scales for repeated use by a doctor with reference to individual patients rather than a "typical patient" (Gillespie, 1989; Gillespie and Bradley, 1988). Sowden used the "typical patient" format but asked health professionals to consider a typical elderly patient with tablet-treated diabetes (Sowden, 1992). The Gillespie work has been considered in some detail and comparison of the results from patient and health professional has been mentioned in the section on positive versus negative outcomes. The availability of scales for health professionals has opened up opportunities for studying matches and mismatches in perceived control between patients and their health professionals. Findings to date have been illuminating. Further investigation of patient-professional mismatches and their consequences is to be encouraged together with evaluations of strategies for reducing such mismatches. Further consideration of the modified forms of the questionnaires is beyond the scope of the present chapter.

DISCUSSION

During the process of developing the perceived control scales for insulin users there were no clear signs that lack of knowledge about diabetes and its management were causing problems with any of the items or scales in the measure. However, responses to the second version of the scales for tablet-treated patients suggested that deficiences in the knowledge of diabetes of many of the patients led to inconsistencies in patient responses, necessitating the exclusion of one of the scenarios and reducing the strength of item-total correlations for some of the ratings, particularly for the scenario "Imagine that you have successfully avoided the complications of diabetes such as problems with your feet". Responses suggested that many patients had no notion of ways in which they personally could reduce the risks of developing complications and Bradley *et al.* (1990) noted that in this same sample it had previously been reported by Lewis *et al.* (1990) that 50% of patients reported having one or more problems that are thought by physicians to be complications of diabetes. Despite this, few of these patients reported having "complications of diabetes". Any lack of awareness of the possibilities of complications associated with diabetes does not seem to have undermined the measure as only the Personal Control measure was affected by inconsistent responses to the "avoiding complications" scenario; the Medical Control and Situational Control measures were unaffected. The sample of patients studied had had little in the way of education about diabetes and its management at that time. In samples of patients from clinics where a diabetes education programme is well established and effective, alpha coefficients may well be increased by more consistent responses.

Principal components analysis of the seven perceived control subscales in the various samples studied, indicated good replicability of the structure of the scales. However, whereas in the first study of insulin users a two-factor solution emerged, three-factor solutions have appeared for subsequent samples of insulin users and tablet-treated patients. In the two-factor solution, Chance and Externality loaded negatively on the same factor on which Internality, Personal Control and Foreseeability loaded positively; Treatment and Medical Control loaded on a second factor (Bradley *et al.*, 1984). In the three-factor solutions Internality, Personal Control and Foreseeability loaded on a separate factor from Externality and Chance. Treatment and Medical Control formed a separate factor as before. Whether three factors emerged or two, the factor structures were similar in their meaning. It is now recommended that three composite scores are calculated rather than two in recognition of the three-factor solution being the one which is most commonly found.

Inclusion of all seven subscales in forming the three composite scales results in highly reliable scales with a broad content domain. The subscales may also be scored separately although it should be noted that some subscales are more reliable than others and the inclusion of only a selection of the subscales at the data collection stage of a study would be to risk finding an unacceptable level of inconsistencies in responses. For those who wish to consider the possibility of excluding a scenario in the interest of brevity, information is provided about the effects of omitting certain scenarios from the insulin users' questionnaire in the section on reliability. Bradley *et al.* (1990) considered and rejected the idea of reducing the number of scenarios from five to four in the tablet-treated patients' questionnaire as this would result in unwanted restriction of the content domain, or excessive reduction of the alpha coefficients on certain scales. The lowest alpha coefficient was obtained for the Treatment subscale and was clearly due to patients' different responses to positive and negative outcomes which were most pronounced for this subscale. As Bradley *et al.* (1984) found, there was considerable reluctance among insulin-treated patients to attribute negative outcomes to Treatment and Medical Control although such attributions for positive outcomes were quite commonly made. Thus, medical factors were not held responsible for problems arising with diabetes management though credit was given to medical factors when outcomes were good.

Mean scores on each of the seven subscales showed a consistent pattern in terms of the strength of the attributions made by insulin-treated patients and by tablet-treated patients. Patients were predominantly internal in their attributions of responsibility and control. They were much more likely to attribute outcomes to themselves than to treatment recommendations and they perceived outcomes to be more under Personal than under Medical Control. Scores on the Externality and Chance subscales were low showing that patients tended to avoid attributing responsibility to other people or circumstances or to chance factors. Stronger attributions were made to Patient Control and Doctor Control when outcomes were positive than when they were negative. In the insulin users, stronger attributions to Externality and Chance for negative outcomes than for positive outcomes had been reported (Bradley *et al.*, 1984) but no such differences were found in the tablet-treated patients studied by Bradley *et al.* (1990). The tablet-treated patients rated negative outcomes as less attributable to Chance and Externality than did the earlier sample of insulin users. Bradley *et al.* (1990) viewed the earlier finding in the broader context of studies of attributions where it is commonly found that individuals tend to make stable attributions e.g. to ability, for expected outcomes while making unstable attributions e.g. to chance factors, for unexpected outcomes. The significantly greater scores on Chance for negative outcomes compared with positive outcomes found previously for insulin users suggested that these patients tended to expect their diabetes to be well controlled whereas the data from tablet-treated patients suggest that the tablet-treated patients did not have the same expectations of good control and associated positive outcomes.

Perceived control scores have proved to be good predictors of important outcomes in diabetes management. Where psychological outcomes of Well-being and Treatment Satisfaction have been measured improved outcomes have been associated with lower scores for Situational Control and/or higher scores for Personal Control (Bradley *et al.*, 1990). Greater expectations of Personal Control and lesser expectations of Situational Control have been associated with improved outcomes including improved metabolic control in tablet-treated patients (Bradley *et al.*, 1990). In insulin-treated patients, Gillespie (1989) reported comparable findings for the Situational Control variable. Furthermore, subscales associated with Personal Control were those which best distinguished between patients experiencing the serious problem of DKA and those who did not have DKA while using CSII (Bradley *et al.*, 1986). Those who had DKA had less sense of personal control over their diabetes prior to starting pump therapy. Had the pump been presented to patients less as a medical solution for controlling their blood glucose levels and more as a mode of treatment that depended for its success on the skill and care of the patient, it is likely that many of the high Medical Control, low Personal Control patients who chose the pumps in the Sheffield study (the Double Externals in the terms of the Wallstons' typology) would have opted for an injection regimen and the high Personal Control, high Medical Control "Believers in Control" would have been more readily attracted to CSII. Thus the pattern of perceived control responses that will be predictive of choice of treatment will depend on what patients understand to be the characteristics and demands of the treatment options. If predicting which patients will use CSII pumps most effectively and with least risk of DKA, we would predict that Believers in Control would fare best and the Double Externals, Pure Medical Control and Pure Situational Control patients would fare worst. Patients need accurate and appropriate information about CSII and what it can and cannot do so that they can judge whether to avoid CSII treatment or whether to increase their levels of personal involvement in managing their diabetes.

It may be that having a greater perception of Personal Control leads to improved glycaemic control, well-being and satisfaction or it may be that the causal relationships (if that is what they are) may be reversed such that better glycaemic control, well-being and/or satisfaction lead to greater feelings of Personal Control. It is quite possible that the causal arrows can go in either direction. The longitudinal studies of insulin users, where perceived control scores obtained at the start of the study predicted subsequent metabolic control and DKA, provide support for the view that different perceptions of control can cause differential changes in metabolic and psychological outcomes. The pattern of findings provides support for the commonly expressed theoretical expectations that a greater sense of personal control will be associated with improved clinical and psychological outcomes in chronic illness, at least in circumstances where opportunities for personal control exist. The pattern of findings for the Situational Control composite score provide complimentary support for what is almost the mirror image of these expectations; that perceptions of Situational Control will be associated with poorer clinical and psychological outcomes.

Perceived Medical Control over diabetes was not, on its own, associated with any of the clinical or psychological outcomes measured in the tablet-treated patients (Bradley et al., 1990) and was not found to relate to metabolic control by Gillespie (1989). This is not surprising given that management of diabetes is so dependent on the day to day decisions and actions of the patient. In combination with other variables, a belief in Medical Control has sometimes been shown to be associated with undesirable outcomes, such as higher GHb levels after twelve months in patients who chose to use CSII in the Sheffield feasibility study (Bradley et al., 1987). Only when the Perceived Control variables were used to type patients, using the framework offered by the Wallstons' typology, did the Medical Control variable combine with other variables to be associated with improved outcomes. "Believers in Control" who scored high on Medical Control while also scoring high on Personal Control and low on Situational Control were the patients with the best outcomes in terms of metabolic control, weight and treatment satisfaction in Bradley *et al.*'s (1990) study of tablet-treated patients, with "Pure Personal Control" types a close second. When high Medical Control was combined with low Personal Control, metabolic and psychological outcomes were poor whether for the "Double Externals" who also had high Situational Control or for the "Pure Medical Control" types who scored low on Situational Control as well as low on Personal Control. Where diabetes is concerned, high levels of perceived Medical Control can be dysfunctional when they are not accompanied by high levels of Personal Control. Because the pattern of scores was in line with predictions the results of the analyses relating to the Wallstons' typology provided support for the initial hypotheses and good evidence for construct validity. For three of the Wallstons' types, no predictions were made. The Wallstons had commented that Type VI individuals (scoring high on both Personal Control and Situational Control but low on Medical Control) are conceptually hard to understand and probably do not exist or are extremely rare. However, Bradley *et al.* (1990) noted that fourteen of their sample could be classified as Type VI and commented that it is a commonly observed form of self-serving bias that people more often attribute positive outcomes to internal factors while attributing negative outcomes more often to chance factors. The Wallstons' Type VI people may be those who show this self-serving tendency more strongly than most. Support for this suggestion was not sought by Bradley *et al.*, but is a hypothesis worth testing.

On the face of it, the Perceived Control of Diabetes Scales for tablet-treated patients would seem to be equally appropriate for use by diabetic individuals treated with diet alone. The Perceived Control of Diabetes Scales have been used with patients treated with diet alone by other research groups who have yet to report their findings. Researchers using the scales with patients treated with diet alone or with patients who differ in other ways, such as education received, from the populations studied to date, need to check the psychometric properties of the scales before going on to use the subscale or composite scores in subsequent analyses.

The scales are likely to prove useful in studies where researchers seek to understand individual differences between patients in their preferences for different treatments and monitoring procedures and the efficacy of those treatments and procedures. Patients' willingness to participate in a clinical trial or in routine treatment/education programmes may also be understandable in terms of information provided about the trial or programme in combination with patients' perceptions of control over their diabetes. The importance of considering psychological processes in designing and conducting clinical trials to evaluate the effects of diabetes treatment and education programmes has been discussed in detail elsewhere (Bradley, 1993).

SUMMARY

The Perceived Control scales have been shown to produce highly reliable composite scores measuring perceived Personal Control, Medical Control and Situational Control over diabetes. Versions are available for insulin-requiring and for tablet-treated patients. The structures of the two versions of the scale were comparable and, in meeting with theoretical expectations, provided evidence for construct validity. Significant and predicted associations of the Perceived Control scores with other variables, including HbA_1 levels, provided further evidence of construct validity. Use of the composite perceived control scores to apply the typology suggested by the Wallstons, proved to be a highly successful method of identifying types of tablet-treated patient who differed significantly in terms of diabetes control, weight and satisfaction with treatment. Evidence for the predictive validity of the scales was provided by studies evaluating the efficacy of different treatment options and the occurrence of diabetic ketoacidosis in CSII pump users. Sensitivity to change data included expected increases in Personal Control following an education programme for tablet-treated patients. The scales are likely to prove useful in studies where researchers seek to understand individual differences between patients in their preferences for different treatments and monitoring procedures and the efficacy of those treatments and procedures.

ACKNOWLEDGEMENTS

I acknowledge with appreciation the contributions of members of the Diabetes Research Group, particularly the work of Kathryn Lewis, Deborah Gamsu and Chris Gillespie and the contributions of other interested colleagues to the development and use of the scales reported in this chapter.

REFERENCES

Alogna, M. (1980) Perception of severity of disease and health locus of control in compliant and non-compliant diabetic patients. *Diabetes Care*, **3**, 533–534

Asher, H. B. (1983) *Causal Modelling*. London: Sage Publications

Bradley, C. (1985) Psychological aspects of diabetes. In K. G. M. M. Alberti and L. P. Krall (eds) *The Diabetes Annual/1*. Amsterdam: Elsevier Science Publishers

Bradley, C. (1989) Psychosocial influences and adjustment: Family and health care systems. In R. Larkins, P. Zimmet, and D. Chisholm (eds) *Diabetes 1988*, Amsterdam: Elsevier Science Publishers

Bradley, C. (1993) Designing medical and educational intervention studies: a review of some alternatives to conventional randomized controlled trials. *Diabetes Care*, **16**, 509–518

Bradley, C., Brewin, C. R., Gamsu, D. S. and Moses, J. L. (1984) Development of scales to measure perceived control of diabetes mellitus and diabetes-related health beliefs. *Diabetic Medicine*, **1**, 213–218

Bradley, C., Gamsu, D. S., Knight, G., Boulton, A. M. J. and Ward, J. D. (1986) Predicting risk of diabetic ketoacidosis in patients using continuous subcutaneous insulin infusion. *British Medical Journal*, **293**, 242–243

Bradley, C., Gamsu, D. S., Moses, J. L., Knight, G., Boulton, A. M. J., Drury, J. and Ward, J. D. (1987) The use of diabetes specific perceived control and health belief measures to predict treatment choice and efficacy in a feasibility study of continuous subcutaneous insulin infusion pumps. *Psychology and Health*, **1**, 133–146

Bradley, C., Lewis, K. S., Jennings. A. M., and Ward, J. D. (1990) Scales to measure perceived control developed specifically for people with tablet-treated diabetes. *Diabetic Medicine*, **7**, 685–694

Brewin, C.R. and Shapiro, D. A. (1984) Beyond locus of control: Attributions of responsibility for positive and negative outcomes. *British Journal of Psychology*, **75**, 43–49

Cronbach, L. J. (1951) Coefficient alpha and the internal structure of tests. *Psychometrika*, **16**, 297–334

Dickens, G. (1979) Treatment compliance in diabetic patients. Unpublished undergraduate project in part-fulfillment of BA in Psychology, University of Sheffield

Ferraro, L. A., Price, J. H., Desmond, S. M. and Roberts, S. M. (1987) Development of a diabetes locus of control scale. *Psychological Reports*, **61**, 763–770

Gamsu, D. S. and Bradley, C. (1987) Clinical staff's attributions about diabetes: Scale development and staff vs patient comparisons. *Current Psychological Research and Reviews*, **6**, 69–78.

Georgiou, A. and Bradley, C. (1992) The development of a smoking-specific locus of control scale. *Psychology and Health*, **6**, 227–246

Gillespie, C. R. (1989) *Psychological variables in the self-regulation of diabetes mellitus*. Unpublished Ph.D. thesis, University of Sheffield

Gillespie, C. R. and Bradley, C. (1988) Causal attributions of doctor and patients in a diabetes clinic. *British Journal of Clinical Psychology*, **27**, 67–76

Jennings, A. M., Lewis, K. S., Bradley, C., Wilson, R. M. and Ward, J. D. (1988) Symptomatic hypoglycaemia in non-insulin dependent diabetic patients treated with oral hypoglycaemic agents, (Abstract). *Diabetic Medicine*, **5** (suppl. 1), 3

Jennings, A. M., Lewis K. S., Murdoch, S., Talbot, J. F., Bradley, C. and Ward, J. D. (1991) Randomised trial comparing continuous subcutaneous insulin infusion and conventional insulin therapy in type II diabetic patients poorly controlled with sulfonylureas. *Diabetes Care*, **14**, 738–744

Kline, P. (1986) *A handbook of test construction: introduction to psychometric design*. London: Methuen

Kohlmann, C.-W., Küstner, E. and Schuler, M. (1991) *IPC-Diabetes-Fragebogen: Version 3.1 für Typ 1-Diabetiker* [IPC-Diabetes Questionnaire: Version 3.1 for Type 1 diabetes patients]. Mainz, Germany: Johannes Gutenberg-Universität, Psychologiches Institut

Kohlmann, C.-W., Schuler, M., Petrak, F., Küstner, E., Krohne, H. W. and Beyer, J. (in press) Associations between type of treatment and illness-specific locus of control in Type 1 diabetes patients. *Psychology and Health*

Levenson, H. (1972) Distinctions within the concept of internal-external control. Proceedings of the 80th Annual Convention of the APA, **7**, 261–262

Lewis, K. S. (1994) An examination of the health belief model when applied to diabetes mellitus. Unpublished Ph.D. thesis; University of Sheffield

Lewis, K. S., Jennings, A. M., Ward, J. D. and Bradley, C. (1990) Health belief scales developed specifically for people with tablet-treated type 2 diabetes. *Diabetic Medicine*, **7**, 148–155

Lowery, B. J. and DuCette, J. P. (1976) Disease related learning and disease control in diabetics as a function of locus of control. *Nursing Research*, **25**, 358–362

Meadows, K. A., Fromson, B., Gillespie, C., Brewer, A., Carter, C., Lockington, T., Clark, G. and Wise, P. H. (1988) Development, Validation and Application of Computer-linked Knowledge Questionnaires in Diabetes Education. *Diabetic Medicine*, **5**, 61–67

Peterson, C., Semel, A., Von Baeyer, C., Abramson, L. Y., Metalsky, G. I. and Seligman, M. E. P. (1982) The Attributional Style Questionnaire. *Cognitive Therapy and Research*, **6**, 287–300

Rotter, J. B. (1966) Generalised expectancies for internal versus external control of reinforcement. *Psychological Monographs*, **80**, 1–28

Sowden, A. J. (1992) Beliefs, policies and health outcomes in diabetes management: the effects of patients' age and mode of treatment. Unpublished Ph.D. thesis, University of London

Wallston, K. A. and Wallston, B. S. (1982) Who is responsible for your health? The construct of health locus of control. In G. Sanders and J Suis, (eds) *Social Psychology of Health and Illness*. New Jersey: Erlbaum. pp. 65–95

Wallston, B. S., Wallston, K. A., Kaplan, G. and Maides, S. (1976) Development and validation of the health locus of control (HLC) scale. Journal of Consulting and Clinical Psychology, **44**, 580–585

Wallston, K. A., Wallston, B. S. and De Vellis, R. (1978) Development of the multidimensional health locus of control (MHLC) scales. *Health Education Monographs*, **6**, 160–170

Weiner, B. (1979) A theory of motivation for some classroom experiences. *Journal of Educational Psychology*, **71**, 3–25

SECTION 5

MEASURES OF BEHAVIOUR
AND COMPOSITE MEASURES

## CHAPTER 14

SOCIAL-ENVIRONMENTAL FACTORS IN DIABETES: BARRIERS TO DIABETES SELF-CARE

RUSSELL E. GLASGOW

Oregon Research Institute, 1899 Willamette Street, Eugene, Oregon, 97401 USA

INTRODUCTION

This chapter has two purposes. The first is briefly to make a case for the importance of social-environmental factors in diabetes, to overview areas in which such work has been conducted, and to outline additional social-environmental research that is needed. The second purpose is to provide an example of this type of research by describing in detail the Barriers to (Diabetes) Self-Care Scale that our research team has developed.

There has been a great deal of research on patient characteristics associated with patient functioning and diabetes outcomes. In particular, psychologists have been active in studying and developing instruments to assess diabetes-related knowledge, beliefs, and attitudes as discussed in other chapters in this book. Medical researchers have investigated a number of biological factors potentially related to diabetes complications and mortality. However, there has been little diabetes-related research on another important set of factors – the social environment in which the patient lives and copes with his or her diabetes (Glasgow & Osteen, 1992). Increased attention to the social context in which patients find themselves could greatly enhance our understanding and prediction of diabetes outcomes. There are at least four important social-environmental influences on patients, which have received varying degrees of attention. The first factor– (1) barriers to diabetes self-care – is the focus of this chapter. Resources to combat self-care barriers come from one or more of the remaining three social-environmental influences: (2) social support from family or peers, (3) interactions with one's health care providers, or (4) community resources and services. Each of these three will be discussed briefly before returning to a more complete discussion of the concept of barriers to self-care and research on this construct.

Social support from family members has been fairly well studied for adolescents with Type 1 diabetes. In general, perceived social support and higher levels of family cohesion are associated with better adherence and glycaemic control (Anderson, 1990; Hanson *et al.*, 1987; Hauser *et al.*, 1990). It also appears that social support may be more related to behaviour change and to outcomes such as weight loss for women than for men (Kaplan and Hartwell, 1987). There has been substantially less research on the role of social support on the functioning of adults with diabetes. Preliminary data, however, indicate that diabetes-specific measures of family support are stronger predictors of diabetes self-care than are more global measures of family functioning, and that positive, supportive family behaviours and negative, nonsupportive behaviours are fairly separate dimensions (Glasgow and Toobert, 1988). Support from non-family members of one's social network has seldom been investigated (Cox and Gonder-Frederick, 1992).

Health care providers are an important source of information and support for overcoming barriers to diabetes self-care, but have been much less studied than family members. The few studies of diabetes patient-provider interactions that have been conducted suggest that the level of patient participation in such interactions is related to self-care (Rost, 1989) and to improvements in glycaemic control and patient functioning (Greenfield et al., 1988). Much more research needs to be conducted in this area. In particular, interactions with different types of health care professionals need to be investigated, including those with nurses and diabetes educators, who often have more direct contact with patients than do physicians.

The level of community resources provided to support recommended diabetes self-care behaviours has received the least attention. Although community-level factors may seem less proximal than family or health care provider interactions, in the long term they may prove equally important. In particular, the accessibility of low-cost or free programmes to reinforce recommended lifestyle changes will be likely to influence the number of patients able to maintain such changes. Programmes to reduce cardiovascular and cancer risks have concluded that it is necessary to change community norms and support to produce lifestyle changes (Farquhar et al., 1990; COMMIT Research Group, 1991). For example, consider the situation of older Type 2 patients recommended to stop smoking, reduce their fat intake, and/or exercise more regularly. Patients living in communities having diabetes support groups, many smoke-free restaurants and public meeting places, an active senior citizens' centre with free recreation facilities, well-maintained and safe walking/jogging paths, and low-cost nutrition education programmes are more likely to be successful at adopting and maintaining such lifestyle changes than are patients who live in communities without such support.

The Concept of Barriers to Self-Care

Support for diabetes self-management from the multiple sources described above is necessary because of the pervasiveness of barriers to self-care or adherence (see the chapter in this volume by Toobert and Glasgow for a discussion of these terms). Barriers to self-care are assessed from the perspective of the patient and include such factors as the cost, time, social pressures, and competing demands and thoughts associated with attempting to follow closely one's recommended regimen.

Diabetes regimens are multifaceted, and each of the several components of the regimen can have its own set of barriers. One of the issues explored later in the chapter is the relationship among barriers to different aspects of the regimen.

The concept of barriers to adherence is part of several theoretical approaches to health behaviour, including both the health belief model (Hess *et al.*, 1986), and social learning conceptualisations of diabetes (Glasgow and McCaul, 1982).

Early work by other research groups on barriers to adherence is briefly reviewed below before turning to a discussion of our barriers instrument. Jenny (1986), using a scale developed for that study, reported the greatest number of barriers to diet and exercise components of the regimen, and the fewest to medication taking, a finding to which we will return later. Hess *et al.* (1986) developed a fourteen-item subscale of their Diabetes Care Profile to assess barriers to adherence. They report a Cronbach's alpha of .69 for the scale, which was inversely related to reports of extent to which subjects followed their meal plan ($r = -.29$, $p < .01$) and positively but quite modestly related to glycosylated haemoglobin level ($r = .14$, $p < .01$). In a related study, Davis *et al.*, (1987) found that the barriers scale of the Diabetes Care Profile was positively correlated with percent of ideal weight for non-insulin-taking NIDDM subjects, but not for subjects taking insulin. In this study, barriers were not related to glycosylated haemoglobin or to hospital admissions. Connell *et al.* (1988), using the same scale, found this barriers measure to be related to concurrently reported regimen adherence in bivariate analyses ($r = -.24$, $p < .05$) but not in multivariate analyses which controlled for the influence of other psychosocial factors.

THE BARRIERS TO SELF-CARE SCALE

The purpose of our Barriers to Self-Care Scale is to identify environmental and cognitive factors that interfere with one or more aspects of diabetes self-care. Our goal was to develop a relatively brief instrument that would assess the patient's perspective on obstacles to several aspects of the diabetes regimen. Over the years, we have used two different versions of the Barriers to Self-Care Scale. Below, I describe the current version of the scale, followed by a discussion of research on both the original fifteen-item scale for insulin users, and on the current longer and more broadly applicable scale.

CURRENT BARRIERS TO SELF-CARE SCALE

Design

The present version of the scale is a thirty one-item self-report instrument that asks subjects to rate how frequently they experience various barriers to self-care (see Figure 1). It was designed to be applicable to adults with non-insulin dependent diabetes and should also be applicable to adults with IDDM, although we do not have data from IDDM patients on this version.

Figure 1 Diabetes Self-Care Education Programme Problem Situations Checklist

Listed below are a number of things that can sometimes make it more difficult to follow one's self-care routine. For each one, please indicate *how often* that situation generally occurs for you, using the scale below. If the particular self-care behaviour does not apply to you (for example, if it asks about medication and you don't take diabetes medication), circle the "0" in the "Does Not Apply To Me" column.

How often do each of the following happen to you?	1 Very rarely or never	2 Once per month	3 Twice per month	4 Once per week	5 Twice per week	6 More than twice weekly	7 Daily	0 Does not apply to me
1. I am not at home and it is time to test my blood glucose level	1	2	3	4	5	6	7	0 I don't test
2. I am not at home when it is time to take my diabetes medication (oral medication or insulin)	1	2	3	4	5	6	7	0 I don't take
3. I am not in a convenient location when it is time to exercise	1	2	3	4	5	6	7	
4. I am at a restaurant or someone else's house at meal times	1	2	3	4	5	6	7	
5. The weather is bad when I would like to exercise	1	2	3	4	5	6	7	
6. I am unsure about the amount of one or more food items I consume	1	2	3	4	5	6	7	
7. I'll say to myself that it won't matter if I don't exercise	1	2	3	4	5	6	7	
8. I'll say to myself that it won't matter if I don't take my diabetes medication	1	2	3	4	5	6	7	
9. I'll say to myself that it won't matter if I don't follow my diet	1	2	3	4	5	6	7	
10. I'll say to myself that it won't matter if I don't check my glucose level	1	2	3	4	5	6	7	

How often do each of the following happen to you?

	1 Very rarely or never	2 Once per month	3 Twice per month	4 Once per week	5 Twice per week	6 More than twice weekly	7 Daily	0 Does not apply to me
11. I am extremely busy	1	2	3	4	5	6	7	
12. I don't have the necessary materials or equipment with me when it is time to take my diabetes medication	1	2	3	4	5	6	7	0 I don't take medication
13. I don't have the necessary materials or equipment with me when it is time to exercise	1	2	3	4	5	6	7	
14. I don't have the necessary materials or equipment with me when it is time to test my glucose level	1	2	3	4	5	6	7	0 I don't test glucose
15. I still feel hungry after finishing a meal	1	2	3	4	5	6	7	
16. I feel sore and stiff	1	2	3	4	5	6	7	
17. I think about how much time it takes to prepare foods the way I should	1	2	3	4	5	6	7	
18. I think about how much time it takes to take my diabetes medication	1	2	3	4	5	6	7	0 I don't take medication
19. I think about how much time it takes to test my glucose level	1	2	3	4	5	6	7	0 I don't test glucose
20. I think about how much time it takes to exercise	1	2	3	4	5	6	7	
21. I have visitors staying with me	1	2	3	4	5	6	7	

How often do each of the following happen to you?

	1 Very rarely or never	2 Once per month	3 Twice per month	4 Once per week	5 Twice per week	6 More than twice weekly	7 Daily	0 Does not apply to me
22. I am still in bed when it is time to take my medication	1	2	3	4	5	6	7	0 I don't take medication
23. I am still in bed when it is time to test my glucose level	1	2	3	4	5	6	7	0 I don't test glucose
24. I feel awkward with other people around when it is time to test my glucose	1	2	3	4	5	6	7	0 I don't test glucose
25. I feel awkward with other people around when it is time to take my medication	1	2	3	4	5	6	7	0 I don't take medication
26. I don't feel well	1	2	3	4	5	6	7	
27. I am around other people who are eating or drinking things I shouldn't	1	2	3	4	5	6	7	
28. I think about the cost of my diabetes medication	1	2	3	4	5	6	7	0 I don't take medication
29. I think about the cost of materials for testing my blood glucose levels	1	2	3	4	5	6	7	I don't test glucose
30. I think about the cost of necessary equipment or fees for exercise.	1	2	3	4	5	6	7	
31. I think about the cost of the the recommended foods to eat according to my meal plan	1	2	3	4	5	6	7	

Scoring

The scale produces an overall barriers score, a modified overall score for patients not on medication for their diabetes, and four subscales for barriers to the regimen areas of glucose testing, diet, exercise, and medication taking.

Both the overall barriers score and the four regimen-specific subscales are calculated by averaging responses across the relevant items. The Dietary Subscale consists of items 4, 6, 9, 15, 17, 27, and 31; the Exercise Subscale consists of items 3, 5, 7, 13, 16, 20, and 30; the Glucose Testing Subscale consists of items 1, 10, 14, 19, 23, 24, and 29; and the Medication Subscale consists of items 2, 8, 12, 18, 22, 25, and 28 (see Figure 1). Thus there are seven regimen-specific items for each regimen area and three general barriers items (#11 – extremely busy; #21 - visitors; and #26 – not feeling well). The overall score is obtained by averaging scores across all thirty one items.

For subjects not prescribed diabetes medication, the overall score is calculated by averaging all items except the seven medication barriers items.

Scale Development

The original barriers scale was developed for use with Type 1 patients aged twelve to sixty five. To obtain a patient perspective and to enhance content validity, procedures from the Behaviour Analytic Model (Goldfried & D'Zurilla, 1969) were employed to construct the questionnaire. The initial item pool was generated by six Type 1 patients and two nurse educators specialising in diabetes who were asked to list as many things as possible that made it difficult to adhere to a Type 1 regimen.

After eliminating redundancies, thirty six unique items were mailed to participants who were asked to rate both the frequency and severity of each problem situation. Following deletion of items that were both infrequent *and* not rated as problematic, and rewording of additional items to remove ambiguities, a fifteen-item scale was created that included at least three items from each of the four regimen areas of diet, exercise, glucose testing and insulin administration. Because of the high intercorrelation between frequency and severity scores, the more straightforward frequency scores have been used in subsequent work.

This scale was then evaluated with sixty five Type 1 patients, twenty seven males and thirty eight females (Glasgow *et al.*, 1986). Mean frequency ratings of barriers varied across different aspects of the regimen. Barriers were reported most frequently to diet and exercise components of the regimen, and least often to insulin administration. Six-month test-retest reliabilities were moderate to good for three of the subscales ($r = .56 - .67$), but low for insulin barriers ($r = .36$). The overall barriers score was more stable ($r = .71$), as would be expected, given the larger number of items.

Both the regimen-specific subscores and the overall score from the original barriers scale significantly predicted regimen adherence in concurrent and six month prospective analyses. In general, glucose testing and exercise adherence were most consistently predicted, with most correlations being in the -.2 to -.3 range (more frequent barriers predicting lower levels of adherence). On more "objective" adherence measures (e.g. self-monitoring logs) the specific barriers subscores for exercise and glucose testing produced stronger correlations than did the overall barriers score (e.g. for glucose testing adherence, the glucose testing barriers subscore correlated $r = -.30$, $p < .005$ with adherence six months later compared to $r = -.15$ (ns) for the overall barriers score). This pattern was not observed on the self-reported adherence measures, on which the overall and regimen-specific scores performed equivalently.

Overall, we felt that results of the initial development work were promising, but that the Barriers to Self-Care Scale would benefit from revision. In particular, we wanted to modify the scale to make it more applicable to persons with Type 2 diabetes (who might or might not take insulin or oral hypoglycaemic agents) and to older adults. We also felt that adding a modest number of items might increase the reliability of the regimen-specific barriers subscores, which performed surprisingly well in the developmental study.

Subject Samples and Procedure

The current version of the scale has been used in two studies (Glasgow *et al.*, 1989, 1989a). The first study was a prospective assessment study of 127 Type 2 patients, and the second an intervention study in which 78 Type 2 subjects were randomized to one of three intervention conditions. The characteristics of subjects in these two studies were similar, and are summarized in Table 1.

Table 1 Characteristics of subjects in Barriers to Self-Care Scale validation studies

Subject Characteristics	Study A	Study B
Average Age	60.8 (40-88)	59.3 (42-75)
Percent Female	66.9%	73.0%
Mean % of Ideal Weight	147.0%	153.0%
Duration of Diabetes	9.1 yr (1-33 yr)	9.3 yr (1-30 yr)
Diabetes Medication:		
Percent on:		
Insulin	30%	39%
Oral Medication	45%	42%
Diet Only	25%	19%

Study A = Assessment Study (Glasgow *et al.*, 1989a)
Study B = Treatment Study (Glasgow *et al.*, 1989)

As can be seen, these patients are fairly representative of middle aged and older Type 2 patients. Over two-thirds were female and most were considerably over-weight (average of 150% of ideal weight). Most had had diabetes for several years (mean of over nine years). Almost half of the sample were on oral agents, another third on insulin, and approximately 20% to 25% were not prescribed diabetes medication.

Descriptive Data

As can be seen in Table 2, there is consistency across the studies in the reported frequency of barriers to different components of the regimen. Both of the studies tabled here, as well as the original barriers questionnaire study, the Jenny (1986) investigation, and the Connell *et al.* (1988) study, reported barriers to dietary self-care occurring most frequently, followed by exercise barriers. Glucose testing barriers are somewhat less frequent, and barriers to medication-taking are reported least often.

Table 2 Psychometric characteristics of current barriers summary scores

Summary Score/Study	# Items	Mean	Standard Deviation	Alpha	Test-Retest Reliability
Overall Score: A	31	2.48	0.90	.86	.74[1]
Overall Score: B	31	2.46	0.87	.84	.58[2]
Dietary Subscore: A	7	2.89	1.18	.55	.68[1]
Dietary Subscore: B	7	3.10	1.26	.63	.56[2]
Exercise Subscore: A	7	2.54	1.23	.66	.58[1]
Exercise Subscore: B	7	2.58	1.15	.59	.47[2]
Glucose Testing Subscore: A	7	1.89	0.91	.61	.49[1]
Glucose Testing Subscore: B	7	1.78	0.73	.39	.32[2]
Medication Subscore: A	7	1.55	0.70	.56	.42[1]
Medication Subscore: B	7	1.53	0.62	.40	.34[2]

A = Assessment Study (Glasgow *et al.*, 1989a)

B = Treatment Study (Glasgow *et al.*, 1989)

[1] Over a 6-month interval

[2] Over a 3-month interval

Reliability

Internal consistency

Table 2 also presents the psychometric characteristics of the current barriers instrument for the two studies. As would be expected from psychometric theory, the full scale, which has a considerably larger number of items (thirty one) than the subscales (seven items each), produces higher estimates of internal consistency. The relatively strong Cronbach's alphas (see the fourth column of Table 2) found in both studies for the overall scale suggest that it is appropriate to conceptualise a general barriers factor. Stated differently, there is consistency across the regimen areas in the extent to which patients experience barriers. Intercorrelations among the subscale scores ranged from $r = .39$ to .72. In general, the larger assessment study produced higher coefficient alphas.

Test-retest reliability

Barriers scores are moderately stable over time, as illustrated in the right-hand column of Table 2. However, the six-month test-retest reliabilities are generally not any higher than those previously reported for the original fifteen-item scale. For reasons which are not entirely clear, test-retest reliabilities tended to be somewhat higher in the study with the longer test-retest interval (six months vs. three months). Given the potential seasonal effects on barriers (e.g. food choices and pressures around holidays, recreational opportunities and obstacles in winter vs. summer), the stability coefficients observed are viewed as moderately strong. Subjects in both studies were assessed throughout the year in roughly equal proportions, thus seasonal effects do not explain why the longer study had better test-retest results. Across studies, the overall barriers score was the most stable, followed by diet and exercise subscores. The glucose testing and medication subscores appear less stable.

Construct Validity: Prediction of Self-Management

The usefulness of the current Barriers to Self-Care Scale in predicting self-management has been most thoroughly evaluated as part of the larger Glasgow *et al.* (1989a) assessment study. Table 3 presents previously unpublished data from this study showing the relationship of scores from the barriers instrument to several different diabetes self-management measures. As can be seen in the top left-hand portion of Table 3, barriers scores were related to concurrently collected self-report measures of dietary and exercise self-management from the Summary of Diabetes Self-Care instrument discussed in the chapter by Toobert and Glasgow in this volume. As can be seen, the regimen-specific dietary or exercise barriers subscale was the best predictor of these respective behaviours, although the overall barriers scale did almost as well. In contrast, the glucose testing barriers score

Table 3 Significant correlations between barriers scales and both self-report and more objective self-management measures

I. Construct Validity: Concurrent Correlations

Barriers Scale	Self-Report Measures			Self-Monitoring/Food Record Measures			
	Diet	Exercise	Glucose Testing	Calories	Fats	Exercise	Glucose Testing
Overall Scale	−.33**	−.25*	—	.29**	.23*	−.26**	.21*
Diet Subscale	−.34**	−.21**	—	.22*	—	−.18*	—
Exercise Subscale	−.26**	−.29**	—	—	—	−.30**	.23*
Glucose Testing Subscale	—	—	—	—	—	—	.28**

II. Predictive Validity: 6-Month Prospective Correlations

Barriers Scale	Self-Report Measures			Self-Monitoring/Food Record Measures			
	Diet	Exercise	Glucose Testing	Calories	Fats	Exercise	Glucose Testing
Overall Scale	−.34**	−.22*	—	.36**	.22*	—	.21*
Diet Subscale	−.26**	−.19*	—	—	—	—	—
Exercise Subscale	−.30**	−.24*	—	.22*	—	—	.25*
Glucose Testing Subscale	—	—	—	.30**	—	—	.23*

$*p < .05$
$**p < .01$
— indicates a nonsignificant correlation

did not predict reported testing frequency. We did not have enough subjects on the same type of diabetes medication to evaluate that barriers subscale.

The four right-hand columns in the top of Table 3 present self-management measures using alternatives to self-report, such as self-monitoring and food records. These results show that the earlier relationships observed between barriers and dietary and exercise behaviours were not due just to shared method variance. In predicting these more 'objective" measures of self-management, the overall barriers scale did as well as or better than the more specific barriers sub-scales. With the exception of the glucose testing self-monitoring measure, on which counter-intuitive results were obtained, these correlations were all in the ex-pected direction (e.g. more barriers associated with less exercise or higher levels of fat consumption).

Correlations between barriers to self-care and glycosylated haemoglobin levels were also conducted. There were no significant correlations in either study be-tween barriers measures and HbA_1. This should not be surprising because some people who encounter barriers will overcome them and others will not.

Predictive Validity

The bottom half of Table 3 presents prospective correlations, predicting self-management behaviours at a six-month follow-up assessment from baseline barri-ers scores. In general, the overall barriers score was the best predictor of both self-reported and more objective dietary adherence measures, as well as of self-reported exercise. Significant relationships were not observed with the more "objective" measure of self-monitored exercise, and once again we obtained the counter-intuitive result of more barriers predicting higher levels of self-moni-tored (but not self-reported) glucose testing.

In summary, both the regimen-specific and the overall barriers scores are mod-erately predictive of dietary and exercise behaviours. Much less consistent and even counter-intuitive relationships are observed for glucose testing. Other stud-ies are needed to examine the predictive validity of medication taking barriers. Given this pattern of results, it would seem parsimonious to use the more reliable overall Barriers to Self-Care Scale score in future applications. Alternative ap-proaches, where applicable, might be to develop considerably longer subscales of barriers to specific aspects of the regimen, as discussed later.

An additional, albeit indirect, indicator of validity is that the rank ordering of frequency of barriers across the different regimen areas (see Table 2) corresponds exactly with the extent to which subjects in other studies have reported difficulty adhering to these different regimen areas (Ary et al., 1986; Orme and Binik, 1989).

Related Research and Future Uses of the Barriers Scale

Recent research has focused on expanding the barriers concept to focus in more detail on particular regimen areas. Irvine et al. (1990) have reported an expanded Environmental Barriers to Adherence Scale (EBAS). This sixty-item scale, as implied by its title, restricts its focus to environmental barriers such as sit-uational factors and has from thirteen to eighteen items for each of the diet, exercise, glucose testing, and medication subscales. The overall scale correlated .63 with our original Barriers to Self-Care Scale, but appears to have somewhat stronger psychometric characteristics (e.g. six-week test-retest of .80, alpha of .94) than our scale. These enhanced reliability scores may be primarily a function of increased scale length (sixty vs. thirty one items), since coefficient alpha is affected by number of items as well as degree of association among items.

Both the overall EBAS barriers score and subscores correlated in predicted directions (rs ranged from .35 to .52) with concurrent self-reports of adherence in all four regimen areas. A change in the response format for the EBAS may be partially responsible for this result. Subjects are asked to rate the extent to which each of the sixty items keeps them from performing their regimen activities (e.g. exercising, eating) as they think they should. Respondents answer using a scale of "never" to "always". This response format seems to blur the distinction between barriers and adherence. The EBAS still appears to be a promising measure, however, and is recommended in cases where its length is not problematic.

Jones (1992, personal communication) has recently developed an eighty three-item questionnaire to assess barriers to glucose testing that is currently being evaluated. Unlike the EBAS, this scale focuses heavily on thoughts and feelings that patients have that may interfere with glucose testing.

Our own current work with the Barriers to Self-Care Scale involves both elaborating and simplifying the current scale to make it more clinically useful to patients and health-care providers. The overall goal is to develop an instrument that can be quickly scored and provide feedback to both parties within the context of a typical office visit. The approach we are taking involves identifying a single regimen area on which to focus until the next visit. Once the patient and health care provider agree upon an intervention target, the relevant regimen-area-specific barriers subscale (e.g. exercise barriers) is administered. We are piloting this assessment using an interactive computer-administered format that automatically scores the instrument and provides a one-page summary feedback sheet to the patient and provider. This print-out summarises both the general types of barriers the patient reports most often (e.g. eating away from home), as well as the specific events or obstacles reported as occurring most frequently. It is hoped that such immediate, personalised feedback will allow the patient and health care team to develop specific plans for overcoming the barriers identified.

An unresolved issue in the assessment of Barriers to Self-Care concerns the response format. In the past we have used both frequency of occurrence and difficulty rating scales. Others such as Irvine et al. (1990) and Hess et al. (1986) have used responses asking how often patients have not followed their regimen because of specific barriers. This type of question seems to demand much more complex judgements from patients. They are required to assess both how often they did not comply (thus blurring the distinction between barriers and adherence) and to attribute the extent to which this noncompliance was due to a particular barrier.

This assessment approach also seems to assume that if something doesn't actually prevent adherence, then it is not a barrier. However, patients may exert considerable effort and resources, and experience substantial discomfort or inconvenience to overcome barriers. This information is important from a quality of life perspective and for answering such questions as, 'How can we make treatment regimens more acceptable for patients?" It is not clear how patients actually make barrier ratings or if they are sensitive to differences in response options, but future research on such issues is clearly indicated.

A second question concerning response options pertains to the time frame that is assessed. Previous work has always asked about past barriers, most often asking in general or "over the past several months". If the goal is to predict and/or prepare patients for future adherence difficulties, it may enhance predictability to ask for estimates of future barriers, as is done with self-efficacy ratings, rather than have patients report on the past.

Future work should combine assessment of barriers with evaluations of support and coping or problem-solving skills. Conceptually, barriers by themselves should not be expected strongly to predict future adherence or self-management. Knowledge of patient coping skills and of family, health care provider, and community support to overcome such barriers are also required to complete the picture. Finally, all research to date has been on barriers as an assessment procedure. The usefulness of barriers as part of an intervention package to prepare patients to cope with obstacles to self-management is an important area that needs to be addressed in future research.

SUMMARY

The Barriers to Self-Care Scale measures the frequency of both environmental (e.g. time, competing demands, social pressure) and cognitive factors that interfere with diabetes self-management. The current scale has been validated on adults with Type 2 diabetes. We believe that the scale is also applicable to adults with Type 1 diabetes, but psychometric properties have not been established for this population (users are encouraged to do so). The barriers scale appears most helpful in identifying factors that interfere with the lifestyle behaviour changes of dietary and exercise adherence. It does not seem to predict glucose testing, and the medication taking scale items have not been thoroughly evaluated. At the present time, the overall barriers score is the most reliable score to use. Persons interested in more regimen-specific barriers may want to use the longer Environmental Barriers to Ahderence Scale (Irvine et al., 1990). Additional research, combining scores from the Barriers to Self-Care Scale with information on coping skills and support for diabetes self-management is indicated.

REFERENCES

Anderson, B.J. (1990) Diabetes and adaptation in family systems. In C.S. Holmes (ed.), *Neuropsychological and behavioral aspects of diabetes.* P. 85–101. New York: Springer-Verlag

Ary, D.V., Toobert, D.J., Wilson, W. and Glasgow, R.E. (1986) A patient perspective on factors contributing to nonadherence to diabetes regimens. *Diabetes Care,* **9,** 168–172

COMMIT Research Group. (1991) Community intervention trial for smoking cessation (COMMIT): Summary of design and intervention. *Journal of the National Cancer Institute,* **83,** 1620–1628

Connell, C.M., O'Sullivan, J.J., Fisher, E.B. and Storandt, M. (1988) Variables predicting adherence and metabolic control among retirement community residents with non-insulin dependent diabetes mellitus. *Journal of Compliance in Health Care*, **3**, 135–149

Cox, D.J. and Gonder-Frederick, L. (1992) Major developments in behavioral diabetes research. *Journal of Consulting and Clinical Psychology*, **60**, 628–638

Davis, W.K., Hess, G.E., Van Harrison, R. and Hiss, R.G. (1987) Psychosocial adjustment to and control of diabetes mellitus: Differences by disease type and treatment. *Health Psychology*, **6**, 1–14

Farquhar, J.W., Fortmann, S.P., Fiora, J.A., Taylor, C.B., Haskel, W.L., Williams, P.T., Maccoby, N. and Wood, P.D. (1990) Effects of communitywide education on cardiovascular disease risk factors, *Journal of the American Medical Association*, **264**, 359–365

Glasgow, R.E. and McCaul, K.D. (1982) Psychological issues in diabetes: A different approach. *Diabetes Care*, **5**, 645–646

Glasgow, R.E., McCaul, K.D. and Schafer, L.C. (1986) Barriers to regimen adherence among persons with insulin-dependent diabetes. *Journal of Behavioral Medicine*, **9**, 65–77

Glasgow, R. E. and Osteen, V. L. (1992) Evaluating diabetes education: Are we measuring the most important outcomes? *Diabetes Care*, **15**, 1423–1432

Glasgow, R.E., Toobert, D.J., Mitchell, D.L., Donnelly, J. and Calder, D. (1989) Nutrition education and social learning intervention for Type II diabetes. *Diabetes Care*, **12**, 150–152

Glasgow, R.E., Toobert, D.J., Riddle, M., Donnelly, J, Mitchell, D.L. and Calder, D. (1989a) Diabetes-specific social learning variables and self-care behaviors among persons with Type II diabetes. *Health Psychology*, **8**, 285–303

Glasgow, R.E. and Toobert, D.J. (1988) Social environment and regimen adherence among Type II diabetic patients. *Diabetes Care*, **11**, 377–386

Goldfried, M.R. and D'Zurilla, T.J. (1969) A behavioral-analytic model for assessing competence. In C.D. Speilberger (ed.), *Current Topics in Clinical and Community Psychology*, **1**. New York: Academic Press

Greenfield, S., Kaplan, S.H., Ware, J.E., Yano, E.M. and Frank, H. (1988) Patients' participation in medical care: Effects on blood sugar control and quality of life in diabetes. *Journal of General Internal Medicine*, **3**, 448–457

Hanson, C.L., Henggeler, S.W. and Burghern, G.A. (1987) Model of associations between psychosocial variables and health-outcome measures of adolescents with IDDM. *Diabetes Care*, **10**, 752–758

Hauser, S.T., Jacobson, A.M., Lavori, P., Wolfsdorf, J.I., Herskowitz, R.D., Milley, J.E., and Bliss, R. (1990) Adherence among children and adolescents with insulin-dependent diabetes mellitus over a four-year longitudinal follow-up: II. Immediate and long-term linkages with the family milieu. *Journal of Pediatric Psychology*, **15**, 527–542

Hess, G.E., Davis, W.K. and Van Harrison, R. (1986) A diabetes psychosocial profile. *Diabetes Educator*, **12**, 135–140

Irvine, A.A., Saunders, J.T., Blank, M. and Carter, W. (1990) Validation of scale measuring environmental barriers to diabetes regimen adherence. *Diabetes Care*, **13**, 705–711

Jenny, J.L. (1986) Differences in adaptation to diabetes between insulin-dependent and non-insulin-dependent patients: Implications for patient education. *Patient Education and Counseling*, **8**, 39–50

Kaplan, R.M. and Hartwell, S.L. (1987) Differential effects of social support and social network on physiological and social outcomes in men and women with Type II diabetes mellitus. *Health Psychology*, **6**, 387–398

Orme, C.M. and Binik, Y.M. (1989) Consistency of adherence across regimen demands. *Health Psychology*, **8**, 27–43

Rost, K. (1989) The influence of patient participation on satisfaction and compliance. *Diabetes Educator*, **15**, 139–143

CHAPTER 15

ASSESSING DIABETES SELF-MANAGEMENT: THE SUMMARY OF DIABETES SELF-CARE ACTIVITIES QUESTIONNAIRE

DEBORAH J. TOOBERT and RUSSELL E. GLASGOW

Oregon Research Institute, 1899 Willamette Street, Eugene, Oregon 97401, USA

INTRODUCTION

Problems with the Assessment of Adherence and Level of Self-Care

Diabetes self-management is of concern because of the assumption that adoption of a healthy lifestyle will produce better metabolic control of diabetes, which in turn will aid in the avoidance of subsequent acute and long-term complications of the disease. Many studies have investigated the links between diabetes self-care and level of diabetes control as well as psychosocial factors which may be predictive of self-care (see reviews by Goodall and Halford, 1991; Glasgow, 1991; Anderson, 1990). However, without adequate means to assess self-care, these relationships may be obscured.

The absence of reliable, valid and unbiased indices to assess level of self-care among individuals with diabetes has other implications for researchers and practitioners alike. It makes it difficult to determine if estimates of self-care vary as a function of actual behaviour or if they are an artifact of the measurement procedure. Without means to determine accurately the frequency or consistency of regimen behaviours it is difficult to formulate self-care improvement strategies. The lack of standard methods for assessing compliance makes it difficult to evaluate compliance to various regimen tasks or to compare the results of different studies aimed at improving adherence.

There are a great many complexities in developing tools to measure adherence and/or self-care behaviour. Glasgow *et al.* (1985) described several problems in conducting research in the diabetes area related to adherence measurement. One central problem concerned the difficulty of measuring the extent to which individuals with diabetes follow their regimen prescriptions. In measuring compliance to a treatment regimen, the critical factor is the comparison of actual behaviour to a known standard. This can be problematic because patients may never have been given a prescription (e.g. exercise) or if they have, it may be nonspecific (e.g. "get some exercise"). Often, measures used to assess adherence (e.g. percent of calories from saturated fat) and the regimen instructions differ (e.g. cut down on red meat). There is an increasing trend to have patients take an active role in regulating their treatment. For instance, if their blood glucose levels are too high,

351

they are told to reduce grams of fat for that day. In this situation, there is not a set prescription against which the patient's behaviour can be assessed. In other cases the prescription may be difficult to extract from medical records, may not be documented by health care professionals, or may simply be unavailable.

There are also more subtle problems associated with measuring diabetes regimen adherence. Investigators may be unable to distinguish between patient error due to skill deficits versus patient nonadherence. It is also difficult to quantify adherence of patients who exceed their prescriptions (e.g. testing blood sugar more frequently than prescribed). In most studies, reliance on subject-reported regimen prescriptions is necessary. Although patient reports of their regimen prescription may not always match actual prescriptions due to patient-provider miscommunication (Johnson, 1992), they probably better represent the goals that individuals try to achieve.

Another complexity is the relative independence of the different components of the diabetes regimen. It has been demonstrated repeatedly (Glasgow *et al.*, 1987; Johnson *et al.*, 1986, 1990; Marquis and Ware, 1979; Orme and Binik, 1989; Schafer *et al.*, 1983; Wilson *et al.*, 1986) that adherence to a given aspect of the regimen is not highly correlated with adherence to other aspects of the regimen. A single global measure of self-care or adherence therefore will likely fail to capture the complexity of adherence behaviours or allow investigation of the separate and combined effects of adherence to different areas of the regimen. Multiple measures of adherence may need to be developed for different components of the regimen (dietary behaviour, exercise, medication taking, glucose monitoring, safety/preventive actions and appropriate integration and timing of all these activities), and even for different dimensions within the same regimen area (e.g. measuring fat intake within the diet area), for different points during the course of the disease, for different types of diabetes (Johnson, 1992) and for different stages of human development (older versus younger adults) (Ary *et al.*, 1986). It is somewhat surprising, given the pivotal role adherence/self-care plays in the larger picture of diabetes control, yet understandable given the complexity of the problem, that new adherence measures are developed each time a new study is initiated (Anderson and Gustafson, 1989; Heiby *et al.*, 1989; Irvine, 1989; Padgett, 1991; Uzoma and Feldman, 1989).

Evolution of the Term "Level of Self-Care"

In light of the complexities outlined above, and because the term compliance or adherence implies one person bending their will to another, or the patient doing what the doctor orders, Glasgow *et al.* (1985) proposed using the term levels of specific self-care behaviours as they occur in relation to specific regimen areas. Others have used the term diabetes self-management similarly (Wing *et al.*, 1986; Goodall and Halford, 1991). We use the term "level of diabetes self-care" for the absolute frequency or consistency of regimen behaviours (e.g. number of days per week on which subjects engage in physical activity, number of calories consumed or number of glucose tests conducted). The terms "adherence", and "compliance" are reserved to compare a patient's behaviour with medical or health advice (Haynes, 1979). Absolute levels avoid such problems as poor prescriptions, or failure to understand or incorrect recall of prescriptions, but have the disadvantage of not being tailored to the individual. For example, caloric intake level measures do not take into account subjects' caloric goals or prescriptions.

Types of Adherence and Level of Self-Care Measures

The measurement of diabetes self-care and adherence varies tremendously in the literature and there are no universally accepted measures of adherence (or level of self-care). Studies have relied on patient self-report (Orme and Binik, 1989), self-monitoring, twenty four-hour recall (Johnson et al., 1990), behavioural observations, global ratings (Heiby et al., 1989), physiological indices, ratings by informed others (physicians, nurses and significant others) (Orme and Binik, 1989) and objective confirmation of self-report. Each type of measurement strategy has strengths and limitations. (For a thorough review of these, we refer the reader to articles by Johnson, 1992; Kurtz, 1990; Orme and Binik, 1989). One solution is to use multiple measures of adherence/self-care to each aspect of the regimen, but due to feasibility issues most studies have relied predominantly upon self-report measures.

The purpose of this chapter is to document the development of the Summary of Diabetes Self-Care Activities (SDSCA) questionnaire and its psychometric properties. Data from three studies were used to: determine the empirical factor structure of the instrument, investigate the reliability and validity of the subscales thus obtained, and examine whether the SDSCA questionnaire is sensitive to changes produced as a result of intervention.

THE SUMMARY OF DIABETES SELF-CARE ACTIVITIES QUESTIONNAIRE

Design

The Summary of Diabetes Self-Care Activities (SDSCA) questionnaire is a self-report measure of the frequency of completing different regimen activities over the preceding seven days. The purpose of developing this instrument was to provide a brief measure of self-care for several different regimen areas that would be feasible for use in most clinical or research settings. Areas of regimen assessed are diet, exercise, glucose testing and medication taking. Many of the questions on this measure were based on a large scale project conducted by the Rand Corporation (Marquis and Ware, 1979) to identify and develop psychometrically acceptable measures of performance of diabetes regimen activities considered to be most important by a panel of experts. The first version of the SDSCA questionnaire was used by Schafer *et al.* (1983) and Glasgow *et al.* (1987). The latest version of the SDSCA scale consists of twelve questions. For each regimen area, items were constructed to measure both absolute levels of self-care behaviour and adherence to individual prescriptions (involving a comparison of self-care behaviours to the perceived prescription).

Adherence and levels of diet self-care are measured by five items as shown in the questionnaire presented in Figure 1. First a five-point adherence item asks "How often did you follow your recommended diet over the last seven days?" The second (adherence) item asks for the percentage of time the respondent successfully limited calories as recommended in healthy eating for diabetes control. These items are referred to as Diet Amount items throughout the rest of this chapter. The last three diet (level) items are concerned with the percentage of meals which included high fibre foods, high fat foods, and sweets and desserts, and are termed Diet Type items. The rationale for employing a seven-day recall period is that self-care behaviour is expected to vary over time, and one wants to obtain a stable estimate. However asking subjects to remember details over longer intervals may result in increased inaccuracies.

Exercise is defined both in terms of absolute activity levels (number of sessions lasting at least twenty minutes, and number of specific exercise sessions in the last seven days) and adherence (percentage of time the respondent exercised the amount suggested by their doctor).

Glucose testing, insulin injections and oral medication taking to control diabetes are examined for both the absolute number (tests, insulin injections or pills) performed/taken in the last seven days as well as the percentage of these activities recommended by the doctor that were actually performed.

Scoring the SDSCA Questionnaire

Studies published by our research group employing the SDSCA questionnaire have routinely used multiple measures having different scales to assess adherence to each regimen component. Raw scores from each measure are converted to standard scores having a mean of zero and a standard deviation of one. These standardised scores are then averaged to form a composite score for each regimen behaviour. The purpose of this procedure is to give items with differing scales equal weighting. For assessing the psychometric characteristics of the SDSCA questionnaire by itself for this chapter, each item within a given regimen area was standardised as described above, and the average of those items was computed. While data were collected on four regimen areas, only three of the four regimen components were analyzed. Medication taking was not analyzed because in our samples, more than a quarter of the subjects were not prescribed

Figure 1 Summary of Diabetes Self-Care Activities

Instructions: Thank you for taking the time to fill this out. The questions below ask you about your diabetes self-care activities *during the past 7 days.*   If you were sick during the past 7 days, please think back to the last 7 days that you were not sick. Please answer the questions as honestly and accurately as you can. Your responses will be confidential.

DIET

The first few questions ask about your eating habits over the last 7 days. If you have not been given a specific diet by your doctor or dietician, answer Question 1 according to the general guidelines you have received.

1. How often did you follow your recommended diet over last 7 days?
   ___ 1. Always   ___ 2. Usually   ___ 3. Sometimes   ___ 4. Rarely   ___ 5. Never

2. What percentage of the time did you successfully limit your calories as recommended in healthy eating for diabetes control?
   ___ 0% (none)   ___ 25% (1/4)   ___ 50% (1/2)   ___ 75% (3/4)   ___ 100% (all)

3. During the past week, what percentage of your meals included high fibre foods, such as fresh fruits, fresh vegetables, whole grain breads, dried beans and peas, bran?
   ___ 0% (none)   ___ 25% (1/4)   ___ 50% (1/2)   ___ 75% (3/4)   ___ 100% (all)

4. During the past week, what percentage of your meals included high fat foods such as butter, ice cream, oil, nuts and seeds, mayonnaise, avocado, deep-fried food, salad dressing, bacon, other meat with fat or skin?
   ___ 0% (none)   ___ 25% (1/4)   ___ 50% (1/2)   ___ 75% (3/4)   ___ 100% (all)

5. During the past week what percentage of your meals included sweets and desserts such as pie, cake, jelly, soft drinks (regular, not diet drinks), cookies?
   ___ 0% (none)   ___ 25% (1/4)   ___ 50% (1/2)   ___ 75% (3/4)   ___ 100% (all)

EXERCISE

6. On how many of the last 7 days did you participate in at least 20 minutes of physical exercise?
   0   1   2   3   4   5   6   7

7. What percentage of the time did you exercise the amount suggested by your doctor? (For example, if your doctor recommended 30 minutes of activity.)
   ___ 0% (none)   ___ 25% (1/4)   ___ 50% (1/2)   ___ 75% (3/4)   ___ 100% (all)

8. On how many of the last 7 days did you participate in a specific exercise session other than what you do around the house or as part of your work?
   0   1   2   3   4   5   6   7

GLUCOSE TESTING

9. On how many of the last 7 days (that you were not sick) did you test your glucose (blood sugar) level?

___ 1. Every day ___ 2. Most days ___ 3. Some days ___ 4. None of the days

10. Over the last 7 days (that you were not sick) what percentage of the glucose (blood sugar or urine) tests recommended by your doctor did you actually perform?

___ 0% (none) ___ 25% (1/4) ___ 50% (1/2) ___ 75% (3/4) ___ 100% (all)

DIABETES MEDICATION

11. How many of your recommended insulin injections did you take in the last 7 days that you were supposed to?

___ 1. All of them ___ 2. Most of them ___ 3. Some of them ___ 4. None of them
___ -8. I do not take insulin

12. How many of your recommended number of pills to control diabetes did you take that you were supposed to?

___ 1. All of them ___ 2. Most of them ___ 3. Some of them ___ 4. None of them
___ -8. I do not take pills to control my diabetes

diabetes medication, and those who were had a wide range of different prescriptions (varying from multiple insulin injections to a single pill per day). In addition, compliance with medication was quite high and the absence of variability on these items was problematic. In our studies (Glasgow *et al.*, 1989a) and in others (Cox *et al.*, 1984) different results have been obtained for insulin and oral medication-taking measures (approximately 90% of the participants taking insulin claimed perfect adherence with medication) so further analyses using these measures were not conducted.

VALIDATIONAL STUDIES ON THE SUMMARY OF DIABETES SELF-CARE ACTIVITIES QUESTIONNAIRE

In this section, validational work on the current version of the SDSCA questionnaire is presented for three samples. This represents an attempt to reach a scientifically acceptable and practically useful set of subscales. First the three samples are described, followed by a description of the procedures for administering the measures in each study. Next, a history and description of the SDSCA questionnaire design is presented followed by analyses of the structure, stability, concurrent and predictive validity and sensitivity to change of the instrument.

Subject Samples

Study 1: Assessment study subjects

Subjects for Study 1 (Glasgow *et al.*, 1989a) were 127 outpatients with Type 2 diabetes mellitus recruited from Lane County, Oregon. Half (51%) of the subjects came from lists of patients provided by the two major diabetologists practicing in the area. Other patients came from lists provided by family practitioners and internists. Selection criteria included having been diagnosed as having diabetes for a minimum of one year and being over forty years of age. Exclusion criteria included major complications that would drastically affect performance of diabetes self-care activities (e.g. end stage renal disease, blindness, pancreatitis); requiring nursing or institutional care, and self-reported severe drinking problems. The clinical criteria recommended by Welborn *et al.* (1983) were used to differentiate Type 2 from Type 1 (insulin-dependent) diabetes. For subjects taking insulin, this method distinguishes Type 2 diabetes on the basis of age at onset, relative weight, and length of time between diagnosis and treatment with insulin.

Of the resulting sample of 127 subjects, two-thirds (66.9%) were female and the mean percent of ideal weight as determined by the National Diabetes Data Group (1979) was 147% (S.D. = 26%). Subjects' ages ranged from forty to eighty eight years with a mean of 60.8, and the average duration of diabetes was 9.1 years (range one to thirty-three years). The average socioeconomic status (Hollingshead, 1975), a combination of occupation and education levels, was 37.9 (S.D. =

12.0), falling in the middle strata of Hollingshead's schema. Almost all participants (98.4%) were white.

Study 1: Assessment study procedures

Subjects attended two sessions one week apart and completed several tasks during the intervening week. The first session lasted 1.5 hours and included a structured interview about subjects' current diabetes regimen, measures of height and
weight, completion of several social learning measures, and participation in
behavioural demonstrations related to diet and social skills. In addition, subjects
were given a packet of measures to be completed at home during the week
between sessions. This packet contained additional social learning measures, and
daily self-monitoring forms for diabetes medication, glucose testing, and physical
activity. Subjects also completed a three-day food record, which was kept for two
weekdays and a weekend day. Toward the end of the week, subjects visited a local
clinic to provide a blood sample for assessment of glycosylated haemoglobin.

At the end of the week, subjects returned for a two hour session that included
review of self-monitoring records completed at home, demonstrations of blood
glucose testing and problem-solving skills, and the SDSCA questionnaire. Finally,
subjects met with the project dietician to review their three-day food records. The
entire procedure was repeated six months later.

Study 2: Nutrition Education study subjects

Seventy-eight outpatients diagnosed by their physician as having Type 2 diabetes
mellitus were recruited from Lane County, Oregon for Study 2 (Glasgow *et al.*,
1989). Inclusion criteria included provision of physician approval, worse than
average glycaemic control (i.e. glycosylated haemoglobin > 9% or physician
judgement of poor control if GHb not available), and meeting the clinical criteria recommended by Welborn *et al.* (1983) for classification of Type 2 (as
opposed to Type 1) diabetes. Subjects ranged from forty two to seventy five years
of age. Seventy-three percent of subjects were women and the average percent of
desirable weight (National Diabetes Data Group, 1979) was 153% (S.D. = 28%).
The mean length of time subjects had diabetes was nine years. Forty-two percent
of the subjects were prescribed oral diabetes medication and 39% took insulin.
Baseline fasting blood glucose levels averaged 175 mg/dl and initial glycosylated
haemoglobin averaged 9.7%.

Study 3: "Sixty Something..." study subjects

Eligibility criteria for the "Sixty Something...." programme (Glasgow *et al.*, 1992)
included being sixty years of age or older, being primarily responsible for one's
own self-care (institutionalised patients were not eligible), meeting the Welborn
et al. (1983) clinical criteria for Type 2 diabetes, and not having major complica-

tions which would interfere with self-care (e.g. legally blind, severe stroke, on kidney dialysis). Subjects meeting these eligibility criteria were required to obtain their physician's permission to participate and to pass a submaximal graded exercise test conducted at the University of Oregon Sports Medicine Laboratory. This exercise test was provided at no charge to participants.

A total of 102 patients completed baseline assessment and were randomised into the study. The average age was sixty seven with 23% of participants over seventy years of age. As would be expected in this age group, there were more women ($n = 64$) than men ($n = 38$) participating. About one-quarter of the participants were treated with insulin and another half were on oral medication for diabetes. Most patients had lived with their diabetes for a number of years (mean = 9.4 years) and 88% also had other chronic diseases, the most common being arthritis and hypertension (both affecting 44% of subjects).

Study 2 and 3: procedures

At an orientation meeting one to two weeks before the regular group meetings began, subjects completed questionnaires about their diabetes regimens including the SDSCA questionnaire. They were also trained to self-monitor their blood glucose by visual inspection of Chemstrip Bg reagent strips in Study 2 and by using a Glucometer M with memory in Study 3. Finally, subjects were given detailed instructions for completing three-day food records and had their height and weight measured.

For Study 2, subjects were stratified by sex, mode of therapy (on insulin or not), and physician, and then randomly assigned to one of three groups: Nutrition Education (NE), Nutrition Education plus Social Learning (NE + SL), or Wait List Control. (For detailed information regarding this intervention, the reader is referred to Glasgow *et al.*, 1989.) The first two groups met weekly for five weeks for meetings of a half hour to two hours duration.

For Study 3, those completing baseline assessment were blocked on type of diabetes medication (insulin, oral medication or no diabetes medication) and then randomly assigned to either immediate or delayed intervention conditions. The intervention consisted of social learning techniques emphasising problem solving, and focused on nutrition, exercise, and glucose self-monitoring (for more information, see Glasgow *et al.*, 1992).

Both studies included post-test and six-month follow-up assessments, at which time the same measures were readministered. In addition, Study 2 included a two month follow-up and Study 3 included a twelve month follow-up.

Changes in SDSCA Questionnaire Over Time

The SDSCA questionnaire has undergone two revisions since its inception. An original eight item scale was originally developed for use with people with Type 1 diabetes (Schafer *et al.*, 1983; Glasgow *et al.*, 1987). It was revised for use with

Type 2 diabetes for the studies presented here. For Studies 1 and 2 eight items were added, two items were dropped, and six of the original items remained the same. The new items included: (a) a global question concerning the percentage of time the patient generally followed his or her doctor's recommendations for controlling diabetes, (b) two adherence items, one for limiting calories and one for exercise, (c) an exercise item asking for the number of exercise sessions in which the respondent participated over the last seven days, d) two blood sugar items and one urine testing item and (e) an item on oral medication. Two urine testing questions were eliminated because of the decreasing percentage of patients using urine as opposed to blood glucose testing. The rest of the items remained intact, however the questionnaire was reorganised so that the global question appeared first, followed by the diet, exercise, glucose testing and then medication taking items.

In the latest version employed in the "Sixty Something..." study, the question-naire was shortened to twelve items. The first change was to eliminate the global question. Our findings, consistent with those of Hanestad and Albrektsen (1991), Israel *et al.* (1986), and Johnson *et al.* (1986) suggested that the global question was not useful or reliable. Other recent revisions were made to adapt the instru-ment for use with Type 2 individuals (e.g. the addition of items about oral medi-cation), to include at least one absolute level of self-care and one adherence item for each regimen component and to enable us to assess the specific dietary behav-iours targeted for change in the "Sixty Something..." programme.

Factor Structure

Factor analysis was used to reveal the empirical structure of the instrument. Three separate principal component factor analyses (Gorsuch, 1983) were con-ducted to evaluate the initial factor patterns of the eight items for studies 1 and 2 and eleven items for study 3. (For reasons explained above, the medication items were not entered into these analyses.) In order to simplify the structure of the factor analytic matrix but to relax the requirement of factor orthogonality (Gor-such, 1983) SPSSX OBLIMIN rotation was employed. Using a criterion of eigen-values greater than one, the overall results suggested three meaningful groupings of variables, which on the average, accounted for between 70% and 80% of the total variance.

The first factor represented self-care/adherence to diet for Studies 1 and 2 and also included fat, fibre and sweets for Study 3 (see Table 1). The second factor con-tained very high loadings for all three exercise items across studies. This factor is also quite similar to the exercise factor reported by Johnson *et al.* (1986) for younger Type 1 patients. The third factor, which also replicated across studies, contained the two glucose testing items.

Table 1 Results of the rotated factor structure for the SDSCA items for each of three studies

Factor

Item	I Diet Factor			II Exercise Factor			III Glucose Testing Factor		
	Study:			Study:			Study:		
	1	2	3	1	2	3	1	2	3
Diet Amount									
Followed diet	.86	.89	.85	—	—	.33	—	—	.30
Limited calories	.86	.86	.80	—	—	—			.35
Ate meals and snacks on time	.64	.34		.34	—		—	—	
Diet Type (included in Study 3 only)									
% of meals which included fibre			.45			.40			—
% of meals which included fats			−.64			—			—
% of meals which included sweets			−.71			—			—
Exercise									
Exercised recommended amount	.45	.42	—	.90	.91	.86	—	—	—
# minutes last 7 days	—	—	—	.91	.91	.93	—	—	—
# sessions last 7 days	—	—	—	.93	.94	.91	—	—	—
Glucose Testing									
Tested recommended amount		—			—				.93
# days tested of last 7	—	—	—	—	—	—	.83	.81	.93
# times wrote down results	—	—	—	—	—	—	.81	.88	

1 = Assessment Study
2 = Nutrition Education Study
3 = "Sixty Something..." Study
— indicates that items loaded ≤.30
empty space indicates that item did not appear on questionnaire for that study

In summary, all items loaded highly on their intended underlying factor in each of the three studies. In addition, all three Diet Amount items and one Diet Type item (fibre) had some loadings above .30 on other factors (see Table 1). One exercise item (exercised recommended amount) loaded on the diet factor in two of the three studies. None of the glucose testing items loaded on other factors. The correlations between the factors were examined for the rotated factor structure matrix, as some degree of factor covariation was expected. The average inter-factor correlation was .16 for Study 1, .16 for Study 2, and .21 for Study 3. As a general conservative criterion, an average inter-factor correlation of .7 or greater would be considered likely to lead to errors in factor interpretation (Nunnally, 1978). The strongest interfactor correlation was between Diet and Exercise in all three studies, and ranged from .27 to .34.

These initial exploratory factor analyses suggested that there exist three mean-ingful and replicable clusters of self-care/adherence items, one associated with each of the three regimen component areas of diet, exercise, and glucose testing. Excellent agreement was obtained across all three studies.

Formation of subscales for the SDSCA

The clustering of items suggested by the oblique solution was employed to form subscales of the SDSCA questionnaire. This was accomplished by standardising and then averaging scores on the items within each regimen area. For Studies 1 and 2 there are three subscales including Diet, Exercise and Glucose Testing; for Study 3 an additional subscale was formed entitled Diet Type which contained the three new diet items specific to this study (e.g. percentage of meals contain-ing high fibre foods, high fat foods and sweets).

Reliability

Internal consistency

Given that the subscales contained in the SDSCA were formed with a small (two to three) and differential number of items, and because the value of Cronbach's coefficient alpha is proportional to the number of items in an index as well as the magnitude of their covariance, average inter-item correlations are presented to assess internal consistency rather than coefficient alpha. The average inter-item correlations within each SDSCA subscale were quite high, generally exceeding .5 (see Table 2). The Exercise items have the highest inter-item relationships. The Diet Type items, which were available only for Study 3 participants had the lowest intercorrelations (average of .20), with Diet Amount and Glucose Testing correla-tions being intermediate.

Test-retest reliability

Of the original 127 participants in the Assessment study, 126 were re-tested six months later, permitting assessment of test-retest reliability. As can be seen in Table 3, these coefficients suggest a moderate degree of self-care behaviour con-sistency (range = .43 to .58) especially given that the follow-up assessment occurred at the opposite time of the year. Retest data are also presented for the two intervention studies. However, given that these two samples received treat-ment during the interval between assessments (in the case of Study 2 a five week intervention; in Study 3 a twelve week intervention) it should be recognised that these correlations represent a mixture of stability of behaviour and response to intervention and it is impossible to separate the two. Generally the results suggest that Diet Amount and Exercise subscales of the SDSCA are relatively stable over

Table 2 Inter-item correlations for each SDSCA subscale for three studies

Subscale	Study 1: Assessment Study	Study 2: Nutrition Study	Study 3: "Sixty Something.." Study
Diet Amount (2 items)	.59	.74	.66
Diet Type (3 items)[a]			.20
Exercise (3 items)[a]	.77	.78	.74
Glucose Testing (3 items)	.38	.54	.76

[a] For subscales containing 3 items, the average inter-item correlation is presented.
Empty space indicates that item did not appear on questionnaire for that study

repeated administrations (median correlations equal to .53 and .50, respectively), while the Glucose Testing subscale is the least stable. The fact that the twelve month test-retest reliabilities in Study 3 were higher than corresponding six month figures suggests that there may be seasonal effects on self-care. Patient dietary and exercise behaviours, in particular, may be more consistent when measured at the same time of year.

Validity

In this section we present data on four types of validity: face and content, concurrent and predictive.

Face and content validity

A diverse group of experts were assembled by the RAND corporation in their original effort to study self-care activities of people with diabetes. Items for review by the group of experts were gathered from the medical treatment literature and research studies of patient compliance. The panel of experts rated the importance of these variables using a consensus-seeking Delphi procedure. Items receiving high ratings included medication-taking, glucose testing, diet, safety and hygiene (see Marquis and Ware, 1979 for further details). The first version of the SDSCA questionnaire was developed by Schafer *et al.* (1983). Their adherence scale was designed for use with people with Type 1 diabetes and consisted of seven questions, five of which were similar to items in the Rand study and concerned diet, insulin injections, and glucose testing (both blood and urine). Schafer *et al.* (1983) developed one item concerning exercise for the first version, since the Rand report did not address this regimen component and they also constructed a measure of frequency of blood glucose testing as the Rand study only addressed urine glucose testing. The instrument has "face validity" in that it inquires only about diabetes-related information and specifically about the areas of the diabetes regimen for which most patients have daily recommended activities.

Table 3 Test-retest reliability for Summary of Diabetes Self-Care Activity Questionnaire subscales for three studies

Subscale	Assessment Study	Nutrition Study		"Sixty Something..." Study		
	From baseline to 6-month follow-up (n=105–127)	From baseline to 2-month follow-up (n=67)	From baseline to 6-month follow-up (n=62–64)	From baseline to post-test (n=101)	From baseline to 6-month follow-up (n=46)	From baseline to 12-month follow-up (n=44)
Diet Amount	.43**	.27*	.45**	.57**	.53**	.70**
Diet Type				.47**	.35*	.59**
Exercise	.55**	.58**	.50**	.51**	.29	.36*
Glucose Testing	.58**	.13	.09	.40**	-.00	.25

*$p < .05$
**$pp < .01$
Empty space indicates that item did not appear on questionnaire for that study

Concurrent validity: levels of self-care measures

Concurrent validity is demonstrated by high correlations between scores on tests measuring the same trait by different methods (Allen and Yen, 1979). Tests of concurrent validity for this report included the correlations of the SDSCA subscale scores with relevant self-monitoring, behaviour inventories, interview and/or reflectance metre measures. To measure convergence for the Diet subscales, average daily caloric intake, average percent of calories from fat, average grams of dietary fibre per day and average percent of calories from sweets were assessed using two procedures for the "Sixty Something..." study and one procedure for the other two studies. Participants in the "Sixty Something..." study completed the dietary history portion of the Block/NCI Health Habits and History Questionnaire (Block, 1988). Data were analyzed using software provided by the National Cancer Institute. In addition, participants in all three studies were instructed in procedures for completing a three-day food record and kept such a record for three consecutive days consisting of two weekdays and one weekend day. Participants received instructions about commonly omitted foods and a sample food record prior to beginning their own food records. Completed records were reviewed with subjects, using food models and household measuring devices to clarify amounts consumed, and analyzed using the Food Processor II Nutrition and Dietary Analysis system (ESHA, 1987). Average daily intake scores on the dietary target behaviours from the diet history and food records were averaged for the "Sixty Something..." study to produce a more reliable score for the analyses reported below. The average daily percent of calories from sweets was obtained from the diet history questionnaire and is available only for the "Sixty Something..." study.

Concurrent validity for the Exercise subscale was assessed for all three studies by asking subjects to record the number of exercise sessions and the number of minutes expended in specific exercise sessions. They were instructed to record only the amount of time they were engaged in continuous exercise activities. In addition, physical activity for subjects in the "Sixty Something...." study was assessed by using the Stanford 7-Day Recall (Blair, 1984). This measure is administered as an interview, consists of questions about the amount of time spent in each of three levels of activity, and is scored to produce a final measure of average kilocalories expended per day.

For validation of the Glucose Testing subscale, subjects in all three studies recorded their blood glucose results and the time and type of test(s) on a weekly blood glucose-monitoring form. In addition, the "Sixty Something..." study participants were provided with a Glucometer M blood glucose monitoring machine with a built in memory metre device. This permitted us to compare the number of blood glucose tests recorded in the patient generated monitoring forms with the number of blood glucose tests retrieved from the memory of the Glucometer M.

Evidence for concurrent validity for *level* of self-care (as opposed to *adherence*) is provided in Table 4. For the Diet Amount subscale there were statistically significant correlations for average self-monitored calories in two of the three studies (Study 1: $r = -.29$, $p < 0.01$; and Study 3: $r = -.23$, $p < 0.05$); and for average percent of calories from fat in all three studies (Study 1: $r = -.21$, $p < 0.05$; Study 2: $r = -.35$, $p < 0.01$; and Study 3: $r = -.35$, $p < 0.01$). The average self-monitored grams of fibre per day was not related to the Diet Amount subscale of the SDSCA. The average percent of calories from sweets (collected only for Study 3) was significantly correlated with the Diet Amount subscale ($r = -.27$, $p < 0.01$).

The Diet Type subscale (available for Study 3 only) was significantly related to average percent of calories from fat ($r = -.25$, $p < 0.05$), not related to average grams of fibre per day, and significantly related to average percent of calories from sweets ($r = -.34$, $p < 0.01$).

All of the correlations between the Exercise subscale of the SDSCA and self-monitored minutes and frequency of exercise sessions are significant and in the expected direction for the two studies for which these data were collected. For the "Sixty Something..." study there was also a smaller, but significant, correlation between the Stanford 7-day Recall Interview measure and the Exercise subscale of the SDSCA.

Analyses of the relationship between the SDSCA Glucose Testing subscale and self-monitored glucose tests produced inconsistent results. In Study 1 there was a strong, significant relationship with self-monitoring data as predicted, but a nonsignificant correlation was found in Study 2 ($r = .51$, $p < 0.01$; $r = .23$, *ns*, respectively). The "Sixty Something..." study failed to reveal a significant relationship between the SDSCA Glucose Testing subscale and either self-monitored or memory meter recorded number of glucose tests conducted.

Table 4 Correlations of SDSCA subscales to self-monitored diabetes self-care behaviours for three studies

Item	Diet Amount Study: 1	2	3	Diet Type Study: 1	2	3
Block/NCI and/or 3-day food record:						
Mean calories per day	−.29**	.03	−.23*			
Mean % of calories from fat	−.21*	−.35**	−.35**			−.25*
Mean grams of fibre/day	.04	.19	.02			.03
Mean % calories from sweets			−.27**			−.34**

Item	Exercise Study: 1	2	3	Glucose Testing Study: 1	2	3
Exercise self-monitoring						
Mean # of exercise sessions for 7 days	.70**		.59**			
Mean minutes of exercise for 7 days	.60**		.46**			
Stanford 7-Day Recall						
Average minutes of activity x intensity			.23*			
Glucose self-monitoring						
Average # of blood glucose tests performed						
1. From self-monitoring records				.51**	.23	−.10
2. From Glucometer M memory						.10

*$p < .05$
**$p < .01$
Study 1 = Assessment Study
Study 2 = Nutrition Education Study
Study 3 = "Sixty Something..." Study
Empty space indicates that item did not appear on questionnaire for that study

In Study 3, we assessed the impact of socially desirable response styles on self-report measurements by correlating each of the SDSCA subscales with the overall score from the Balanced Inventory of Desirable Responding (Paulhus, 1984). Three of the four subscales were significantly related to this measure including Diet Amount ($r = .35$, $p < .01$), Diet Type ($r = .29$, $p < .01$), and Glucose Testing ($r = .30$, $p < .01$). Therefore, partial correlations, which controlled for social desirability, were computed for all of the Study 3 results presented above. This adjustment did not meaningfully alter the results obtained. Of the twelve validity coefficients involved, there was a median change of $r = −.02$, ranging from a .12 increase to a −.10

decrease. The correlation between the Exercise subscale and the Stanford 7-Day Recall Interview measure became nonsignificant (r decreased from .23 to .13), while two correlations reached higher levels of statistical significance, and the interpretation of the others remained unchanged.

Concurrent validity: adherence

In the 'Sixty Something..." study, we also had information on regimen prescription, and thus were abe to study *adherence* in addition to the level of self-care analyses reported above. To examine the relationship between the self-reported adherence items from the SDSCA questionnaire and self-monitored adherence, we computed two adherence scores for each adherence item. Information was obtained from each patient's physician concerning their specific prescription for the patient (i.e. recommended number of daily calories, recommended length and frequency of exercise sessions and recommended frequency of blood glucose testing). The number of physicians who provided this information ranged from sixty five to seventy depending on the self-care area. Patients were asked to provide identical information. Two adherence scores for each adherence item on the SDSCA questionnaire were calculated, one based on the physician prescription and one based on the patients' memory of their prescription. Adherence scores were calculated by dividing the patients' self-monitored frequency of each regimen behaviour by the patient or physician version of the prescribed regimen.

As can be seen in Table 5, there were moderate but significant correlations for the SDSCA questionnaire adherence items with their two respective adherence scores – physician and patient versions of the prescription – with the exception of adherence to recommended calories based on physician prescription and adherence to recommended number of glucose tests, based on both versions of the prescription. The correlations ranged from .10 for adherence to number of glucose tests performed (based on physician's version of the regimen) to .51 for adherence to number of exercise sessions (based on physician's prescription). Although it was not a focus of this chapter, we found moderately high and significant correlations between the patient and physician versions of regimen prescription (r's were .85, .65, .33 and .73 for adherence to calories, exercise minutes, exercise sessions and glucose testing respectively; $p < .01$ in each case with the exception of exercise sessions: $p < .05$).

Predictive validity

Predictive validity is the degree of correspondence between a measure and a criterion variable. In order to assess this correspondence, a standard with which to compare the measure is required. This is very difficult or impossible with diabetes self-management (Israel *et al.*, 1986; Johnson, 1992) because no one behavioural variable approximates what is normally considered the criterion variable (i.e. GHb). The literature tends to utilise diabetes control as a measure of adherence (Johnson, 1992; Clarke *et al.*, 1985). However, these two constructs need to

Table 5 Correlations of SDSCA adherence items with self-monitored adherence scores for "Sixty Something..." study

Self-Monitored Adherence Based Upon:	SDSCA Adherence Item			
	Calories	Exercise Minutes	Exercise Sessions	Glucose Testing Frequency
Physician version of prescription:				
Calories	−.22			
Minutes of exercise		.49**		
Exercise sessions			.51**	
Glucose testing frequency				.10
Patient version of prescription:				
Calories	−.22*			
Minutes of exercise		.35*		
Exercise sessions			.36**	
Glucose testing frequency				.14

* $p < .05$
** $p < .01$

be kept conceptually distinct. Many variables, in addition to self-care, contribute to level of metabolic control including: (a) the appropriateness of prescribed regimens; (b) patient-physician interaction; (c) the type and duration of disease; (d) temporal factors (self-care behaviours and GHb reflect different time periods); (e) the presence of other illness conditions; (f) drug interactions or changes in medication; (g) individual differences in psychophysiologic responses to stress; (h) social support; and (i) heredity (Johnson, 1992; Glasgow *et al.*, 1989a; Glasgow, 1991; Jacobson *et al.*, 1990). This leaves us with the question of what to use for a standard against which to compare our measures of self-care.

With these caveats in mind, we computed correlations between the subscales of the SDSCA questionnaire and three physiological endpoints: desirable weight, glycosylated haemoglobin and fasting blood glucose, for all three studies. Three of the SDSCA subscales, Diet Amount (Study 2: $r = -.26$, $p < .05$), Diet Type (Study 3: $r = -.21$, $p < .05$) and Exercise (Study 1: $r = -.23$, $p < .01$ and Study 2: $r = -.31$, $p < .01$) were correlated significantly with desirable weight and all correlations were in the predicted direction. However none of the relationships held up across all studies. The Diet Amount subscale for Study 2 and the Diet Type subscale for Study 3 were each correlated with fasting blood glucose ($r = -.27$, $p < .05$ and $r = -.22$, $p < .05$, respectively). There were no SDSCA subscales significantly associated with glycosylated haemoglobin.

Sensitivity to Change

A series of paired comparison t-tests were used to evaluate change from pretest to post test on individual items from the SDSCA for treated subjects in Studies 2 ($n = 23$) and 3 ($n = 52$). As can be seen in Table 6, there was post-test improvement on the Diet Amount items of "percentage of time generally followed diet" for both studies, and for "percentage of time limited calories" for Study 2. For both studies, all of the individual items forming the Glucose Testing subscale indicated that intervention produced significant increases from pretest. These individual items included "number of days tested" (both studies), "number of tests that were recorded" (Study 2) and "percentage of glucose tests recommended by doctor that were actually performed" (Study 3). There were no significant pretest to post test changes on the individual items from the Exercise subscale for either study. Exercise, however, was not targeted for change in Study 2. Finally, with the exception of 'percentage of meals which included fibre", there were no significant changes on the individual items from the Diet Type subscale.

Curiously, reported dietary fibre intake significantly decreased from baseline. This finding is not convergent with either the self-monitored (three day food record) or food frequency measures of the same behaviour. In fact, there were non-significant increases in average daily grams of dietary fibre from pre to post test on both of these measures. It is possible that fibre was not a familiar concept to subjects at baseline and therefore, in responding to a global question about fibre intake (as opposed to keeping track of specific foods and not being required to label them as to type), their criteria for what they considered high fibre foods changed over time.

DISCUSSION

The findings reported in this chapter provide support for the reliability and validity of the SDSCA questionnaire, a brief self-report instrument to assess both adherence and level of self-care for each of four diabetes regimen areas. Despite the inherent difficulties in measuring self-reported adherence, the results of the three studies reported here indicate that the SDSCA subscales are moderately stable over time (with the exception of glucose testing).

Structure of the SDSCA Questionnaire

When the eight items common to all three studies were submitted to a principal-component factor analysis and oblique rotation, three consistent and relatively independent factors resulted, accounting for a significant portion of the variance. The initial structure determined by factor analysis and the replication of these factors on a second and third sample indicate that this instrument is internally consistent but not unidimensional. This level of internal consistency is considered unusually high given the brevity of the scale. It is therefore suggested that the SDSCA questionnaire should not be used to provide a total adherence/level of self-care score but rather summary scores for each regimen area. This confirms the findings of other investigators (Johnson et al., 1986; Orme and Binik, 1989) that the components of diabetes management are relatively unrelated to each other, even when assessed by similar (self-report) methods.

Table 6 Sensitivity to change: Pretest and post-test on SDSCA items for intervention subjects in two studies

	Mean (and Standard Deviation)			
	Pretest		Post-test	
Diet Amount				
Nutrition Study (Study 2)				
Followed diet	3.6	(0.8)	4.0	(0.5)*
Limited calories	58.0	(28.2)	69.3	(20.3)*
"Sixty Something..." Study (Study 3)				
Followed diet	3.8	(0.9)	4.1	(0.6)*
Limited calories	63.9	(21.2)	68.3	(20.5)
Diet Type				
"Sixty Something..." Study (Study 3)				
% meals with fibre	79.8	(17.2)	72.1	(23.0)*
% meals with fats	26.4	(15.2)	25.5	(19.5)
% meals with sweets	16.4	(14.8)	15.4	(19.3)
Exercise				
Nutrition Study (Study 2) (Changes in exercise not targeted)				
"Sixty Something..." Study (Study 3)				
% exercised recommended amount	62.5	(33.0)	65.6	(31.1)
Days in last 7 days	4.6	(2.4)	4.6	(2.1)
Sessions in last 7 days	4.2	(2.5)	4.5	(2.1)
Glucose Testing				
Nutrition Study (Study 2)				
# days tested in last 7	2.9	(1.1)	3.8	(0.6)**
# tests recorded results	3.3	(1.3)	4.0	(0.0)*
"Sixty Something..." Study (Study 3)				
Tested recommended amount	80.8	(31.6)	96.6	(14.9)***
# days tested in last 7	3.4	(1.0)	3.9	(0.2)***

$*p < .05$
$**p < .01$
$***p < .001$

Concurrent Validity

Evidence for concurrent validity of the SDSCA questionnaire was also obtained. Concurrent validity for levels of self-care, as measured by other self-monitoring and interview measures, was strong for the Diet Type and Amount subscales. Twelve of the thirteen correlations for diet were in the expected direction. Although the absolute magnitude of these correlations was not particularly high (e.g. .20 to .35 generally), they should be interpreted in the context of the difficulty of assessing diet and the generally low correlations among different dietary assessment methods (Block, 1982). The lack of relationship between the SDSCA fibre item and dietary fibre self-monitoring was not unexpected for several reasons – those stated above as well as the fact that this is a new item and perhaps needs further development.

All three measures of exercise (frequency and duration of exercise sessions, as well as the average kilocalories expended per day for the Stanford 7-Day Recall) were significantly associated with the Exercise subscale of the SDSCA.

The Glucose Testing item concerning average number of tests performed and the self-monitoring measures of this construct were strongly correlated in Study 1. However, the glucose testing item was not validated in Studies 2 and 3. The lack of a consistent relationship between the SDSCA and self-monitored glucose testing adherence items is somewhat surprising, given the discrete nature of the behaviour and short recall period (past seven days) on which subjects were reporting.

The present set of analyses suggest that an individual's self-reported adherence to both perceived and physician-validated regimen activities was associated with self-monitored measures of the same behaviours. In addition, the intercorrelations of physician-reported regimen prescriptions with the patient-perceived regimen prescriptions were statistically significant and in the expected direction. These are unusual findings in that others have reported much weaker relationships between patient recall and actual regimen recommendations (Page et al., 1981; Rost et al.,1990).

Predictive Validity

The relationships between the SDSCA subscales and physiological endpoints were briefly addressed in this chapter. Although these analyses revealed significant relationships between desirable weight and fasting blood glucose for some of the studies, a relationship between metabolic control as measured by GHb and the SDSCA subscales was not obtained. A possible explanation for this is that physiological endpoints may not be the standard to employ for predictive validity. Other measures such as patient functioning (Kaplan, 1990), quality of life (Hanestad and Albrektsen, 1991) or changes in medication prescription may be more appropriate. Level of metabolic control is dependent on factors other than adherence. For example, some patients may find that they can maintain low levels of GHb without adhering to their recommended regimens, while others may find that their GHb levels are high despite close adherence. Such variability may be due to differences in endogenous insulin secretion, stress reactivity, appropriateness of regimen prescription, medication effects, autonomic neuropathy, adequacy of response to blood glucose test results, and other self-care skills not currently measured. It may also be that there is a subset of patients for whom self-care is strongly related to GHb, and others for whom it is not, as Wing *et al.* (1985) have suggested for responsiveness to diet.

Research and Clinical Utility

According to Alpher *et al.* (1987) the more specific an instrument is, the more discriminative power and practical utility it is likely to have. The SDSCA questionnaire provides researchers with a diabetes-specific, brief (most patients will complete it in seven minutes or less), self-administered instrument. This is an advantage given that we recommend that the SDSCA questionnaire be included with other measures of self-care. However, as Johnson (1992) points out, we may be over-concerned with the length of the instruments we administer. The solution to the paradox between length of overall instrument and reliability concerns may lie in the specificity and range of the components within regimen areas. In particular, it may be necessary to assess a broader range of activities related to diet. Moreover, use of more items, provided they tap into a similar construct and are statistically related to one another, could also serve to increase the reliability of this measure. In any event, we do not recommend that this instrument be used in place of more comprehensive data collection procedures such as self-monitoring of diet.

The SDSCA questionnaire appears to show practical utility as a change measure. The results presented in this chapter demonstrate that the SDSCA questionnaire is fairly sensitive to interventions designed to influence the dietary and glucose testing (but not exercise) self-care behaviours of people with Type 2 diabetes. The SDSCA questionnaire may prove useful both as a brief screening instrument to identify those patients who may be currently experiencing difficulty with one or more of the diabetes self-care areas, and to measure improvements as a result of patient education. We have computerised and are currently piloting the SDSCA questionnaire as part of a brief assessment/intervention during a routine office visit with their physician that is designed to identify problems patients experience with diabetes self-care.

Limitations of the SDSCA Questionnaire

The twelve-item scale reported in this chapter does not measure all aspects of adherence/self-care for adults with Type 2 diabetes. Relevant measures which appear to be promising for future validational work but are not included in the SDSCA questionnaire consist of foot care, safety, and insulin self-regulation. We hope future research efforts will address these important diabetes regimen areas.

An interpretive problem concerns distortions in reporting as a result of the tendency to see oneself in a desirable light. It would be optimal to develop revised scales that are less sensitive to social desirability, but given the complexities of that task, a feasible alternative might be to use a measure of social desirability as a covariate when using the SDSCA and other self-report instruments (e.g. Glasgow *et al.*, 1992).

Another limitation of these findings has to do with the problem of relying on correlations rather than structural coefficients to test validity. Usually the correspondence between a measure and its criterion variable is measured by their correlation. The absolute value of this correlation has been referred to as a validity coefficient by Lord and Novick (1968). Bollen (1989) argued, however, that the "closeness" of the measure and its criterion variable depends on factors other than the magnitude of this validity coefficient. The validity coefficient is affected by the relation between the "observed" measure and its accompanying unobserved construct or "latent variable", the relation between the latent variable and the criterion variable, and the degree of random measurement error variance in both the measure and its criterion variable. This situation is exacerbated when several criterion-related measures are used. Bollen (1989) stated that "even with no change in the measure's association with the 'construct' or latent variable, we are led to different values of validity, depending on the criterion variable's relation to the construct". Further validation studies with larger samples will permit use of more sophisticated statistical techniques such as structural equation modelling to explore and clarify these relationships.

SUMMARY

In summary, measurement of adherence/self-care behaviour is a complex, multidimensional task, of which measurement of diet is often the most difficult component. Efforts to improve these measures should focus on not just the brevity of the instrument but on interpretability, reliability, validity, and utility. Overall, the pattern of results provides initial support for the validity of the SDSCA subscales. The factors representing the diabetes self-care areas measured by the SDSCA subscales appear to be replicable, and were relatively invariant across three moderately large samples of adults with Type 2 diabetes. This investigation has also shown that subjects' self-reports of self-care behaviour on the SDSCA are associated with self-monitoring and interview measures of the same behaviours.

We suggest that additional measures for the separate subscales identified in this report be developed so that multiple indicators can be employed in future investigations. Development of finer grained measures of the components of a regimen area (e.g. more carefully measured fibre intake; assessing patient responses to high blood glucose readings) should further enhance the measurement of adherence and level of self-care. We hope researchers will be encouraged by these positive preliminary findings which demonstrate the potential utility of the SDSCA questionnaire. Additional research is clearly necessary to develop adherence/self-care level measures that are predictive of health status and acute and/or long-term complications associated with chronically elevated blood glucose.

REFERENCES

Allen, M.J. and Yen, W.M. (1979) *Introduction to measurement theory.* Monterey, California: Brooks/ Cole Publishing Company

Alpher, V.S., Blanton, R.L. and Nunnally, J.C. (1987) Multifactor measurement of bodily feelings: Conceptual development, scale construction, and empirical validation. *Journal of Psychopathology and behavioural Assessment,* **9**, 403–421

Anderson, L.A. (1990) Health-care communication and selected psychosocial correlates of adherence in diabetes management. *Diabetes Care,* **13**, 66–76

Anderson, J.W. and Gustafson, N.J. (1989) Adherence to high-carbohydrate, high-fibre diets, *The Diabetes Educator,* **15**, 429–434

Ary, D.V., Toobert, D., Wilson, W. and Glasgow, R.E. (1986) Patient perspective on factors contributing to nonadherence to diabetes regimens. *Diabetes Care,* **9**, 168–172

Blair, S.N. (1984) How to assess exercise habits and physical fitness. In J. D. Mattarazzo, *et al.* (eds), *Behavioural health: A handbook of health enhancement and disease prevention.* New York: Wiley

Block, G. (1982) A review of validations of dietary assessment methods. *American Journal of Epidemiology,* **115**, 492–505

Block, G. (1988) *Health Habits and History Questionnaire: Diet History and Other Risk Factors.* Washington, DC: National Cancer Institute, National Institutes of Health

Bollen, K.A. (1989) *Structural equations with latent variables.* New York: Wiley

Clarke, W.L., Snyder, A.L. and Nowacek, G. (1985) Outpatient pediatric diabetes - I. Current practices. *Journal of Chronic Disease,* **38**, 85–90

Cox, D.J., Taylor, A.G., Nowacek, G., Holley-Wilcox, P. and Pohl, S.L. (1984) The relationship between psychological stress and insulin-dependent diabetic blood glucose control: Preliminary investigations. *Health Psychology,* **3**, 63–75

ESHA Research (1987) *The Food Processor II, IBM and compatible version.* Salem, Oregon

Glasgow, R.E. (1991) Compliance to diabetes regimens: Conceptualization, complexity and determinants. In J.A. Cramer and B. Spilker, (eds), *Patient compliance in medical practice and clinical trials.* New York: Raven Press

Glasgow, R.E., McCaul, K.D. and Schafer, L.C. (1987) Self-care behaviours and glycemic control in Type I diabetes. *Journal of Chronic Disease,* **40**, 399–412

Glasgow, R.E., Toobert, D.J., Hampson, S.E., Brown, J.E., Lewinsohn, P.M. and Donnelly, J. (1992) Improving self-care among older patients with Type II diabetes: The "Sixty Something..." Study. *Patient Education and Counseling,* **19**, 61–74

Glasgow, R.E., Toobert, D.J., Mitchell, D.L., Donnelly, J.E. and Calder, D.C. (1989) Nutrition education and social learning interventions for Type II diabetes. *Diabetes Care,* **12**, 150-152

Glasgow, R.E., Toobert, D.J., Riddle, M., Donnelly, J., Mitchell, D.L. and Calder, D. (1989a) Diabetes-specific social learning variables and self-care behaviours among persons with Type II diabetes. *Health Psychology,* **8**, 285–303

Glasgow, R.E., Wilson, W. and McCaul, K. (1985) Regimen adherence: A problematic concept in diabetes research. *Diabetes Care,* **4**, 96–98.

Goodall, T.A. and Halford, W.K. (1991) Self-management of diabetes mellitus: a critical review. *Health Psychology,* **10**, 1–8.

Gorsuch, R.L. (1983) Factor analysis. Hillsdale, NJ: Lawrence Erlbaum Associates

Hanestad, B.R. and Albrektsen, G. (1991) Quality of life, perceived difficulties in adherence to a diabetes regimen, and blood glucose control. *Diabetic Medicine,* **8**, 759–764

Haynes, R.B. (1979) Introduction. In R.B. Haynes, D.W. Taylor, D.L. Sackett, (eds), *Compliance in Health Care.* Baltimore, Md: Johns Hopkins Press

Heiby, E.M., Gafarian, C.T. and McCann, S.C. (1989) Situational and behavioural correlates of compliance to a diabetic regimen. *Journal of Compliance in Health Care,* **4**, 101–116

Hollingshead, A.B. (1975) *Four factor index of social status.* Unpublished manuscript, Yale University

Irvine, A.A. (1989) Self-care behaviours in a rural population with diabetes, *Patient Education and Counseling*, **13**, 3–13

Israel, C., Berndt, D.J. and Barglow, P. (1986) Development of a self-report measure of adherence for children and adolescents with insulin-dependent diabetes. *Journal of Youth and Adolescence*, **15**, 419–428.

Jacobson, A.M., Adler, A.G., Wolfsdorf, J.I., Anderson, B. and Derby, L. (1990) Psychological characteristics of adults with IDDM. *Diabetes Care*, **13**, 375–381

Johnson, S.B. (1992) Methodological issues in diabetes research: Measuring adherence. *Diabetes Care*, **15**, 1658–1667

Johnson, S.B., Freund, A., Silverstein, J., Hansen, C.A. and Malone, J. (1990) Adherence-health status relationships in childhood diabetes. *Health Psychology*, **9**, 606–631

Johnson, S.B., Silverstein, J., Rosenbloom, A., Carter, R. and Cunningham, W. (1986) Assessing daily management in childhood diabetes. *Health Psychology*, **5**, 545–564

Johnson, S.B., Tomer, A., Cunningham, W.R. and Henretta, J.C. (1990) Adherence in childhood diabetes: Results of a confirmatory factor analysis. *Health Psychology*, **9**, 493–501

Kaplan, R. M. (1990) behaviour as the central outcome in health care. *American Psychologist*, **45**, 1211–1220

Kurtz, S.M.S. (1990) Adherence to diabetes regimens: Empirical status and clinical applications. *The Diabetes Educator*, **16**, 50–56

Lord, F.M. and Novick, M.R. (1968) *Statistical Theories of Mental Test Scores.* Reading, MA: Addison-Wesley

Marquis, K.H. and Ware, J.E. (1979) *Measures of diabetic patient knowledge, attitudes, and behaviour regarding self-care: Summary report.* (Contract No. 200-77-0722). Santa Monica, California: RAND

National Diabetes Data Group (1979) Classification and diagnosis of diabetes mellitus and other categories of glucose intolerance. *Diabetes*, **28**, 1039–1057

Nunnally, J.C. (1978) *Psychometric theory.* 2nd ed. New York: McGraw-Hill

Orme, C.M. and Binik, Y.M. (1989) Consistency of adherence across regimen demands. *Health Psychology*, **8**, 27–43

Padgett, D.K. (1991) Correlates of self-efficacy beliefs among patients with non-insulin dependent diabetes in Zagreb, Yugoslavia. *Patient Education and Counseling*, **18**, 139–147

Page, P., Verstraete, D. G., Robb, J. R. and Etzwiler, D. D. (1981) Patient recall of self-care recommendations in diabetes, *Diabetes Care*, **4**, 96-98.

Paulhus, D.L. (1984) Two-component models of social desirable responding. *Journal of Personality and Social Psychology*, **46**, 598–609.

Rost, K., Roter, D., Quill, T. and Bertakis, K. (1990) Capacity to remember prescription drug changes: deficits associated with diabetes. *Diabetes Research and Clinical Practice*, **10**, 183–187

Schafer, L.C., Glasgow, R.E., McCaul, K.D. and Dreher, M. (1983) Adherence to IDDM regimens: Relationship to psychosocial variables and metabolic control. *Diabetes Care*, **6**, 493-498

Uzoma, C.U. and Feldman, R.H.L. (1989) Psychosocial factors influencing inner city black diabetic patients' adherence with insulin. *Health Education*, **20**, 29–32

Welborn, T.A., Garcia-Webb, P., Bonser, A. *et al.* (1983) Clinical criteria that reflect C-peptide status in idiopathic diabetes. *Diabetes Care*, **6**, 315–316

Wilson, W., Ary, D.V., Biglan, A., Glasgow, R.E., Toobert, D.J. and Campbell, D. R. (1986) Psychosocial predictors of self-care behaviours (compliance) and glycemic control in non-insulin-dependent diabetes mellitus. *Diabetes Care*, **9**, 614–622

Wing, R.R., Epstein, L.H., Nowalk, M.P., Koeske, R. and Hagg, S. (1985) behaviour change, weight loss, and psychological improvements in type II diabetic patients. *Journal of Consulting and Clinical Psychology*, **53**, 111–122

Wing, R.R., Epstein, L.H., Nowalk, M.P. and Lamparski, D.M. (1986) behavioural self-regulation in the treatment of patients with diabetes mellitus. *Psychological Bulletin*, **99**, 78–89

SECTION 6

USE AND ABUSE OF
PSYCHOLOGICAL MEASURES

CHAPTER 16

ADAPTING SCALES AND PROCEDURES: THE LIMITS OF RELIABILITY AND VALIDITY

CLARE BRADLEY

Department of Psychology, Royal Holloway, University of London, Egham Hill, Egham, Surrey, TW20 0EX, UK.

USING QUESTIONNAIRES WITH NEW POPULATIONS

Researchers often describe the questionnaires they have used as having "established reliability and validity". They may then provide a reference to a paper reporting the psychometric properties of the scale developed for an entirely different population from the one to which the scales have subsequently been applied. For example, the Beck Depression Inventory (BDI) was developed as a measure of depression in the general population and was not developed specifically for people with diabetes. However valid and reliable a measure of depression the BDI may be with a general population sample, it cannot be assumed that it will be equally valid or reliable if used with respondents who have diabetes. Indeed, there are good reasons to suggest that the BDI is not a valid measure of depression in people with diabetes as several symptoms of depression in non-diabetic populations are symptoms that in diabetic populations may well arise from poor diabetes control rather than from depression (Bradley and Lewis, 1990). These issues are considered in more detail in Chapter 6 on the Well-being Questionnaire included in this volume.

When a questionnaire is used with a different population from that which provided the data for the scale development work, we cannot assume that it will retain the psychometric properties it originally demonstrated. If, nevertheless, the user judges that the questionnaire is likely to work equally well with the new population being studied, the onus is then on the user to support this judgement with evidence for the psychometric properties of the measure when used with the new population.

MODIFYING QUESTIONNAIRES

If we modify a questionnaire, we can no longer count on the psychometric properties remaining unchanged even though we use it on a similar population. Modifications may include omission of certain items, changes to the instructions asking respondents to consider a longer or shorter time period than that which was originally specified. The psychometric properties of a questionnaire may even be changed by altering the format or typeface used. It may be that such changes can be made without reducing reliability or validity but this cannot be assumed.

The Case for Modifications

If the scales are inappropriate for the intended sample then they will be of dubious value unless changes are made. Clearly it would be inappropriate to give a questionnaire written in Finnish to a population of patients in the UK. Few if any of the patients would understand the questions and it would have no validity in such circumstances. It is less obvious that a questionnaire designed for Americans with diabetes may need modification before it could be used with people with diabetes in the UK. I recently modified a "Diabetes Hassles" scale designed by Kanner and Jacobson and modified by Gonder-Frederick, Cox and colleagues at the University of Virginia (Cox, personal communication, 1992). Careful consideration of the instrument revealed that some items would not be familiar to a British sample, some items would not be relevant, and some would have different meanings. For example, the American term 'shots' was used in several items and was changed to 'injections', the term used by British patients. Other items were concerned with issues of payment for health care which are less relevant for users of the British National Health Service (NHS) than for users of the American health care system. Thus the American item 'Not enough money to buy medical supplies' was changed to 'Not enough money to buy the food needed to follow my diet' in the British translation. British NHS patients with diabetes have to buy their own food but do not have to buy most of their medical supplies. Similarly, 'Having trouble paying your doctor's bills', was not generally relevant for a British population and was replaced with a substitute item.

Thus, when planning to use American scales in Britain or British scales in America, some items will need translation before use while others may need to be omitted. It is possible that additional items may need to be added to improve content validity for the new population. For example, we might consider adding items concerned with NHS waiting times or other problems with the service which might be common concerns for British patients though less relevant to American patients.

Modifications will be needed if units of measurement are used which patients will not understand. The DKN scales to measure knowledge of diabetes described by Beeney et al., in Chapter 9 refer to blood glucose levels in mmol/l which would be incomprehensible to American patients used to mg/100mls and would need adapting to refer to ranges of blood glucose that would make sense in mg/100mls. Units of length and weight are currently a cause of confusion within the UK. Children are now being taught in metric units while adults are more likely to be familiar with yards, feet and inches, stones, pounds and ounces than with metres and centimetres, kilograms and grams. A questionnaire intended to be appropriate for adolescents as well as adults should include both units of measurement if such measurements are required. The Summary of Diabetes Self-Care Activities measure presented by Toobert and Glasgow in Chapter 15 provides response options in both percentages and fractions which is likely to make the questionnaire comprehensible to a larger proportion of respondents than would be the case if percentages or fractions were used alone.

With any measure of "knowledge" the potential user needs to consider what is being taught to patients in the clinic where the questionnaire may be used. As well as changing units of measurement to correspond to local use, it may be that terminology needs adapting or that brand names may need changing. Some items in the DKN scales ask about which "'diabetic' food items are approved by the diabetic clinic?". It should be established that local recommendations correspond appropriately before such items are used unmodified. Indeed, it would be good practice to ask each of the health professionals, involved in a diabetes clinic, to study the questionnaires and to indicate which items they regard as acceptable in order to identify difficulties which may call for modifications to be made to the questionnaire before use with patients. Disagreements among health professionals need to be openly discussed and resolved between members of the diabetes care team in order to ensure that any modifications made are appropriate. Toobert and Glasgow's Summary of Diabetes Self-Care Activities instrument (Chapter 15) would also need to be considered in the context of local recommendations. For example, items concerned with doctors' specific recommendations about the amount of exercise to be taken may not be appropriate for use in clinics where patients are not offered any clear recommendations concerning exercise.

Omission of Items

Items that are clearly inappropriate in a local context, undermine face validity and are far better omitted than included unmodified. However, the implications for other psychometric properties need to be considered. When items are omitted from short scales it may be that reliability, in the form of internal consistency, will be compromised. Sometimes authors of scales can advise on the likely consequences of omitting one item. The authors may have data from reliability analyses which include information about the effects on alpha coefficients of removing each item. The greater the resulting reduction in alpha, the more important it is to include that item for the internal consistency of the measure. On the other hand, items that can be dropped without serious reduction in alpha may be considered for exclusion in future work though the implications for other psychometric characteristics, particularly content validity, need also to be considered. Lewis and Bradley in Chapter 12 provide information about the minimal effects on alpha of omitting one item that refers to tablet taking from the scales concerned with benefits of and barriers to treatment. The item on tablet taking is clearly inappropriate for patients who do not take tablets. The information from the reliability analyses suggested that adequate reliability would be retained if the scales were modified for patients treated with diet alone by dropping the one item concerned with medication.

In Chapter 13 on the Perceived Control of Diabetes scales, information is provided about the consequences for alpha of omitting specific scenarios. This is useful information for a researcher wishing to estimate the risks attached to shortening the instrument or for those concerned about the functioning of an item in a particular local context. For example, in a diabetes clinic where some patients were not informed about the risks of complications of diabetes or where patients were not given the evidence for improved diabetes control reducing those risks, patients might be bewildered, shocked or upset by an item concerned with perceived control over complications of diabetes. Such an item would be better omitted until a suitable diabetes education programme has been introduced.

Additional Items

It is often desirable to append additional items to an instrument known to be reliable and to have validity with the population to be studied but where additional or more detailed information is needed on issues of particular relevance. For example, researchers may wish to add further items to the DQOL measure of quality of life described by Alan Jacobson and colleagues in the Diabetes Control and Complications Trial Research Group in Chapter 5 or to the DTSQ measure of treatment satisfaction described in Chapter 7. The authors of the DQOL suggested that additional questions or questionnaires might be needed for specific circumstances where a treatment being evaluated might be expected to have particular consequences, for example, consequences for sexual function. The DQOL would not provide the coverage of this issue which might be needed in specific circumstances. Additional instruments might be used in conjunction with the DQOL or additional items might be designed and developed for inclusion within the DQOL. It should be noted however, that it is not sufficient to design items in the same format as those in the DQOL or DTSQ and assume that they can be added in to the total score along with the other items. The new items should either be treated as stand-alone items for which scores are considered separately or they should be submitted to psychometric development procedures with a view to developing a new subscale or a new extended version of the original questionnaire. In these cases where a new subscale or scale is constructed, evidence must be provided for the reliability and validity of each new measure.

Psychometric Analyses Recommended Following Modifications

Chapter 3 considered the challenges faced by those wishing to translate questionnaires for use in other languages or cultures and emphasised the importance of investigating the psychometric properties of each new translation as if it were a completely new instrument. As with a newly designed instrument, sample size permitting, factor analysis may be used to examine the factor structure and the nature of any subscales and alpha coefficients may be calculated to estimate internal consistency. Where sample size is insufficient for such analyses, correlation matrices may be used to determine relationships between items and between sub-scales and to seek confirmation of the expected pattern of interrelationships. Questionnaires to which other kinds of modification have been made should also be treated as if they were new instruments for which reliability and validity cannot be assumed. Where modifications are minor or carefully designed, there is every likelihood that the new version of the questionnaire will have similar levels of reliability and validity as its forerunner but reliability and validity should not be assumed. Evidence should be sought from correlations, factor analyses and reliability analyses. A problem arises when researchers wish to modify scales for use in studies involving only small numbers of patients where there is little scope for psychometric analyses to confirm the adequacy of the modified measure. The scales may work as predicted in small-scale studies but if the scales do not work as expected it is difficult to judge where the problem lies. Consider, for example, the case of a researcher shortening the DTSQ measure of satisfaction with treatment to three items and using this newly shortened version in a study evaluating the effects of changing treatment from insulin injections to continuous subcutaneous insulin infusion (CSII) pumps. The researcher may expect to find increased satisfaction scores following change to CSII as has been found in previous studies and reported in Chapter 7. If no significant changes are found, there may be several possible explanations. It may be that these patients were already more satisfied at the start of the study with their injection treatment and no further improvement was needed or it may be that further improvement was hard to demonstrate given the restricted range of scores on this shortened scale. Thus the findings may be providing a valid indication of patients' experiences or they may be a reflection of the reduced sensitivity of the modified scale. If the scores obtained leave room for improvement in satisfaction scores following change to CSII, a lack of any such change using an untested modification of a scale may be the result of a serious reduction in the reliability of the measure rather than a reflection of patients' views. A large enough sample size to allow investigation of reliability is needed to choose between such explanations. (Chapter 2 provides further information on reliability assessment).

If modified scales fail to work as expected when they have been translated, shortened, added to or used in a different context from those in which they have previously been shown to have reliability and validity, the original scale should not be criticised. It is the responsibility of the researcher who modifies the scale to establish the psychometric properties of any new version.

Reporting Studies Using Modified Scales

When disseminating findings of studies which have used modified scales, it is important to acknowledge the authors of the original scale. Failure to do so may give rise to charges of plagiarism. It is also important to describe clearly the modifications made to the questionnaire. The modifications should be specified precisely enough to allow the modified questionnaire to be reconstructed and the modified questionnaire should be made available on request.

There are many questionnaires in circulation which do not include a copyright statement or any other indication of ownership. This does not mean that they can be copied freely. Someone will own the copyright and although they may well be willing to give permission for widespread use, this should not be assumed. It is important to track down the source of the questionnaire before using it, partly to avoid the risk of being sued for breach of copyright and partly because the questionnaire may have been superceded by an updated version. It is accepted practice to modify other authors' questionnaires or to extract part of a questionnaire, perhaps a single subscale, provided that appropriate acknowledgement is given to the source. Examples of this practice are provided in the following section on short forms.

Short Forms of the Measure

There is great demand among potential users of scales for shorter questionnaires than those available. Authors of scales sometimes go on to develop short forms of their scales on the strength of experience gained from using the original measure. For example the ATT39 described by Welch *et al.* in Chapter 11 has given rise to the short form ATT19. Sometimes other researchers select items from longer instruments with a view to developing a shorter measure. For example the Depression and Anxiety subscales that are included in the Well-being Questionnaire in Chapter 6 were derived from much longer measures developed by Zung (1965, 1974). Warr and Parry (1982) reported evidence for the validity of the Depression subscale and Warr *et al.* (1985) went on to derive and use the Anxiety subscale along with the Depression subscale.

Sometimes authors of scales can advise on the likely effects of omitting a single item as described in the section above. However, users may wish for a more substantial reduction in the length of a questionnaire. Where a much shorter questionnaire is needed, it may be possible to identify a subscale which may be taken out of a much longer scale. Although such a strategy will reduce the breadth of a measure, it may have the advantage of preserving the reliability of the subscale. This strategy was used when the audit working group of the Royal College of Physicians and the British Diabetic Association wanted to include a short measure of well-being in a National Study of audit of diabetes care. The twenty two item measure described in Chapter 6 was judged by the physicians involved to be too long for audit purposes. The measure might have been shortened sufficiently by selecting two or three items from each subscale. This would have preserved the breadth of content with items from the Depression, Anxiety, Energy, and Positive Well-being scales covering the range of considerations relevant to well-being. However, the newly-shortened measure might not have been reliable. Had there been time, funding, and a qualified research worker available to work on existing data sets to identify the most promising items for inclusion in a short form, it would have been useful to try to develop a short form with the breadth of content of the original twenty two-item measure. In the absence of such resources, the low-risk strategy was adopted of selecting one subscale from the four available in the original measure. The Depression subscale was selected as it measures the aspect of Well-being that was of most particular concern to the audit working group. In addition, the opportunity was used to explore the value of a separate newly modified subscale to measure diabetes-specific depression in a questionnaire which included only twelve items in two six-item subscales. Data are now being collected using this Depressed Well-being Questionnaire which has been described in an early publication from the audit working group (Wilson *et al.*, 1993).

Researchers may select one reliable subscale from a longer questionnaire and, in order to retain some of the breadth of content provided by the original, they may choose in addition to include single items from other subscales which may provide useful supplementary information scored and treated as individual items.

Finally, having considered the work involved and the risks attached to shortening an already developed questionnaire, potential users would do well to re-examine the original questionnaire. They may then decide that it is not too long after all.

THE DEVELOPMENT OF RESEARCH MEASURES FOR CLINICAL USE

Most of the questionnaires presented in the *Handbook* chapters were originally designed for research purposes rather than for routine clinical use. However, several of the research measures meet the criteria for scales suitable for clinical use. They are short, easily administered, straightforward to score and interpret and are suitable for repeated administration (Wilkin *et al.*, 1992). The quality of life, well-being and satisfaction measures described in Section 2, which includes a measure of fear of hypoglycaemia, are examples of measures with direct clinical applications. One possible exception, the DCCT Diabetes Quality of Life measure, is regarded by many physicians as too lengthy for routine clinical use. There is some evidence for sensitivity to change in response to major changes of treatment but it is not yet clear whether the DCCT measure would be sensitive to smaller, but potentially important, changes such as efforts to tailor a treatment regimen to a particular patient's needs. The Well-being Questionnaire, DTSQ Measure of Satisfaction, and the Fear of Hypoglycaemia Scale are shorter than the DCCT measure and there is more evidence for the scale structure to support the scoring methods proposed. However, the scale scores need to be interpreted within a broader context of other measures. While scores indicating low levels of well-being or satisfaction or high levels of fear clearly indicate that there is a problem; scores suggesting that well-being and satisfaction levels are high and that there is little fear of hypoglycaemia do not necessarily mean that all is well. For example, patients may have an excellent sense of well-being and be satisfied with their treatment but their blood glucose control may be such that they risk serious complications in the future. Such a pattern of outcomes is not uncommon and may be a reflection of patients' lack of knowledge about the effects of blood glucose on risks of future complications. Alternatively the same pattern of findings might occur in a well-informed patient who has decided to take the increased risk of future complications rather than meet the demands of a complex treatment regimen which has been recommended. If the reasons for the pattern of outcomes can be established, appropriate educational interventions and modifications to the treatment regimen may lead to an improvement in diabetes control without undue reduction in well-being or satisfaction levels. The scores on the questionnaires need to be interpreted in the wider context of other measures of processes (e.g. knowledge) and outcomes (e.g. glycosylated haemoglobin levels) in diabetes management.

The measures of cognitive function and knowledge described in Section 3 have direct clinical applications. Providing the items are compatible with information given within a particular clinic, the DKN knowledge scales are short enough and suitably straightforward to administer, score and interpret to be useful for many clinical purposes. Measures of cognitive function generally require the specialist skills of an experienced test administrator and interpreter and, given that the measurement of cognitive function is only occasionally appropriate for clinical purposes, such measurement is best conducted by psychologists trained in such testing.

The measures of self-care behaviours and barriers to self-care described in Section 6 may need modification to suit particular local requirements but they clearly have direct clinical applications which are now being explored and charted.

Section 5 measures are best regarded as research instruments. The Diabetes-Specific Health Belief scales and the Perceived Control of Diabetes scales are lengthy instruments, and are more complex to score and interpret than other measures in this *Handbook*. Although the ATT39 developers can offer a short enough form of the measure in the ATT19, interpretation is not straightforward. It is far from clear that one set of ATT39 beliefs, or even the ATT19 beliefs, is indicative of good adjustment across different clinics in different cultures. Clinical research would be needed to explore the clinical uses and limitations of the ATT19 within a particular clinic before considering routine clinical use.

Although I would not advise use of the Diabetes-Specific Health Beliefs scale or Perceived Control of Diabetes scales as clinical tools, the theoretical frameworks which guided the construction of those questionnaires can be very helpful in conducting interviews with patients to gain insight into their problems. Exploration of patients' perceptions of control of their diabetes may, for example, reveal feelings of helplessness and unrealistic expectations of the diabetes care team or the insulin delivery technology which may be an important cause of inappropriate self-care behaviour and inadequate blood glucose control. Exploration of patients' beliefs about the risk of complications may reveal that complications are regarded as inevitable and therefore that there is little reason to strive to improve blood glucose control any more than is necessary to keep acute symptoms at bay.

A similar lack of motivation may follow when patients are ignorant of any risk of complications associated with chronically raised blood glucose levels.

If used clinically, the questionnaires to measure attitudes and beliefs would be likely to raise more questions than they can answer. Such beliefs can be elicited without the use of questionnaires in the context of a consultation where patients' concerns can be directly addressed, information can be provided when needed, alternative perceptions of events and their causes can be suggested and constructive strategies for improving outcomes negotiated. Questionnaires are not a substitute for listening to patients. While there is clearly an important role for reliable and valid questionnaire assessment of psychological outcomes and processes, there are limits within which those questionnaires can be expected to be useful within clinical settings.

The questionnaires to measure quality of life, well-being and satisfaction are those for which there is currently the greatest demand from clinicians who wish to use the measures for routine evaluation of psychological outcomes alongside clinical measures of diabetes control and complications. The Diabetes Control and Complications Trial Research Group reported at the American Diabetes Association annual conference in June 1993, that intensified insulin treatment reduces the risk of retinopathy. This finding has widespread implications for patients' and health professionals' beliefs and behaviour as well as for patients' psychological well-being. It becomes increasingly important to ensure that when improvements in blood glucose control are strived for, it is not at the expense of reduced quality of life, well-being and satisfaction. The monitoring of psychological outcomes is an essential first step in improving such outcomes (Bradley, 1994). The challenge we face now is to evaluate the use of our psychological measurement instruments in a clinical context and establish the limits of their reliability and validity and their sensitivity to change in clinical use. For clinical purposes, norms are needed to assess the meaning of individual patients' scores. Clinical research is needed to establish cut-off points and guidelines about when intervention is likely to be effective and the nature of the intervention needed for different profiles of outcomes.

We have come a long way in the last decade in developing and documenting a wide selection of psychological measures which have proved to be valuable instruments in diabetes research. The continuing work on research tools provides a valuable foundation on which to build tools designed for clinical use.

SUMMARY

In this chapter it is emphasised that existing questionnaires will not always be suitable for the population or circumstances to be studied. There are however, times when modifications can usefully be made. Examples are given of cases where it is appropriate to omit items or to add new items. The value of short forms of questionnaires is acknowledged and strategies are suggested for shortening instruments with the least risk of reducing reliability to unacceptable levels. The validity and reliability of the original instrument cannot be assumed to be retained when modifications have been made or when the questionnare is used with a different population. The psychometric properties of any modified scale must be re-examined and assessed. Finally, the clinical potential of the measures described in the *Handbook* is considered. While some of the instruments are unsuitable for clinical purposes, many have direct clinical applications and warrant further development and use in the context of ongoing clinical research.

REFERENCES

Beck, A.T., Ward, C.H., Mendelson, M., Mock, J. and Erbaugh, J. (1961). An inventory for measuring depression. *Archives of General Psychiatry*, 4, 561–571

Bradley, C. (1994) Contributions of Psychology to Diabetes Management. *British Journal of Clinical Psychology*, 33, 11-21

Bradley, C. and Lewis, K.S. (1990) Measures of Psychological Well-being and Treatment Satisfaction developed from the responses of people with tablet-treated diabetes. *Diabetic Medicine*, 7, 445–451

Warr, P.B., Banks, M.H. and Ullah, P. (1985) The experience of unemployment among black and white urban teenagers. *British Journal of Psychology*, 76, 75–87

Warr, P.B. and Parry, G. (1982) Depressed mood in working-class mothers with and without paid employment. *Social Psychiatry*, 17, 161–165

Wilkin, D., Hallam, L. and Doggett, M.A. (1992) *Measures of need and outcome for primary health care.* Oxford: Oxford University Press

Wilson, D.D.R., Home, P.D., Bishop, A., Bradley, C., Brown, K.J.E., Hargreaves, B. and Members of a Working Group of the Research Unit of the Royal College of Physicians and British Diabetic Association (1993) A dataset to allow exchange of information for monitoring continuing diabetes care. *Diabetic Medicine*, 10, 378–390

Zung, W.W.K. (1965) A self-rating depression scale. Archives of General Psychiatry, 12, 63–70.

Zung, W.W.K. (1974) The measurement of affects: Depression and anxiety. In P. Pichot and R. Olivier- Martin (eds), *Psychological Measurements in Psychopharmacology.* Basle: Karger

APPENDIX

ADDITIONAL MEASURES INCLUDING RECENTLY
DEVELOPED AND NEWLY DESIGNED SCALES

APPENDIX

ADDITIONAL MEASURES INCLUDING RECENTLY DEVELOPED AND NEWLY DESIGNED SCALES

The chapters of the *Handbook* provide a selection of the many scales available for a wide range of purposes in diabetes research and clinical practice. Authors of the chapters provide references to many of the other instruments that have been used. Information about developed scales that are documented in publications referred to in the chapters of the *Handbook* can be found by referring to the *Handbook* index or by reading the introduction and discussion sections of chapters concerned with similar measures. Those measures referred to earlier in the *Handbook* are not included here. This appendix is reserved for developed scales that have not been referenced elsewhere in the *Handbook* and for newly designed instruments for which there may be little documented evidence of psychometric properties.

Potential users are advised to review any available publication or reference to associated work before contacting the author of the instrument for further information. It should be noted that authors of newly designed scales are likely to be in the early stages of establishing the scales' reliability and determining appropriate methods of scoring. Potential users need to consider how they will score the instrument and how they will justify their scoring method on the evidence currently available.

Although many of the appendix entries have been constructed using information provided for this purpose by the authors of the instrument, others are derived from published information. It cannot, therefore, be assumed that authors of instruments continue to be involved in their development and are able and willing to provide further information.

There are, undoubtedly, measures I have overlooked that would have been useful additions. I welcome information about such measures and invite any authors or users of such measures to send me details which may provide the foundations for an even more comprehensive second edition of the *Handbook*.

QUALITY OF LIFE, WELL-BEING AND SATISFACTION MEASURES

Audit of Diabetes-Dependent Quality of Life (ADDQoL)

Summary   This measure has been newly designed to identify domains of life important to the individual, the quality of which is impaired by diabetes and its management. The questionnaire includes fourteen items at present and is undergoing pilot work in three centres prior to more extensive development work as part of the British Diabetic Association / Royal College of Physicians National Study of Audit of Diabetes Care.

Authors   C. Bradley, C. Todd and E. Symonds

Address   Dr Clare Bradley, Director, Diabetes Research Group, Department
                 of Psychology, Royal Holloway, University of London, Egham Hill,
                 Egham, Surrey TW20 0EX, UK

Reference   Todd, C., Bradley, C. and Symonds, E. (1993) Psycho-social mea-
                 surement in the audit of diabetes services. *Audit Trends*, **1**, 141-143

The Depressed Well-Being Questionnaire (DWBQ)

Summary   The twelve-item DWBQ was designed for routine use in a study of
                 audit of diabetes care. Its purpose is to identify individuals with
                 depressed mood and to determine the extent to which that
                 depressed mood is general or is specific to diabetes and its man-
                 agement. The first six items are the Depression subscale from the
                 Well-Being Questionnaire described by Bradley in Chapter 6. The
                 second six items are specific to diabetes and were adapted from
                 Meadows' Diabetes Health Profile (also included in these appen-
                 dices).

Author   Clare Bradley and colleagues

Address   Dr Clare Bradley, Diabetes Research Group, Department of Psy-
                 chology, Royal Holloway, University of London, Egham Hill,
                 Egham, Surrey TW20 0EX, UK

Publication   Wilson, A.E., Home, P.D. for the Diabetes Audit Working Group of
                 the research Unit of the Royal College of Physicians and the Brit-
                 ish Diabetic Association (1993) A Dataset to Allow Exchange of
                 Information for Monitoring Continuing Diabetes Care. *Diabetic
                 Medicine*, **10**, 378–390.

Diabetes Clinic Satisfaction Questionnaire (DCSQ)

Summary   The DCSQ was designed to assess patients' satisfaction with diabe-
                 tes health care delivery. Initially called the review of Diabetes Care
                 Service Questionnairee, the DCSQ is a one-page questionnaire
                 suitable for routine use in auditing of diabetes care services. The
                 eighteen items concern waiting times, privacy, continuity of care,
                 aspects of treatment recommendations, information, communica-
                 tion and other aspects of relationships with doctors, nurses and
                 other clinic staff. Items are rated on a four point scale labelled

"Not applicable", "Satisfied", "Slightly Dissatisfied", "Dissatisfied". Additional open-ended questions invite patients to mention any additional problems and request comment and suggestions for improvements. Items are currently treated separately for the purpose of analysis.

Authors   Clare Bradley and colleagues

Address   Dr Clare Bradley, Director, Diabetes Research Group, Department of Psychology, Royal Holloway, University of London, Egham Hill, Egham, Surrey TW20 0EX, UK

Publication   Wilson, A.E., Home, P.D. for the Diabetes Audit Working Group of the research Unit of the Royal College of Physicians and the British Diabetic Association (1993) A Dataset to Allow Exchange of Information for Monitoring Continuing Diabetes Care. *Diabetic Medicine*, **10**, 378–390.

Diabetes Hassles Scale

Summary   Newly designed questionnaire modified from a scale originally designed by Kanner and Jacobson. The Diabetes Hassles scale measures frequency of experience of hassles associated with diabetes and its management. The instrument includes 93 items which are each rated for how much of a hassle they were in the last four weeks on a 4-point scale from "none or not applicable" to "a great deal".

Authors   Linda Gonder-Frederick, Daniel J. Cox and William L. Clark.

Address   Linda Gonder-Frederick, Research Associate Professor, Department of Behavioral Medicine and Psychiatry, Blue Ridge Hospital, Drawer F, Charlottesville, Virginia 22901, USA.

Reference   Kanner, A.D., Lee. D.K., Rountree, L. and Wilson, A.M. (1986). Relationship of psychological stress and glycaemic control in diabetic children. *Diabetes*, **35** (Suppl. 1) 443, p. 112A.

Problem Areas in Diabetes Survey (PAIDS)

Summary   This measure is currently being developed to provide a brief self-report instrument to assess diabetes-specific distress. It comprises twenty four items, each representing an area of diabetes-specific distress. These include difficult feelings about diabetes, interpersonal problems, and frustration with aspects of the regimen. On a six point Likert scale, patients rate the degree to which each item is currently problematic for them, from 1 ("no problem") to 6 ("serious problem"). A total scale score is computed by averaging the twenty-four item scores.

Authors   William H. Polonsky and colleagues.

Address   c/o Dr William H. Polonsky, P.O. Box 2148, Del Mar, CA 92014, USA

Reference   Polonsky, W.H., Anderson, B.J., Lohrer, P.A. and Schwartz C. Assessment of Diabetes-Specific Distress. Manuscript in preparation available from Dr Polonsky.

HEALTH STATUS AND SYMPTOM MEASURES

Diabetes Impact Measurement Scales (DIMS)

Summary   The DIMS was designed to measure health status in adults with diabetes (Type 1 or 2). Forty-four Likert scale items, some of which were taken directly from the well-known Rand scales, were selected or designed to measure: 1) symptoms; 2) diabetes-related morale; 3) social role fulfilment; 4) well-being. The factor structure empirically derived did not support the hypothesised four subscales but instead identified one main factor. The self-administered questionnaire takes 15-20 minutes to complete.

Authors   G. Steven Hammond and Thomas T. Aoki

Address   Thomas T. Aoki, MD, University of California, Davis, Division of Endocrinology, 4301 X Street, Building FOLB II-C, Sacramenta, CA 95816, USA

Publication Hammond, G.S. and Aoki, T.T. (1992) Measurement of Health Status in Diabetic Patients: Diabetes Impact Measurement Scales.

Edinburgh Hypoglycaemia Scale

Summary   A structured questionnaire to identify those symptoms which may
                be experienced during a hypoglycaemic reaction. Factor analysis
                of 295 insulin-treated outpatients identified eleven key hypogly-
                caemic symptoms loading highly on one of three clear factors:
                autonomic (sweating, palpitation, shaking and hunger), neurogly-
                copenic (confusion, drowsiness, odd behaviour, speech difficulty
                and incoordination) and malaise (nausea and headache). This
                three-factor model was replicated in a second sample. The authors
                used a binary response format which they suggested was sufficient
                for retrospective research, while alternative response formats were
                suggested for a seven-point scale, or a visual analogue scale may be
                used recording current experience of symptoms.

Author   Dr I. J. Deary

Address   Department of Psychology, University of Edinburgh, 7 George
                Square, Edinburgh EH8 9JZ, Scotland, UK

Publication   Deary, I.J., Hepburn, D.A., MacLeod, K.M. and Frier, B.M. (1993)
                Partitioning the symptoms of hypoglycaemia using multi-sample
                confirmatory factor analysis, *Diabetologia*, **36**, 771–777.

Seven Sexual Symptoms (SSS)

Summary   This measure has been developed for use as a screening test to dif-
                ferentiate between organic and psychogenic impotence and
                reduce the need for nocturnal penile tumescence (NPT) monitor-
                ing. The measure was developed with a sample of sixty diabetic
                men with impotence: 17 were categorised by NPT as having
                organic impotence and 17 as having psychogenic impotence. Of
                the 18 sexual symptoms investigated, 7 were identified as most
                effectively differentiating between cases of organic and psy-
                chogenic impotence categorised by NPT monitoring.

Authors   Gene G. Abel, Judith V. Becker, Jerry Cunningham-Rathner, Mary
                Mittelman, and Marshall Primack

Address   c/o Dr Gene G. Abel, New York State Psychiatric Institute, 722 W.
                168 Street, New York, NY 10032, USA

Reference   Abel, G.G., Becker, J.V., Cunningham-Rathner, J., Mittelman, M. and Primack, M. (1982) Differential Diagnosis of Impotence in Diabetics: The Validity of Sexual Symptomatology. *Neururology and Urodynamics*, **1**, 57–69.

KNOWLEDGE

Patient Knowledge Test

Summary   This test was developed by Etzwiler and associates at the International Diabetes Center, Minneapolis in 1984 to assess diabetic patients' knowledge in seven separate content areas. It is a fifty item, multiple-choice test, consisting of a total score and seven subscores based on seven content categories: nutrition, insulin, general knowledge, methods of control, pattern control, exercise, and complications.

Authors   Etzwiler and associates, International Diabetes Center, Minneapolis, MN, USA

Address   c/o Judy Ostrom Joynes, International Diabetes Center, 5000 West 39th Street, Minneapolis, MN 55416, USA

Reference   Garrard, J., Joynes, J.O., Mullen, L., McNeil, L., Mensing, C., Feste, C. and Etzwiler, D.D. (1987) Psychometric Study of Patient Knowledge Test. *Diabetes Care*, **10**, 500–509.

MEASURES OF ATTITUDES AND BELIEFS

Diabetes Attitude Scale (DAS) for Health Professionals

Summary   The purpose of the scale is to measure attitudes of health care professionals (including doctors, nurses and dieticians) toward diabetes and its treatment. A national panel of seventeen diabetes experts generated the initial pool of items. The thirty one items are scored using a five-point Likert scale indicating extent of agreement or disagreement with each statement. Eight subscales were identified using principal components analysis. Acceptable reliabilities for the subscales were reported and they were labelled as follows; special training (7 items), control/complications (4 items), patient autonomy (5 items), compliance (3 items), team care (4 items), non-insulin dependent diabetes (3 items), difficult to treat (3 items), outpatient education (2 items).

Author   Robert M. Anderson EdD

Address   Michigan Diabetes Research and Training Center, Towsley Center for Continuing Medical Education, Room G-1201, Box 0201, Ann Arbor, MI 48109-0201, USA

Reference   Anderson, R.M., Donnelly, M.B., Gressard, C.P. and Dedrick, R.F. (1989) Development of Diabetes Attitude Scale for health care professionals. *Diabetes Care*, **12**, 120–127.

Diabetes Onset Locus of Control (DOLoC) Scales

Summary   The DOLoC scales were developed for use with adults at risk of developing diabetes with a view to predicting their health-related behaviour in response to an educational intervention. A twenty four item questionnaire was designed to measure locus of control beliefs specifically about development of diabetes. Items included were modelled on those used by Wallston *et al.* (1978) in the Multi-dimensional Health Locus of Control Scale and those used by Georgiou and Bradley (1992) in the Smoking Locus of Control Scale. Psychometric analyses included a series of repeated factor and reliability analyses which resulted in sixteen of the original items being retained to represent four four-item subscales labelled Internality; Chance; Powerful Others; Significant Others. Satisfactory alpha coefficients of internal reliability were obtained for each subscale.

Authors   Dr Clare Bradley and colleagues

Address   Dr Clare Bradley, Director, Diabetes Research Group, Department of Psychology, Royal Holloway, University of London, Egham Hill, Egham, Surrey TW20 0EX, UK

References   Wallston, K.A., Wallston, B.S. and De Velliis, R. (1978) Development of the multidimensional health locus of control (MHLC) scales. *Health Education Monographs*, **6**, 160–170.
Georgiou, A. and Bradley, C. (1992) The development of a smoking-specific locus of control scale. *Psychology and Health*, **6**, 227–246.

Doctor Attitudes to the Management of Diabetes Scale

Summary   The purpose of the scale is to measure doctors' attitudes to their involvement in non-technical aspects of diabetes management. An initial pool of ninety-nine items was generated from various sources, including responses of ninety-eight Australian diabetes-specialist physicians to open-ended pilot questions. Theoretical models of health behaviour guided item selection and the instrument is designed with seven subscales to measure self-efficacy, non-compliance, consultation style, management of patient psychological problems, complications, perceived impact of diabetes, and biomedical orientation. Pilot testing reduced the measure to forty eight items which are scored using a five-point Likert scale ('disagree completely' to 'agree completely').

Authors   Linda J. Beeney and Dr Stewart M. Dunn

Address   Medical Psychology Unit, Department of Medicine, University of Sydney, NSW 2006, Australia

Publication   Beeney, L.J., Dunn, S.M. and Turtle, J.R. (1991) Medical Responses to Non-adherence: Who's Frustrated? *Diabetes*, **40** (Suppl. 1), 542A.

Health Belief Model Scale (HBM11): Short form of Given *et al*.'s seventy-six-item measure

Summary   This eleven-item Health Belief Model scale, providing a shorter alternative to the original HBM76, designed and developed by Given *et al.* (1983; see Chapter 13 for reference and details), has been developed for use by diabetes educators to determine the psychological readiness of individuals using insulin to self-manage their diabetes. Using a five point Lickert scale (1= strongly agree and 5 = strongly disagree), high scores equate with psychological readiness to undertake diabetes self-care actions. The items divide into three factors: low barrier, high benefit and seriousness.

Author   Dr Ann C. Hurley, RN, DNSc

Address   61 Babcock Street, Apt.3-A, Brookline, MA 02146, USA

Reference   Hurley, A.C. (1990) The Health Belief Model: Evaluation of a Diabetes Scale. *The Diabetes Educator*, **16**, 44–48.

Personal Models of Diabetes Interview (PMDI)

Summary   The PMDI is a fifty-item structured interview that includes questions about a person's beliefs and feelings concerning the cause, symptoms, treatment, course and consequences of their diabetes. The form provides detailed instructions to the interviewer. Open-ended responses are coded with categories supplied on the interview form. Other questions are responded to on rating scales or by choices supplied by the interviewer. The interviewee's responses are coded on the interview form during the interview. Data may be taken directly from the completed form for computer entry and analysis.

Author   Sarah E. Hampson

Address   Oregon Research Institute, 1899 Willamette Street, Eugene, OR 97403, USA

Publication Hampson, S.E., Glasgow, R.E. and Toobert, D.J. (1990) Personal models of diabetes and their relations to self-care activities. *Health Psychology*, **9**, 632–646.

MEASURES OF COPING

The Appraisal of Diabetes Scale (ADS)

Summary   The ADS is a seven item measure, with Likert-type scales, designed to assess adult patients' appraisal of their diabetes. Items are concerned with: degree of upset caused by diabetes; perceived amount of control over diabetes; degree of uncertainty; perceived vulnerability to worsening of diabetes; personal control over diabetes; self-efficacy in coping with diabetes; and effect of diabetes on life goals. The scale takes five minutes or less to complete and may be useful as a brief screening instrument for adjustment to diabetes. Scale development work published by Carey *et al.* (1991) studied only male patients but provided substantial evidence for reliability and preliminary evidence for validity with this selected sample.

Author   Michael P. Carey

Address   Department of Psychology, 430 Huntington Hall, Syracuse University, Syracuse, New York 13244-2340, USA

Publication   Carey, M.P., Jorgensen, R.S., Weinstock, R.S., Sprafkin, R.P., Lantinga, L.J., Carnrike, C.L.M. Jr., Baker, M.T. and Meisler, A.W. (1991) Reliability and Validity of the Appraisal of Diabetes Scale. *Journal of Behavioral Medicine,* **14**, 43–51.

Diabetes Coping Measure

Summary   A measure of cognitive and behavioural coping specific to diabetes. The Diabetes Coping Measure has emerged from the item and factor analyses of sixty-seven items compiled from several sources including the ATT39 described in Chapter 11 and items (rewritten) from the Medical Modes Coping Questionnaire (Feifel *et al.,* 1987, 1987a). Five point Likert scales range from "Agree strongly" to "Disagree strongly". Analysis of responses of 310 insulin-using patients showed three clear replicated factors involving 44 items described as follows: 1) a positive Confrontation of diabetes and a tackling spirit (13 items); 2) Avoidance/passive-acceptance of diabetes (15 items); 3) a Grief reaction to the diabetes expressed as resentment, anger and depression (16 items). Factors 1 and 2 provided some empirical support for the medical coping concepts described by Feifel *et al.* Internal reliability for the total test and three subscales were ≥0.71 ≤0.85.

Author   Dr Garry Welch

Address   National Institutes of Health Postdoctoral Fellow, Mental Health Unit, Joslin Diabetes Centre, One Joslin Place, Boston, Mass 02215, USA

References   Feifel, H., Strack, S. and Nagy, V. T. (1987) Degree of life threat and differential use of coping modes. *Journal of Psychosomatic Research,* **31**, 91–99.
Feifel, H., Strack, S. and Nagy, V. T. (1987a) Coping strategies and associated features of medically ill patients. *Psychosomatic Medicine,* **49**, 616–624.

MEASURES OF BEHAVIOUR

Diabetes Family Behaviour Checklist (DFBC)

Summary   The DFBC is a measure of family interaction for use by individuals between the ages of twelve and sixty four with insulin-dependent diabetes mellitus (IDDM) and their family members, and concerns behaviour specific to the diabetes self-care regimen. It assesses family behaviours that may support or interfere with the appropriate conduct or timing of four regimen behaviours: insulin injection, glucose testing, diet, and exercise. The numbers of items assessing family behaviour considered by the researchers to be supportive and nonsupportive are approximately equal.

Authors   Lorraine C. Schafer, Kevin D. McCaul and Russell E. Glasgow

Address   c/o Dr Kevin D. McCaul, Department of Psychology, Programs in Health and Behavior, North Dakota State University, Fargo, North Dakota 58105, USA

Publication   Schafer, L.C., McCaul, K.D. and Glasgow, R.E. (1986) Supportive and Nonsupportive Family Behaviors: Relationships to Adherence and Metabolic Control in Persons with Type I Diabetes. *Diabetes Care*, **9**, 179–185.

The Diabetes Self-Care Scale (DSC)

Summary   The DSC was developed to be a self-report measure of the constellation of self-care activities carried out in the home setting by individuals who require insulin. Reliability by internal consistency for subjects in the follow-up component of the test phase was considered adequate (scale total alpha = .89). The DSC scale contains three subscales that were also internally consistent in this study: general (6 items), diet (7 items) and insulin (9 items). Two exercise and two foot care items make up the remainder of the DSC scale total.

Author   Dr Ann C. Hurley, RN, DNSc

Address   61 Babcock Street, Apt.3-A, Brookline, MA 02146, USA

Reference   Hurley, A.C. (1990). The Health Belief Model: Evaluation of a Diabetes Scale. *The Diabetes Educator*, **16**, 44–48.

Self-Care Inventory

Summary   This measure concerns how well respondents have followed their
                prescribed regimen for diabetes care in the past month and con-
                sists of a fourteen-item questionnaire using a six-point scale: 1
                (Never) to 5 (Always) and NA (not applicable). Questions cover
                four topics: blood glucose regulation; insulin and food regulation;
                exercise; emergency precautions.

Author   Annette M. La Greca

Address   Professor of Psychology & Pediatrics, Director, Child Psychology
                Division, University of Miami, PO Box 248185, Coral Gables, FL
                33124, USA

Publication   La Greca, A.M., Follansbee, D. and Skyler, J.S. (1990) Develop-
                mental and Behavioral Aspects of Diabetes Management in Young-
                sters. *Childrens Health Care*, **19**, 132–139.

PROFILE MEASURES

Diabetes Educational Profile (DEP)

Summary   The DEP is a self-administered questionnaire containing seventy-
                five items designed for use by diabetes clinicians to document the
                psychosocial adjustment of patients with diabetes. The ultimate
                purpose is to achieve more effective educational and behavioural
                interventions and facilitate patient adjustment and adherence.
                The constructs measured closely resemble constructs in the
                Health Belief Model (Becker, 1974). Six factors have been identi-
                fied: Control Problems, Social Problems, Barriers to Adherence,
                Benefits of Adherence, Regimen Complexity, and Risk of Compli-
                cations.

Authors   Wayne K. Davis, George E. Hess, R. Van Harrison and Roland G.
                Hiss.
Address   c/o Wayne K. Davis, Department of Postgraduate Medicine and
                Health Professions Education, Office of Educational Resources
                and Research, G1113 Towsley Center, Box 057, University of Mich-
                igan Medical School, Ann Arbor, MI 48109, USA

Reference   Davis, W.K., Hess, G.E., Van Harrison, R. and Hiss, R.G. (1987) Psychosocial Adjustment to and Control of Diabetes Mellitus: Differences by Disease Type and Treatment. *Health Psychology*, **6**, 1–14.

Diabetes Health Profile (DHP)

Summary   The Diabetes Health Profile (DHP-1) is a forty-four item self-completion questionnaire for identifying psychosocial dysfunction in people with insulin-requiring diabetes mellitus. The DHP covers three domains: 1) lowered mood (18 items); 2) eating restraint failure (10 items); and 3) activity-restricting anxiety (10 items). Conference reports of initial factor analysis on data from 234 patients supported the hypothesised domains. Evidence for satisfactory internal consistency for each domain and test-retest reliability was reported. Completion time is approximately fifteen to twenty minutes. The DHP has been used in several studies including a study of Outcome Measures in Ambulatory Care (OMAC) conducted by the Centre for Health Services Research, University of Newcastle and publications are awaited.

Author   Keith A. Meadows

Address   Department of Public Health Medicine, University of Hull, Cottingham Road, Hull, HU6 7RX, UK

Publication   Meadows, K.A. and Wise, P.H.W. (1992) A national profile of knowledge and psychosocial status in 2239 Type 1 diabetic patients. *Diabetic Medicine*, **9**, (Suppl.1), 48A.

Diabetes Interview Schedule (DIS)

Summary   The Diabetes Interview Schedule (DIS) is a semi-structured interview guide developed for use by diabetes health professionals for the identification of management and psychosocial problems in patients with insulin-requiring diabetes and as a means of raising sensitive issues for discussion between patients and health professionals. The DIS covers fifteen key areas including: adequacy of diabetes management, disease impact on social and leisure activities, level of social support, family interactions, general and diabetes-related anxiety and depression, self-esteem and body image. Provisional reliability and validity of the DIS has been reported in conference presentations.

Author   Keith A. Meadows

Address   Department of Public Health Medicine, University of Hull, Cot-
                  tingham Road, Hull, HU6 7RX, UK

Publication   Meadows, K.A., Thompson, C., Brown, K., Sensky, T. and Wise,
                  P.H. (1991) The Development of the Diabetes Interview Schedule
                  (DIS) for the Identification of Psychosocial Problems in IDDM
                  patients. *Diabetes*, **40**, (Suppl.1), 539A.

AUTHOR INDEX

SUBJECT INDEX